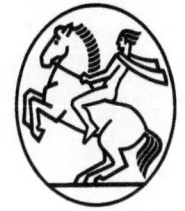

Modern Concepts in Neurotraumatology

First Scandinavian Symposium
on Neurotraumatology
May 20–23, 1985, Göteborg, Sweden

Edited by Sten Lindgren

Acta Neurochirurgica
Supplementum 36

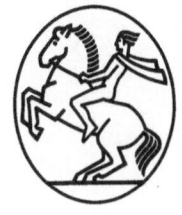

Springer-Verlag Wien New York

Sten Lindgren, M.D., Professor of Neurosurgery
Department of Neurosurgery, Sahlgren's Hospital, Göteborg, Sweden

With 67 Figures

Library of Congress Cataloging-in-Publication Data. Scandinavian Symposium on Neurotraumatology Head Injuries (1st: 1985: Göteborg, Sweden). Modern concepts in neurotraumatology. (Acta neurochirurgica. Supplementum; 36.) 1. Head—Wounds and injuries—Congresses. 2. Nervous system—Wounds and injuries—Congresses. I. Lindgren, Sten, 1920– . II. Title. III. Series. RD593.S348 1985. 617'.48044. 86-17713.

ISBN-13: 978-3-211-81931-9   e-ISBN-13: 978-3-7091-8859-0
DOI: 10.1007/978-3-7091-8859-0

Preface

It has become increasingly difficult for the single clinician to cover the whole area of traumatology and particularly neurotraumatology. This is now a science with various specialized fields of research. The results are published in different and special journals, proceedings and books often not easily available to those responsible for the daily practical management of the patients with head injuries.

Epidemiological investigations are necessary to evaluate the severity and frequency of accidents and injuries. Such studies will stress the importance of analysis of the causes and also the importance of prevention. They are useful for evaluation of the effects of injuries despite management.

Moreover, the researchers of the different aspects may need some knowledge of other links in the chain of events at and after an impact. This is particularly evident with respect to the problems of accident and injury, their prevention, reduction, management and the presentation of the most important clinical features in each case for international comparisons.

Therefore it is appropriate to let the different specialists briefly discuss and present their aspects of the subject. Moreover, it may facilitate and stimulate the clinicians in studying special fields of interest.

This was the intention behind the "Scandinavian Symposium on Neurotraumatology" held in May 1985 in Gothenburg:

— To accumulate wider knowledge for the neurosurgeon and better understanding between the researchers in various fields to the benefit of the coming and present patients.

Sten Lindgren

Contents

VIII   Contents

Clinical Assessment of Consciousness

Practical Assessment of Patients with Head Injuries

Outcome

Pathophysiology and Pathomorphology

Treatment and Prognosis

Acta Neurochirurgica, Suppl. 36, 1–6 (1986)

Introduction

S. Lindgren

Department of Neurosurgery, Sahlgren's Hospital, University of Göteborg, Sweden

In the beginning of research on the mechanics of head trauma, its severity was more related to the characteristics of the impacting object such as its velocity, mass, shape, contact surface etc than to the response of the impacted head. In Fig. 1 the biomechanical course of a head injury is summarized.

Axisymmetric impacts with the direction through the center of gravity of the head result in so-called translational (or linear *skull-head*) *acceleration* (m/sec^2) on which the physical head injury criterion (HIC) was based.

A simple illustration of the time course magnitude relationship of acceleration, velocity, and length (referrable also to deformation and displacement) is seen in Fig. 2.

However, *oblique impact* to the head can cause rotational or angular (mixed translational and rotational) movements—with the center of their axes moving during and after impact loading (boxing); similar movements also occur at indirect impulsive loading (battered children, whiplash).—The velocity and acceleration of such head movements are often measured in "*radians*"/sec and /sec^2.

At direct trauma to the head the duration of an impact loading of the skull is usually less than 20 msec. A slow direct loading of more than 200 msec, between big masses, will cause crush-fractures of the skull and, in the beginning, less damage to the intracranial contents.

However, impulsive loading often during some hundred msecs will particularly cause an *intracranial response* (see Fig. 1).

The severity of resulting injuries has been studied with *clinical "injury scaling"* such as AIS (Fig. 1); some suggestions for improvement are also mentioned (considering age and impact site—EIS) as is "scaling 2 weeks" after trauma. The relation between "acute injury scaling" and residual disability is also discussed in the supplement.

The described mechanics of impact and of tissue response with probable clinical effects can be seen in Fig. 3: Effects—of contact with skull deformation—of translation—of rotational movements and—of violent head-neck tension are mentioned. The anatomical tissues involved and resulting symptoms, immediate, early and late are summarized.

The *site of direct impact* such as occipital, temporoparietal, frontal or vertex impacts is important; contrecoup contusions often occur in the frontal and temporal lobes at the first two impact sites. Diagnostic localization of skin (scalp) injuries may facilitate the approach to the "combined head injury concept".—Brain tissue damage may occur due to different intracranial response (movements) in the different compartments, particularly in relation to the shape of skull and dural folds, including the tentorium and its opening.

The mechanics and the importance of the tissue material properties for the intracranial response and experimental research are particularly considered.

Systemic effects of trauma (Fig. 4) occur particularly at multiple injuries to the body, but also as intrathoracic consequences of head injury and of unconsciousness.

It must be remembered that each surgeon and neurosurgeon has the most excellent opportunity of studying the relationship between the resulting injury and the eliciting impact in *each patient* coming under their acute care. This will also contribute to the knowledge and information concerning possibilities to decrease not only the frequency of accidents but also of the severity of injuries; the very important prediction of intracranial complications may also be facilitated.—

Direction	Skull response Tolerance curves? "injury criteria"? (HIC)	Intracranial response (compartmental) forces, pressures, deformations	Injury site, nature grading (AIS, EIS)
	deformational,—skull contact—local propagated—local total volume change	local tissue displacem. at skull deform, fracture, modified by anatomy (hemisph. etc) cavitation?	+ surface hemorrhages: extra- intradural focal brain lesions ? damage
Axisymmetric			
Impact — Site	translational, accel., veloc.	accel, pressure pattern— ("steady")—impact directional (cavitation—supporting?) transversal displacement?: in ant. post. imp.—at for. magn. in vertex imp.—at tentorium	0? +? (magnitude?) +? axial (coma?)
Oblique Impulsive loading			
	angular, accel., veloc. before, during, after impact	different tangential (and radial) forces related to rot. axis. compartmental movements—rot. centers, CSF modifications	+ brain surface, veins lesions, hemorrhages + Axial (coma?)
	cranio-spinal movements	brain axis—deformation?	?

Impact: see text.
Skull response: Impact, particularly axisymmetric impact, produces skull deformation—see Fig. 3.
Intracran. resp.:   Oblique direct head impact and impulsive loading are often combined with the most important mechanical cause of injury:
                     brain tissue deformation, influenced by the compartment anatomy.
                     So-called cavitation includes phenomena of implosion, turbulence, etc.
Injury: AIS—EIS see text and Fig. 6. Coma is denoted for "concussion". Axial: diencephalon—medulla.

Fig. 1. Head injuries. Biomechanical research pattern

The eliciting factors leading to the chain of events resulting in accident and injury must be elucidated.

The pathology, particularly the acute forensic *intra-cranial neuropathology* is described. Except for skull deformation and fracture related to extradural hematomas it is particularly the angular movements that may cause intracranial hematomas. Lesions of venous but also of arterial origin or focal contusions within the brain tissue may occur; both types of vessels may cause acute subdural hematoma probably with different prognosis and surgical results. Such lesions often produce lateralizing signs of "focal" neurological deficits. The brain tissue may also suffer from mechanics causing mainly petechial hemorrhages in those dying at the accident. In those surviving longer axonal injury may appear in the white matter subcortically or mainly in the upper pontine region. These microscopically revealed types of lesions have been called "diffuse injury", but the symptom in common is the impairment

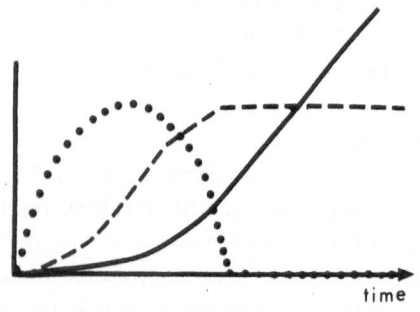

Fig. 2. Relative time course of magnitude: .... Accleration (l/t^2).
– – – – Velocity (l/t). ———— Length (l) (with respect to movement-deformation)

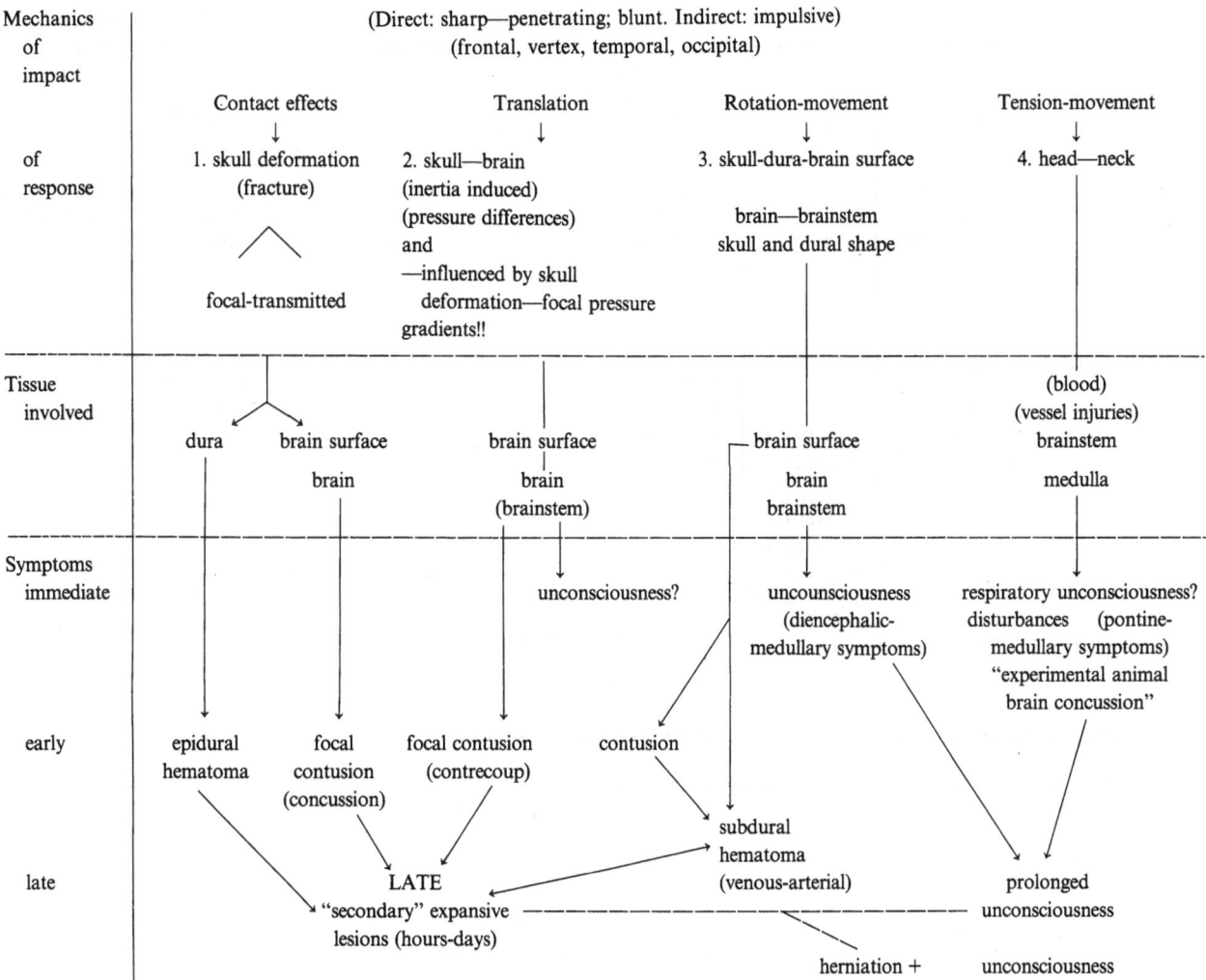

Mechanics of impact

(Direct: sharp—penetrating; blunt. Indirect: impulsive)
(frontal, vertex, temporal, occipital)

of response

Contact effects	Translation	Rotation-movement	Tension-movement
↓	↓	↓	↓
1. skull deformation (fracture)	2. skull—brain (inertia induced) (pressure differences) and —influenced by skull deformation—focal pressure gradients!!	3. skull-dura-brain surface brain—brainstem skull and dural shape	4. head—neck

focal-transmitted

Tissue involved

(blood) (vessel injuries) brainstem

dura   brain surface   brain surface   brain surface

brain   brain (brainstem)   brain brainstem   medulla

Symptoms immediate

unconsciousness?   uncounsciousness (diencephalic-medullary symptoms)   respiratory unconsciousness? disturbances (pontine-medullary symptoms) "experimental animal brain concussion"

early

epidural hematoma   focal contusion (concussion)   focal contusion (contrecoup)   contusion

late   subdural hematoma (venous-arterial)

LATE   prolonged

"secondary" expansive lesions (hours-days)   unconsciousness

herniation +   unconsciousness

Effect on CNS *related* 1. *to* impact direction, site and skull deformations. 2. *to* former position. 3. *to* surroundings. 4. *to* neck (S Lindgren, Lancet 1: 1964, 1251–1253. S Lindgren *et al.*, Injury 1973, p 31–34)

Fig. 3. Trauma to the head. Impact and response mechanics—clinical effects

of consciousness and of "coma", which can be readily recognized clinically.

Before description of these acute events at trauma, briefly summarized here, the symposium reviewed *varying epidemiological approaches* and methods of studying accidents and head injuries (see also Fig. 5) related to the time of accident and usually called "precrash", "crash" and "postcrash" periods. Information about prevention is also very important (Fig. 5) and investigators may in the future try even more to reveal the initial and real causes of accidents and resulting injuries.

The practical care in the *acute phase of head injuries* at the accident site, during transport and in hospitals without neurosurgical specialists is particularly discussed. The need of *resources* for mild, moderate and severe head injury patients is described as well as the *management levels* at the three different types of hospitals, organized in each geographical region in Sweden. Including the availability of CT scanning these resources considerably influence the distribution of patients.

The clinical course and type and severity of symptoms and nature and location of lesions are extremely important for increasing our possibilities to analyse the single case. Therefore, the general *diagnostic terminology* of head injury was particularly discussed in the symposium with reference both to severity and duration, resulting in a modified *diagnostic classification* as a proposal for *ICD 10*. The system of severity classification of *AIS* lends itself rather easily to the contents of diagnostic terminology in a modernized form.—

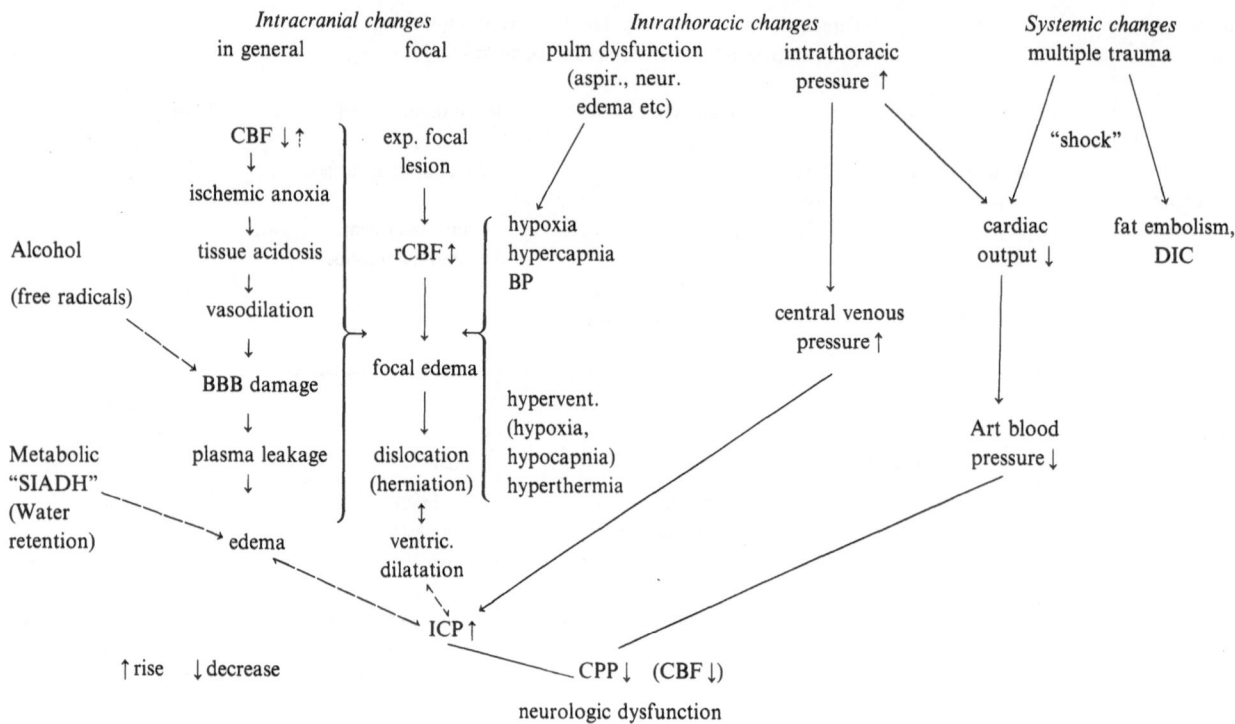

(Regarding "pulmonary dysfunction" *cf.* Popp JA *et al.* (1982) J Neurosurg 57: 784–790.

Fig. 4. Head injury and multiple trauma. (Posttraumatic effects S. Lindgren 1978)

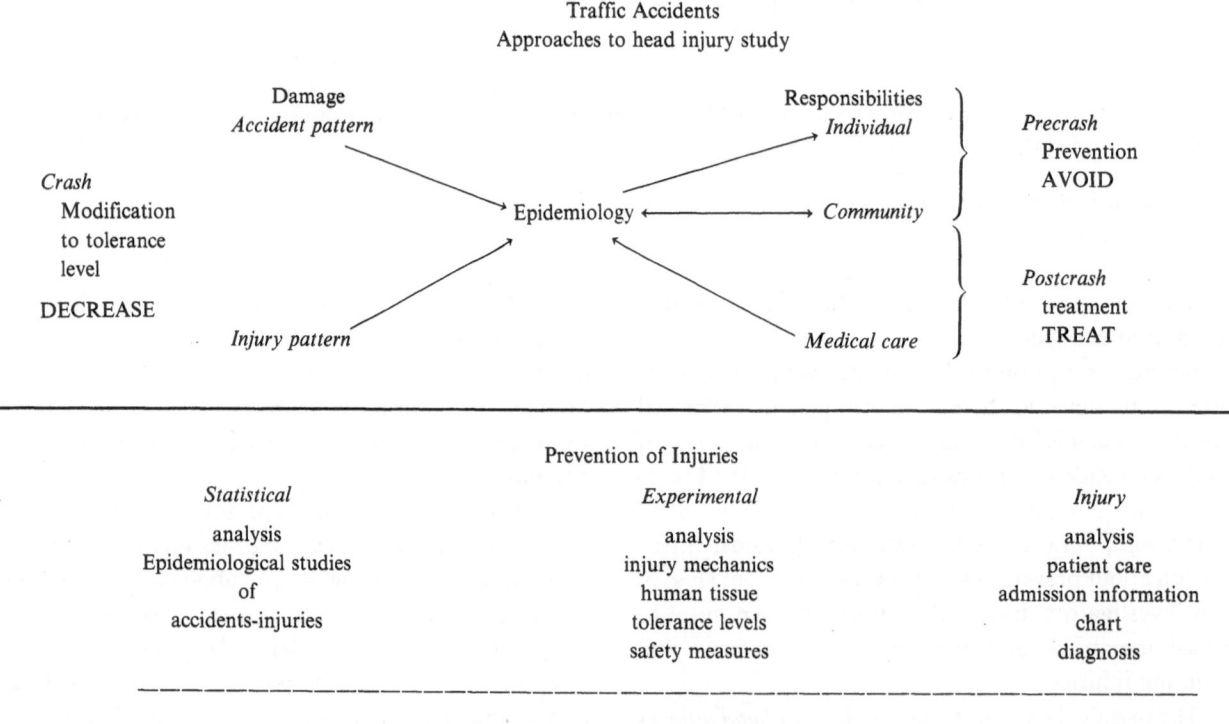

Fig. 5. Traffic accidents. Approaches to head injury study

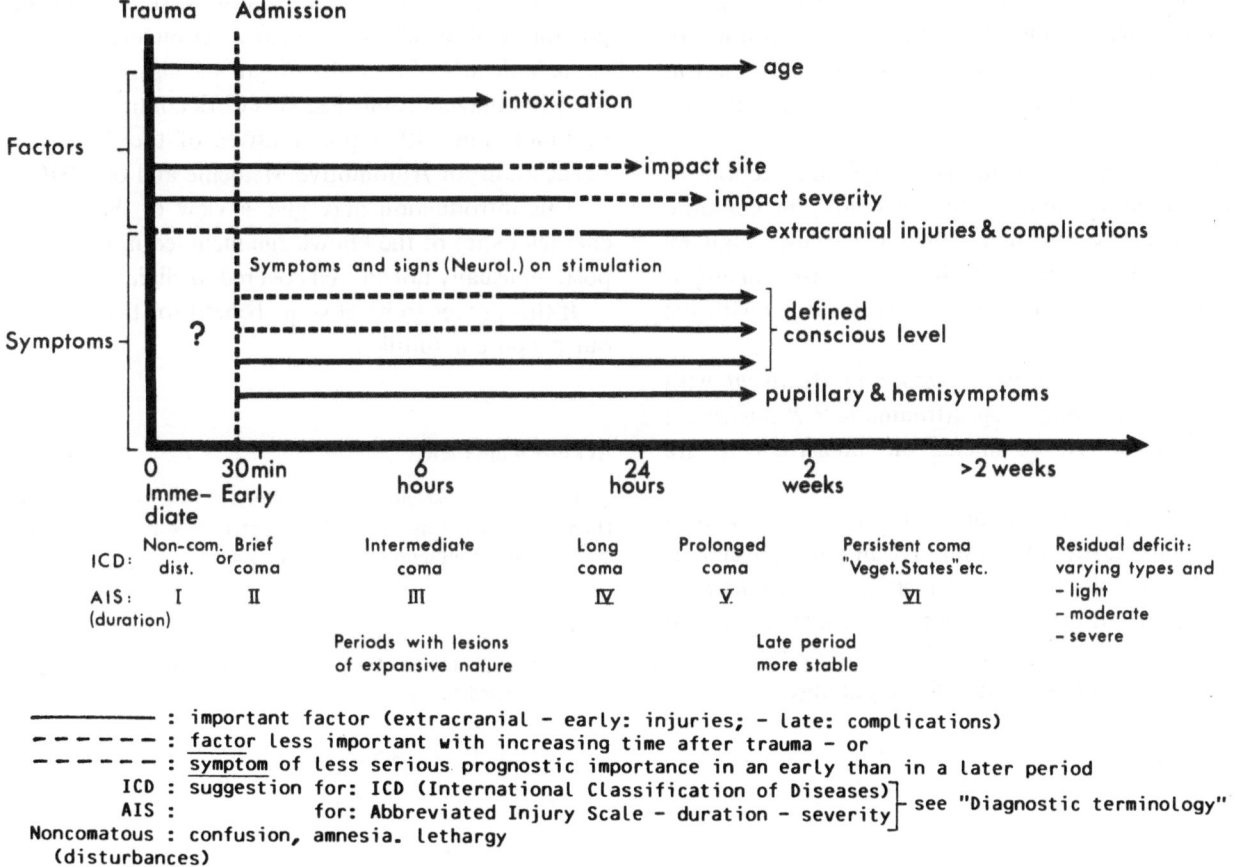

Fig. 6. Acute head injuries. Time related significance of evaluation parameters

Posttraumatic non-comatous disturbances and impairment of consciousness—with the *lack of adequate terminology* in humans—are discussed.

The most important symptom and finding after head injury is unconsciousness. The physiological aspects in animals and in man related to consciousness and arousal, wakefulness and awareness are reviewed and discussed. A short comment is given on electrophysiological assessment of conscious levels. Varying aspects on coma or reaction level scales are reported as well as practical examples on *management charts* for admission or observation.

Figure 6 shows the course of a head injured patient where also such factors as age, intoxication, impact site, impact severity and extracranial injuries and complications are mentioned; regarding the extracranial injuries the non-interrupted part of the arrow in the beginning means influence of "multiple injuries" and later the additional extracranial complications: pneumonia, urinary infection etc.

In Fig. 6 as well as later in the supplement five various durations of coma periods are mentioned as

degrees of "duration—severity" indicating "severity" of the nature of injury in regaining conscious states. The reason for the different time limits is given in the discussion of "diagnostic terminology". It seems as the verbal terms for these five durations can represent the diagnostic contents for ICD 10 as well as duration—severity degrees in Roman numerals related to the AIS-code; the AIS itself may be added with their incidentally noted clinical severity codes as well. This might reduce the need for the numerous and varying diagnostic terms used at present.

The neurological symptoms and signs on stimulation, here mostly related to the attempts of defining the appropriate "*conscious level*" was particularly discussed in the symposium. The question of "coma level" is also analysed, partly towards a background of the use of sum scores and single line scales. Among the latter particularly RLS (Reaction Level Scale 1–8) is mentioned.

Factors restricting the use of *coma scales* as well as *prediction of outcome* are extensively reported on. Possible mechanisms of "*vegetative state*" in terms of different degrees of involvement of arousal and of awareness are considered. Posttraumatic symptoms of dizziness and *vertigo* are discussed as well as abnormalities of *sympathetic regulation* after cervical cord lesions.

The more extensive and very important sections of pathophysiology and pathomorphology in common medical reviews are here covered in some detail by highly qualified specialists in *biochemistry, neuropathology, cerebral blood flow* and *brain edema* with the most recent information.

Finally, the possible *evaluation of treatment* with help of enzyme analyses, posttraumatic *ICP monitoring* as well as a few comments on intensive care are mentioned.

Craniofacial surgery for trauma with modern concepts from plastic surgery and recent pathophysiological aspects on the different traumatic *intracranial hematomas* and their treatment are considered. Special features of *head injuries in children* are discussed with relations to anatomy and pathophysiology.

The symposium ended with a discussion about the possibility of the use of a similar reaction level scale or coma scale and of a similar diagnostic classification in the Scandinavian countries. This work continues partly in connection with representatives of the American Association for Automotive Medicine and of WHO.

This introduction may give a view of the special characteristics of the knowledge included in this symposium, usually not so well covered in clinical reviews.

If this proves to be of some benefit for the readers, our purpose is fulfilled.

Acknowledgement

I would like to acknowledge the efforts of Mrs. H. Eliasson, G. Hilmarch, I. Sandberg and D. S. Lindgren in editing, typing and arranging the manuscripts for this supplement.

Author's address: Professor Dr. S. Lindgren, Department of Neurosurgery, Sahlgren's Hospital, University of Göteborg, S-41345 Göteborg, Sweden.

Acta Neurochirurgica, Suppl. 36, 7–9 (1986)

Epidemiology of Accidents in the Field of Traffic Medicine

P. G. Hansson

Department of Orthopedic Surgery, Länssjukhuset, Halmstad, Sweden

Summary

Epidemiological studies of accidents are based on the methods used in studying contagious diseases together with time factors. Essential is the understanding of the interrelations between these factors. Difficulties in obtaining a complete material must be considered as all sources used today have limitations.

Keywords: Head injuries; accidents; epidemiological principles.

The term epidemiology of accidents and injuries was probably coined around 1940, but (1949) John Gordon[3] has the credit of giving a background and a system to this aspect. A modern and dynamic approach to the study of accidents is to use the methods developed and adopted in the field of public health for the study and control of epidemic disease. Accidents may be interpreted as resulting from something more than the agent directly involved, but resulting from the total forces and conditions involved in the competition between man and his environment.

The three factors usually considered in the study of infectious diseases, host, agent and environment have their parallels in the study of accidents.

Host	Agent	Environment
Road user	Vehicle	Road and surrounding
Worker	Machine	Factory
House wife	Ladder	Kitchen
Football player	Football	Field

The first step in an epidemiological approach to accidents involves a study of their distribution in terms of who had the accidents, and when, where and how they occurred with regard to different classes of accidents, of agents and mechanisms of injury. This descriptive phase of epidemiology has often been used in a rather static way. In studying traffic accidents it is often said that 80% of the accidents are due to the road user, and 10% each to the vehicle and environment. This is a static way of looking into the problem. If 80% of the accidents are due to the road user, usually a driver, the vehicle and environment are probably too difficult to handle for the poor human being.

A more dynamic way is to consider the epidemiological factors as parts of a system, where the factors are dependent on each other. If there is a disturbance in the system, the result may be an accident or a near-accident. Another way of looking into accidents is to consider the time factors. The periods most often used are the Pre-accidental or Pre-crash period, the Accidental or Crash period and Post-accidental or Post-crash period. When using both the epidemiological and time factors a matrix can be made for systematizing the study and finding ways to prevention. An example is given in Fig. 1.

William Haddon[4] has considered energy damage and different countermeasure strategies to prevent damage in a wider sense. Besides accidents and injuries to human beings he includes all kind of damage to living and non living material (*cf.* Tab. 1).

	PRECRASH	CRASH	POSTCRASH
HOST			
AGENT			
ENVIRONMENT			

Fig. 1. Matrix of investigations on relation between time course and epidemiological factors

Table 1. *Prevention or Reduction of Accident and Injury*. Based on Haddon's ten Strategies (1973)

		Avoid Accident	
			ex. traffic inj.
1.	Prevent the generation of energy: kinetic, thermal ionizing and electrical		speed limits
2.	Reduce amount of energy	Precrash	speed limits
3.	Prevent release of energy		road safety, alcohol regul.
4.	Modify rate of release		car—damping properties
		Decrease Injury	
5.	Separate energy and susceptible structure—in space or time		
6.	Separate energy and structure with interposition of material		alcohol control
7.	Modify contact surface shape and hardness	Crash	car internal safety
8.	Reduce damage—strengthen structure		personal phys. safety
		Treat Injury	
9.	Emergency alarm, care transport	Postcrash	roadside care ambulance
10.	Reparative and rehabilitative measures		care hospital

(*Haddons ten strategies*. J of Trauma 13: 321–331, 1973) modified.

Reliability of Traffic Accident Statistics

Epidemiological models can also be used to study the role and responsibility of different parts of society (Fig. 2). The models can be more or less complex[2].

Official statistics on road traffic accidents and injuries are issued in most developed countries. They are used for international comparisons, to find out differences between countries and regions, to get a picture of the overall situation and to compare the situation from time to time. They also constitute an instrument for introduction and follow-up of traffic safety measures.

In Sweden official statistics on road traffic accidents are compiled by National Central Bureau of Statistics (SCB) from police reports. Accident, seriousness of injury and vehicle are defined according to recommendations given by Economic Commission for Europe (ECE). Several reports from Sweden, Scandinavia and some other countries have shown deficiences in official statistics. In a study from Halmstad[5] it was found that fatalities were correctly reported, that seriously injured were reported in 43% and slightly injured reported in only 29%. Injuries to unprotected road users were less correctly reported than injuries to protected road users and collision accidents were better reported than single accidents. The official statistics thus did not only underestimate the number of traffic victims, but gave a distorted picture of the overall situation. This is the more serious as the statistics are used as a basis for preventive measures. Figures similar to this have also been given in other Swedish studies as well as in other countries[1, 7, 8].

Another way of obtaining injury materials is to use hospital materials. Hospitalized patients in Sweden are registered according to WHO's International Classification of Diseases (ICD). A special code is used for cause of injury—E-classification. Outpatients are exceptionally registered by diagnosis or cause of injury.

A third source are traffic injury materials collected from insurance companies. A prerequisite for this is that at least one of the participants in the accident is insured. There is probably a risk for underestimation of accidents with unprotected road users and of single accidents.

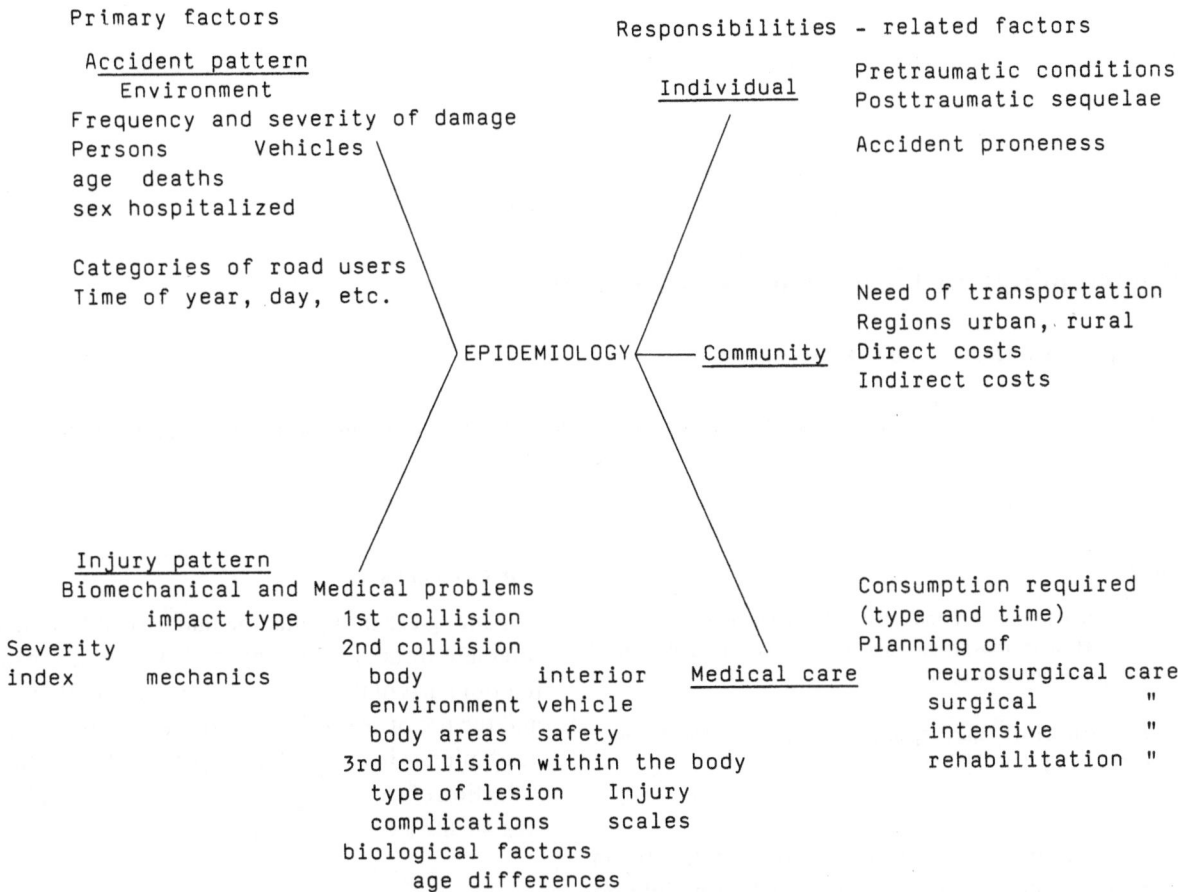

Fig. 2. Traffic accidents: Approaches to head injury studies. Related factors include the person or organizations with most obvious responsibility

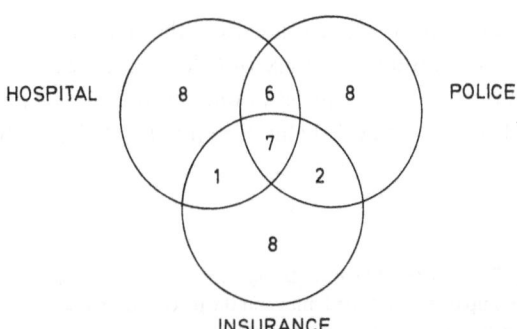

Fig. 3. Reports of 40 injured persons from three different sources; only seven persons reported in all sources

In a pilot study from Östergötland, a county in Sweden where 40 injured were studied it was found that only 7 of the victims could be traced in all three sources—hospital, police and insurance companies (Fig. 3). Probably no material can be totally correct in all respects. Therefore careful consideration must be given to the quality of the material in an accident study.

References

1. Bull JP, Roberts BJ (1973) Road accident statistics—a comparison of police and hospital information. Accid Anal Prev 5: 45–56
2. Carlsson S, Silverbåge Carlsson G, Hansson P *et al* (1973) Epidemiology of head injuries. In: Proceedings International Conference on the Biokinetics of Impacts. Amsterdam, pp 131–152
3. Gordon JE (1949) The epidemiology of accidents. Am J Public Health 39: 504–515
4. Haddon W (1973) Energy damage and the ten countermeasure strategies. J Trauma 13: 321–331
5. Hansson PG (1974) Road traffic causalties in a surgical department. Acta Chir Scand (Suppl) 442 (Thesis)
6. Nygren Å (1984) Injuries to car occupants—some aspects of the interior safety of cars. Acta Otolaryngol (Suppl) (Stockh) 395 (Thesis)
7. Sande J, Thorson J (1975) An evaluation of the official Swedish statistics on seriously injured in road traffic accidents. Scand J Soc Med 3: 5–11
8. Tolagen A, Trafikskadade i Östergötland. Thesis 1977. University of Linköping, No 46

Author's address: P. G. Hansson, M.D., Department of Orthopedic Surgery, Länssjukhuset, S-30185 Halmstad, Sweden.

Acta Neurochirurgica, Suppl. 36.10–12 (1986)

Epidemiology of Head Injuries in Sweden

Å. Nygren, C. Tingvall, and **H. Gustafsson**

Division for Research and Development, The Folksam Group, Stockholm, and Chalmers University of Technology, Göteborg, Sweden

Summary

The estimated number and cause of head injuries in Sweden are discussed. Head injuries are common in many activities and the need of head protection is stressed.

Keywords: Head injury; epidemiology; traffic accidents; sports accidents; occupational injuries.

Head injuries are common. According to statistics in Sweden 25,000–30,000 persons meet with head injuries each year[1]. Most of the head injuries are caused by trauma directly to the head and occur in 70% of the cases in connection with traffic. Table 1 shows the frequency and causes of head injuries in Sweden. The incidence of head injuries is 3–3.6/1,000. (Sweden: population 8 millions.) Head injury is here defined as an injury to skull and brain as reported by medically educated people.

Head Injuries in the Traffic

Every year 600–800 persons are fatally injured in the traffic. In 70% of the cases the main cause of death is a head injury. 2,400 persons are permanently disabled, > 10%, in the traffic and 500 sustain a head injury.

Table 1. *Head Injuries—Frequency and Causes (Sweden 1983)*

Cause of head injury	Number
Traffic	15,000
Industry	6,000
Other	3,000–8,000
Total	25,000–30,000

Car Occupants

Among car occupants the majority of head injuries originate from violent contacts between the head and interior parts of the car. Increased interior safety of cars and the use of seat belts have decreased the number of head injuries in cars[8]. Nygren (1984)[8] showed that the reduction of classified head injuries due to seat belt use was 40–80% (see Table 2).

Unprotected Road Users

Motor Cyclists

Among unprotected road users the main cause of death is head injury. The use of helmets has decreased the number of head injuries among motor cyclists and mopedists. Motor cycle helmets reduce head injuries by 60–70%[1].

Table 2. *Types of Head Injuries Among Surviving Car Drivers*. Belted drivers compared to unbelted ones and the percentage reduction due to seat belt use

Type of injury	Injury frequency among drivers		Reduction in %	Sign. level
	Belted N = 3,059	Unbelted N = 412		
Hematoma	0.2	1.5	86.7	.
Observation susp. concussion	9.6	16.3	41.1	...
Cerebral concussion	3.7	13.3	70.6	...
Abrasion/laceration of the scalp	10.2	17.7	42.4	...
Skull fracture	0.6	1.2	50.0	N.S.

Cyclists

The total number of bicycle accidents with head injuries amounts to 4,000–6,000 a year. The fatal outcome is estimated at 1 : 100,000. In 1985 Lind[5] showed from a hospital material that head injuries are common in bicycle accidents. In single accidents 37% of the cyclists had head injuries and in collisions 53%.

At a fall from a height of 2 m the head impacts the ground at a speed of 18 km/h. This fact, the use of high speed bicycles and statistics strongly advocate the use of a helmet when cycling.

Pedestrians

Head injuries among pedestrians are also common and occur from violent contact between the head and the exterior parts of a car or ground. Among injured pedestrians 60–70% suffered from head injuries[5].

Occupational Injuries

In 1981 about 100,000 persons were injured in occupational accidents. 7% of these persons sustained head injuries, *i.e.* 6,000–7,000 in the industry per year. One fourth of the industrial head injuries occurred due to falls from heights, another third was caused by moving objects hitting the head, 10% was due to falling objects and the rest to falls from tripping on things.

Sports Injuries

For injuries due to sport activities it is difficult to get appropriate figures. The main part of the sports

Table 3. *Estimated Number of Head Injuries in Sport Accidents Leading to Permanent Disability and the Relative Frequency of Head Injuries Correlated to the Total Number of Persons with Permanent Disability (1–100%), 1976–1983*

Type of sport	Estimated number of head injuries in sport accidents leading to permanent disability	Relative frequency of head injuries correlated to total number of persons with permanent disability in %
Football	25	5.9
Ice-hockey	23	27.0
Bandy	—	—
Handball	3	5.9
Basket-ball	—	—
Long distance racing	2	10.5
Cycling	9	75.0
Rugby	3	3.3
Total	65	10.1

organizations in Sweden are insured with Folksam. A presentation of the result of the insurances was made in 1985[10]. The number of persons receiving compensation for permanent disability was presented as well as the number of persons having received compensation for medical care.

In Table 3 the estimated number of persons with head injuries leading to permanent disability is presented for different sports during 1976–1983.

Table 4. *Estimated Number of Head Injuries in Different Sports, 1983*

Type of sport	Estimated number of head injuries in sport accidents	Relative frequency of head injuries correlated to the number of injuries (percentage)
Football	218	10.1
Ice-hockey	61	11.5
Bandy	12	14.0
Handball	38	8.4
Basket-ball	6	5.4
Long distance skiing	14	18.0
Cycling	10	41.0
Wrestling	5	10.2
Rugby	1	5.3
Total	365	10.4

Table 4 shows the number of persons who had compensation for medical care due to injuries in sport accidents in 1983. It can be seen that cycling and ice-hockey are the two sports where head injury is an important part of the injury pattern leading to permanent disability. There is room for increased use and improvement of helmets. Brain concussion occurred in every 27th match in the highest Swedish division of ice-hockey and knock outs in young amateur boxing in 1–4% of all matches[6].

As a comparison can be mentioned that brain concussion occurs in American football in 19/100 active players per year and in Soccer to 5/100.

Riders

Riding has been increasingly popular during the past decades. The increased number of riders means an increased number of injured riders. This has been shown in Sweden by Ingemansson and by Dittmer *et al.* in Germany (1977)[2].

Most sports involve an injury risk for their pracisers, but fatal injuries are rare. Riding is an exception with

Table 5. *Riding Frequency and Accidents (Sweden)*

Active riders	250,000
Horses	70,000
Riding occasions	10,000,000
Total humber of accidens with injuries	7,000
Fatal outcome	5
Total number of accidents with head injuries	1,200
Head injuries with fatal outcome	3

approximately 4 victims every year in Sweden. Inge-mansson (1983)[3] also showed a high number of serious injuries, *e.g.* head injuries in 66% of those fatally injured, for survivors the proportion of head injuries was 17%.

It is obvious that a well functioning helmet is an important protection of a rider.

Downhill Skiers

Collision accidents among downhill skiers have increased[9]. These accidents have another injury pattern compared to single accidents. Head injuries are more frequent in collision accidents.

Folksam has studied the effect of helmet use among skiers, 1–14 years old. The usage rate of helmets is fairly high in this group. In the Folksam material[9]. 45.9% used a helmet at the accident. Table 6 shows the number of injuries to the head and other parts of the body among helmet users and nonusers.

Table 6. *Number of Injuries Among Downhill Skiers, 1–14 Years, With and Without Helmet*

Helmet use	Head injury	Other injury	Proportion of head injuries correlated to total number of injuries in %
Users	15	151	9
Nonusers	27	118	18

There was a statistical reduction of head injuries due to helmet use, especially in collision accidents.

Comments on the Epidemiology of Head Injuries in Sweden

Head injuries are a problem in many activities. It is important to evaluate the problem in the different areas. In cycling for example it is important to increase the helmet use. At many places of work the need for helmet use should be studied. In other activities it seems important to improve the head protection.

Even slight head injuries with a short period of unconsciousness can give long-term consequences and disability. More knowledge about how to treat slight head injuries is necessary. *All sports* should have similar restrictions for the participants for attending further training and competition as in the most careful rules in boxing for young amateurs.

References

1. Aldman B, *et al* (1979) The protective effect of crash helmets. A study of 96 motorcycle accidents. IV IRCOBI Conference on Biomechanics of Trauma, Bron, France, 1979. Proceedings, pp 63–74
2. Dittmer H, Wubbena J (1977) Eine Analyse von 367 Reiterunfällen. Unfallheilkunde 80: 21–26
3. Ingemansson H (1983) Ridskador. En studie i samband med ridning och handhavande av hästar. Thesis. University of Uppsala
4. Franksson C, *et al* (1981) Kirugi. AWE Gebers, Almqvist Wiksell, Uppsala
5. Lind M (1985) Personal communications. Karolinska Hospital, Stockholm
6. Ludwig R (1985) Personal communication
7. Nygren Å, Tingvall C, Gustafsson H (1985) Injuries among pedestrians. (In press)
8. Nygren Å (1984) Injuries to car occupants. Some aspects of the interior safety of cars. Acta Otolaryngologica [Suppl] 395
9. Rapporterade skadefall vid SLAO-anläggningar. Folksam, 1985
10. Sports Injuries 1976–1983. Folksam, 1985

Authors' address: Å. Nygren, M.D., Ph.D., Division for Research and Development, The Folksam Group, Stockholm, Sweden.

Acta Neurochirurgica, Suppl. 36, 13–15 (1986)

Head Injuries in a Population Study

G. Silverbåge Carlsson

Department of Neurosurgery, Sahlgren's Hospital, University of Göteborg, Sweden

Summary

In a population study of altogether 1,112: 60-, 50-, and 30-year-old men performed in Göteborg, Sweden, data on head injuries suffered during life were obtained by personal interview. Two head injury concepts were used, one wide definition to cover all sorts of head injuries (HI-w) and one restricted only to delineate head injuries with evidence of presumed brain involvement (HI-r).

24% of the 60-year-old men, 21% of the 50-year-old men and 23% of the 30-year-old men reported at least one head injury with unconsciousness. When taking only the 3 first decades of life into account a significantly higher proportion of men in the youngest cohort had been unconscious than in the older ones, and the youngest men also had a significantly higher incidence of both HI-w and HI-r than the older men.

Accidents at home, in roads and in sports/recreational areas dominated in childhood, place of work in adult age. HI-r accidents occurred somewhat more often in roads and sports/recreational areas than HI-w accidents. Falls, traffic and blows/impacts were the most common causes. Falls dominated in childhood. Motor vehicles were more often involved in childhood accidents in the youngest cohort than in the two older ones.

The proportion of self-care decreased due to a strong secular trend. Out-patient care increased due to both a secular trend and to the age of the victim. The proportion of in-patient care increased with the age of the victim but showed no evident secular trend. $1/5$ to $1/3$ of all head injuries with unconsciousness were not medically attended.

Keywords: Head injuries; accidents; epidemiology; morbidity.

Introduction

The epidemiology of head injuries deals with a wide range of injuries from minor injuries not medically attended to severe ones causing the death of the patient. The design of epidemiological studies therefore may vary according to the purpose the data are intended for.

For a study of possible sequelae of head injuries it seemed necessary to know all types of head injuries people had suffered, even those not medically attended. It was also considered important to cover the whole life time.

Study Populations and Methods

The present study is a population study of altogether 1,112 60-, 50-, and 30-year-old men, performed in Göteborg, Sweden. The study population has been described in detail before[4]. The two oldest cohorts were sampled from the population register of Gothenburg. This register covers the entire population and must by law be kept up-to-date.

The third cohort, the 30-year-old men, were sons of the 60-year-old men and are thus, as opposed to the two oldest cohorts, not necessarily representative of the corresponding age-sex segment of the general population.

These men were invited to an examination at Sahlgren's Hospital. Data on head injuries suffered during life were obtained by interview performed by a physician during this examination. More detailed information on the methodology has been given elsewhere[4].

Injury Concepts

Two head injury concepts were used:

Wide concepts (HI-w)

1. head trauma which caused restricted activity for one day or more;
2. head trauma for which the participants had sought medical attendance;
3. head trauma with loss of consciousness.

Restricted Concept (HI-r)

head trauma with loss of consciousness and/or posttraumatic amnesia and/or neurologic signs of brain involvement and/or skull fractures.

Results

Incidence of Head Injuries

Figure 1 shows the incidence of accidents with head injuries (HI-w) related to age at the time of the accidents in the three cohorts. There was a peak incidence in childhood and adolescence, and there was a tendency to higher incidences in younger cohorts with

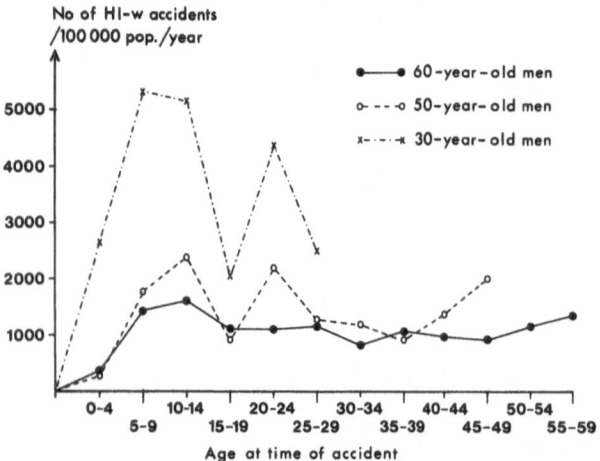

Fig. 1. Incidence of head injuries (wide concept) in relation to age at the time of accident in three male cohorts

peak incidences of about 1,500 accidents/100,000 population/year for the 60-year-old men, around 2,000 for the 50-year-old men and approximately 5,000 for the 30-year-old men.

The corresponding incidence curves for HI-r were very similar but with a lower incidence level, with peak incidences of about 1,000/100,000 population/year for the two older cohorts and over 2,000/for the youngest one. The incidence curves for head injuries with loss of unconsciousness were almost identical to those for HI-r. 24% of the 60-year-old men, 21% of the 50-year-old men and 23% of the 30-year-old men reported at least one head injury with loss of consciousness during life.

Multiple Injuries

Multiple injuries were analyzed from three different aspects. The term may be used, in a longitudinal study like this, to indicate that a person has sustained more than one head injury during life, for instance one at 2 years of age, one at 17 and one at 49 years of age. In that sense 3–7% of the populations reported multiple injuries with a maximum of 7 HI-r accidents/person.

Multiple injuries may also mean that more than one head region was injured in a certain accident. The multiplicity will then depend on how many regions were used in the registration of injuries. In this study the head was subdivided into 3 regions; skull, face and eyes. Thus, face did not include eyes and not the part of the face covering the skull, i.e. the forehead. In 62% of the HI-w accidents isolated skull injuries were reported, isolated face injuries in 27% and isolated eye injuries in 7%. Multiple regions were involved in 4%.

In HI-r accidents isolated skull injuries dominated

(85%). 9% of the accidents comprised isolated face injuries and 7% included multiple injuries.

A third possible sense of multiplicity could mean a combination of head injuries and injuries to other parts of the body at a certain accident. Here, too, the proportions are influenced by the definition of the body regions used for registration. We used a total of 15 body regions[4]. Defined in this way there was a higher proportion of injuries to other body regions combined with a head injury the older the victim was at the time of the accident.

Place of Accident and Cause of Injury

Figure 2 illustrates place of accident for HI-w accidents. Home accidents dominated in childhood and road accidents and accidents in sport/recreational areas were also more common in young ages. In the adult part of life place of work was reported as place of accident in almost half of the accidents. There were no important differences in place of accident in HI-w accidents compared to HI-r accidents, even though road and sport/recreational accidents were somewhat more common in HI-r accidents.

Falls, traffic and blows/impacts, registered according to the International Classification of Diseases[1], were the most common causes of head injuries. Falls were most common in childhood. Falls and traffic were more common in the youngest cohort compared to the two older cohorts both for HI-w and HI-r.

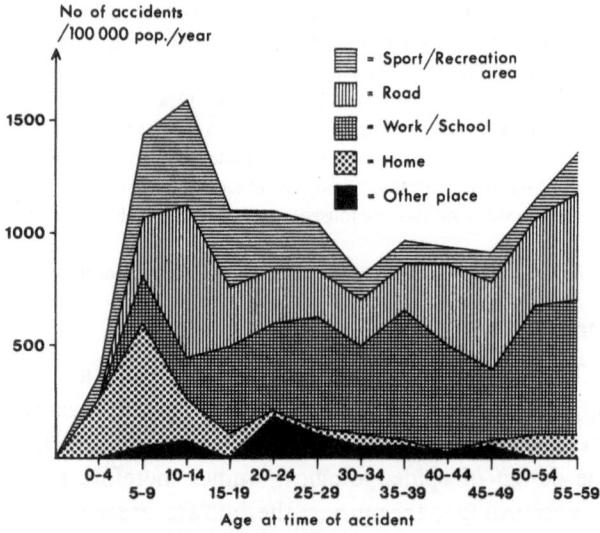

Fig. 2. Incidence of head injuries (wide concept) in relation to age at the time of the accident and subdivided into its components according to place of accident. Thus the top curve shows the total number of accidents per 100,000 population per year. Men 60 years of age at interview

The category of injured road user is influenced by age of the victim and of secular trends with for instance increasing motorization. Children victims were more often pedestrians than adults and this was more pronounced in the youngest cohort. Bicyclists become traffic victims in young ages but in decreasing proportion with increasing motorization and higher ages. Motor vehicles were more often involved in the youngest cohort and in this cohort no bicyclist was injured after the age of fifteen.

Type of Care

During the studied period the proportion of self-care decreased due to a strong secular trend. Out-patient care increased due to both a secular trend and to the age of the victim whereas the in-patient care did not show any evident secular trend but increased with age of the victim. Overall 20–33% of head injury accidents with unconsciousness were not medically attended in the three cohorts.

Concluding Remarks

This study has yielded a comprehension of the occurrence of defined head injuries in three male samples from the general population.

The reported incidences are minimal ones on account of memory default[2], other causes of underreporting[4], and non-participation (non-participants having a higher incidence of head injuries[3]).

In spite of these possible sources of bias the incidences of injuries comparable to HI-r reported here are higher than those reported from hospital studies. This is probably due to the fact that the two oldest cohorts in this study are representative of the general population and that this study also covers injuries not medically attended. As far as I know this is the first published estimate on non-attendance of defined head injuries in adult populations.

References

1. International Statistical Classification of Diseases, Injuries and Causes of death, 1965 revision adapted for indexing of hospital records and morbidity statistics. Swedish National Health Board, 1973
2. Silverbåge Carlsson G (1983) Validity of injury data collected by interview: a Study of Men Born in 1913 and 1923. J Neurol Neurosurg Psychiatry 46: 818–823
3. Silverbåge Carlsson G, Svärdsudd K (1985) Comparison of participants and non-participants in a population study of injuries. Scand J Soc Med 13: 15–22
4. Silverbåge Carlsson G, Svärdsudd K, Carlsson S, Tibblin G (1986) A study of injuries during life in three male populations. J Trauma 26: 364–373

Author's address: G. Silverbåge Carlsson, Department of Neurosurgery, Sahlgren's Hospital, University of Göteborg, S-413 45 Göteborg, Sweden.

Acta Neurochirurgica, Suppl. 36, 16–17 (1986)

Acute Injury Statistics—a True Picture?

Å. Nygren[1], P. G. Hansson[2], C. Tingvall[1], and H. Gustafsson[1]

[1] Folksam Research and Development Division, Stockholm, Sweden
[2] Department of Orthopedic Surgery, County Hospital, Halmstad, Sweden

Summary

The official data on traffic victims are based on police-reported accidents. Many authors have shown that these data are not fully representative. In order to obtain reliable accident statistics, it is suggested that these be based primarily on injured persons with long-term consequences.

Keywords: Accident statistics; police-reported accidents; insurance material; hospital material.

In Sweden, as in other countries, the official statistics on road traffic accidents rely on police reports. Many studies have shown that when based on this source, the accident figures are underrepresented.

In 1974 Hansson compared official statistics with hospital data, and found that fatally injured traffic victims were correctly reported, while this was true for only 43% of seriously injured and 29% of slightly injured victims[1]. Tolagen, in 1977, found similar figures[2]. In a report from 1983 Nilsson and Thulin[3] compared three sources of statistics: the number of injured persons admitted to hospital, victims of police-reported accidents, and victims of accidents reported to the insurance companies. The material was small, but it was evident that the three sources reciprocally did not cover all accidents. Thus, among accidents reported to the insurance companies, single-car accidents and car-pedestrian accidents were underrepresented, and the same was true among police-reported accidents; moreover, all injured persons did not visit a doctor.

In another study Nilsson and Thulin (1982) investigated traffic safety on the basis of the statistics of the National Board of Health and Welfare covering hospitalized patients injured in road traffic accidents.

They reported that in total the official statistic covered 45% of the road casualties in the patient statistics. Injured cyclists and pedestrians were found to be underrepresented in the official statistics as compared with the number of patients admitted to hospitals in Sweden.

This was probably the reason why young people were underrepresented in the official statistics, as a large proportion of this group are unprotected road-users.

What is the Best Source of Accident Statistics?

Accident statistics are required for the follow-up of traffic safety in a country. They are important for hospital planning, for education of road-users, for construction of new cars, for evaluations concerning insurance risks, and for the planning of streets and cities, and so on. From the previously mentioned studies it may be concluded that we have three main sources of information to deal with. In addition there are a number of ad hoc studies, but in no cases is complete information provided. In a national report on traffic accidents and statistics in 1975 it was concluded that the basis for statistics on traffic accidents should be police-reported accidents complemented with information from insurance companies and hospitals.

In the last calculation of the costs of traffic accidents in Sweden (1982), an estimation was made on the basis of police-reported accidents supplemented with hospital data.

Injuries with Long-term Consequences Should be the Primary Basis in Studies of Injury Statistics

The cost to the society as a result of traffic accidents can be divided into costs for hospital care, costs for sick leave and costs for loss of production, and in 1982 was estimated at 2,509.5 million SEK. More than 63%

(1,605 mill) was attributable to production loss for persons with serious consequences. The total costs to the society for fatally injured and permanently disabled persons were estimated at 2,056.6 million SEK. To this figure should be added the cost for loss of human dignity, which includes suffering and sorrow. This sum is difficult to assess but should be included in the calculation. In Sweden this sum is set at 3.7 million SEK for each fatally injured and 1 million SEK for each disabled person.

As the accident statistics are incomplete and the costs of obtaining appropriate figures are too high[5], it seems reasonable to try to get relevant figures for fatally injured persons and for persons who suffer permanent medical disability.

Fatally Injured

The correct figures for fatally injured persons can be obtained from police reports on accidents complemented with figures from the National Bureau of Statistics (SCB).

Permanent Medical Disability

The number of persons with permanent medical disability due to traffic accidents could be evaluated from insurance material. This should include all compensation for injuries paid by the traffic insurance industry as well as all compensation for accidents during commuting paid by the National Social Insurance Board. Some of the underreporting of single-car accidents and accidents to unprotected road-users should probably be covered by the statistics for commuting accidents administered by the National Social Insurance Board.

Conclusion

1. It is important to have reliable statistics on traffic accidents in order to follow trends.

2. Traffic accident statistics are valuable in hospital planning, for education of road-users, for construction of new cars, for evaluations concerning insurance risks, and for planning of streets and cities.

3. The three main sources of the statistics are police reports on accidents, hospital data and insurance data, none of which is complete.

4. It is suggested that more appropriate figures would be those concerning traffic victims with long-term consequences (fatally injured and persons with permanent medical disability) as they represent the majority of the costs and a great deal of suffering, which means that measures taken would hopefully have a good cost-benefit ratio.

5. An insurance material of traffic accident victims consists of both police data and hospital data and contains valuable information on those who are permanently disabled. For improvement of traffic safety, these records are therefore suggested as a good source of accident statistics.

References

1. Hansson PG (1974) Road traffic casualties in a surgical department. Acta Chir Scand (Suppl) 442
2. Tolagen A (1977) Trafikskadade i Östergötland. En undersökning av skadade i trafiken i Östergötlands län under 1½ års tid. Linköping University Medical Dissertations No 46, Linköping
3. Nilsson G, Thulin H (1983) Trafikolyckor och trafikskadade i Östergötland under två veckor i mars och två veckor i oktober 1982. VTI Meddelande nr 348
4. Nilsson G, Thulin H (1982) Beskrivning av trafiksäkerhetsläget med hjälp av Socialstyrelsens patientstatistik. VTI Rapport no 237
5. Trafikolyckor och statistik. Betänkande av trafikolyckskommittén. Statens offentliga utredningar (SOU) 1975: 40
6. Nygren Å (1984) Injuries to car occupants—some aspects of the interior safety of cars. Acta Otolaryngol (Stockh) (Suppl) 395
7. Hoot K, Persson U (1985) Vad kostade 1982 års vägtrafikolyckor. IHE Meddelande 1985: 3. ISSN 0349-7631

Author's address: Å. Nygren, M.D., Ph.D., Folksam Research and Development Division, Stockholm, Sweden.

Acta Neurochirurgica, Suppl. 36, 18–20 (1986)

HIC—the Head Injury Criterion

Practical Significance for the Automotive Industry

H. Mellander

Volvo Car Corporation, Product Development Department 95205, PVN, S-40508 Göteborg, Sweden

Summary

Efforts to decrease the losses in human lifes on the roads during fifties led to an increased research into the biomechanics of head impact. A break-through was made with the introduction of the Wayne State Tolerance Curve. This curve was interpreted and a weighted injury criterion was developed. This criterion was later transformed into the Head Injury Criterion (HIC) and used in a proposed legislation to improve the crashworthiness of cars. Although heavily criticized the HIC-criterion still is the most established method to assess head injury in automotive impact conditions.

Keywords: Head injury criterion; head trauma; automotive trauma; biomechanics.

During the late fifties and the early sixties physicians and epidemiologists began to focus the problem of head injuries in traffic accidents. It became obvious that it was not enough to diagnose and treat head injuries. It was necessary to prevent or mitigate violence to the head. This contributed to the birth of a new science; the Biomechanics of Impact.

The biomechanician, often an engineer or physician, faced a multidisciplinary task which involved cooperation with physicians, physiologists, biologists and engineers. Aeromedical and defense research formed the platform from which the science was developed. Universities and a few automobile manufacturers followed suit and activities were started around the world. Information about the effect of trauma to the head was gathered from suicide attempts (free falls), experiments with volunteers, cadavers and animals.

It was found that injuries to the head and brain could be divided into two groups: 1) inertia related injuries where the visceral brain matter is displaced causing internal bleedings, diffuse injuries or injuries to the nerves, 2) localized or penetrating trauma causing the skull to fracture and thereby exposing the brain to damage.

From a car manufacturers viewpoint the most important work is definitely the research conducted at the Wayne State University during the fifties. A variety of different experiments were performed with heads from human cadavers and dogs in conditions similar to those found in the automobile environment. It was found that head injury (defined as the occurrence of a linear fracture) correlated with the magnitude of linear acceleration and pulse duration (angular acceleration was not measured).

These data and data from tests with volunteers for low g—long duration exposure were plotted in the same graph and the famous Wayne State curve was drawn up, see Fig. 1.

Charles W Gadd analyzed the curve and by plotting the data on log-log paper he found that a straight line approximated the curve quite well[1].

The equation for this line is

$$\bar{a}^{2.5} \cdot T = 1,000$$

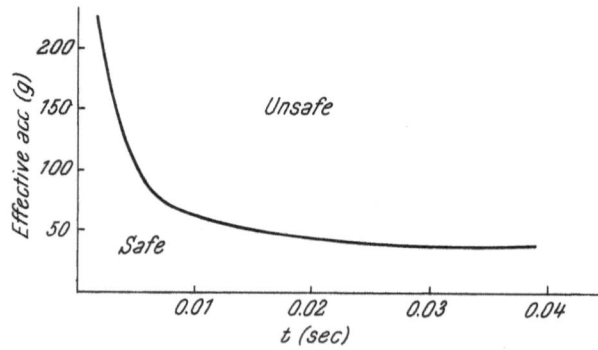

Fig. 1. Wayne State Curve

where $\bar{a}$ is average acceleration in g

T is duration in seconds.

He also gave this expression a general form

$$I = \int\limits_{\Delta t} \bar{a}^n \, dt$$

n = weighting factor > 1

and called it the Gadd Severity Index.

This equation had a tremendous impact on the scientific and legal communities. It was subjected to many alterations and was finally adopted by the legislators in U.S.A. in the format shown here.

$$HIC = \left[\frac{\int\limits_{t_1}^{t_2} a \, dt}{(t_2 - t_1)} \right]^{2,5} \cdot (t_2 - t_1)$$

a = resultant acceleration in centre of gravity of head
$t_2 - t_1$ = the time interval which maximizes the function.
2,5 = n.

It was denominated the HIC (Head Injury Criterion). In a proposed standard, Federal Motor Vehicle Safety Standard 208, from 1976 it was required that a car should be crash-tested into a fixed barrier at 50 km/h with test dummies as occupants. The HIC-values calculated from accelerometer readings in the heads of the dummies were not to exceed 1,000. It was stated that HIC ≤ 1,000 ensured "most of the population from a serious to fatal injury".

The automotive industry was in need of some biomechanical threshold values and the HIC-criterion was soon widely used and perhaps misused in a way that no one could have foreseen.

The HIC-criterion was developed as an impact criterion and was never intended for inertia loadings such as when forces are transmitted through the neck as in the case of a belted occupant with no head impact. Regardless of this and in lack of something better it was and still is used for all impact conditions and without consideration of the direction of impact.

The exponent 2.5 in the Gadd equation was selected for the forehead (skull) and not for facial impacts. However, no matter where an impact occurs on a dummy head the effect has been estimated with HIC!

Researchers in biomechanics also began questioning the analytical approach and the experimental technique in the original work[2].

Regardless of its pros and cons the HIC-criterion has led the automotive industry in the right direction and the cars of today are vastly improved compared with those of the early sixties.

In 1979 the legislators in America were once again trendsetters as they introduced crashworthiness rating of passenger cars. The rating test is performed at 35 mph and HIC among other criteria is calculated. The test data are reported to the consumer who can by himself judge from the guiding figures which car he wants to buy.

This has led to a competition in low HIC-values which has little scientific relevance.

Recent cadaver experiments in France on brains with ink perfusion have resulted in data which suggest a threshold value of 1,500 instead of 1,000[4]. This work has led to a new debate of the HIC-criterion but both legislators and researchers seem to hesitate to change the old level of 1,000.

It is worth mentioning the common misunderstanding that a HIC of 999 means you are "safe" and 1,001 means you are "dead". Anyone with a little knowledge about the scatter among individuals and their susceptibility will understand how wrong this is. A much better approach is to talk about the risk of being injured. Recent statistical studies have given methods to analyze biomechanical data in order to compute risk functions. The use of such functions has a much better scientific meaning and it is up to the legislators to choose a level for their protection criterion.

Most biomechanicians are today convinced that brain injury is a result of three different injury mechanisms, angular acceleration[3], linear acceleration and local deformation of the skull. This makes the current HIC-criterion rather obsolete and limited efforts are made around the world to come up with a better alternative.

Thus, the "scientific beauty" of the HIC-criterion has still to be challenged but however, heavily criticized the HIC-criterion will continue to be the most important parameter in rating of the crashworthiness of passenger cars but not of passengers. Money and resources put into biomechanical research are scarce and it will probably take a long time before any breakthrough for a new criterion can be made. In the meantime it is important that the users understand the origin and the limits of the HIC-criterion so that HIC values will be objectively judged, put in their right perspective, and not regarded as some "magical values".

References

1. Gadd Ch W (1966) Use of a Weighted—Impulse Criterion for Estimating Injury Hazards SAE, 660793, Stapp Car Crash Conference 1966, pp 164–174

2. Newman JA (1975) On the use of the Head Injury Criterion (HIC) in Protective Headgear Evaluation SAE 751162, Stapp Car Crash Conference 1975, pp 615–640

3. Ommaya AK (1985) Biomechanics of head injury. In: Melvin J, Nahum AM (eds) Experimental aspects in the biomechanics of trauma. Appelton-century-Crofts, pp 245–269

4. Walfish G, Fayon A, Tarriere C, Chamouard F (1981) Tolerance to impact: influence of the jerk (rate of onset of linear acceleration) on the occurrence of brain injuries, Ircobi Conference 1981, pp 286–296

Author's address: H. Mellander, Volvo Car Corporation, Product Development Department 95205, PVN, S-40508 Göteborg, Sweden.

Acta Neurochirurgica, Suppl. 36, 21–22 (1986)

Injury Scaling

P. G. Hansson

Department of Orthopedic Surgery, Länssjukhuset, Halmstad, Sweden

Summary

AIS and ISS are the scales almost exclusively used today in accident research for estimating severity of injury and mortality. The limitations in these scales are discussed. These limitations are considered in the new Probability of Death Score (PODS).

Keywords: Injuries: head injuries; severity scaling; threat to life.

One of the difficulties in earlier traffic medicine work was the lack of agreement on how the severity of injuries should be judged. One simple injury scale is used in official statistics on traffic accidents and injuries. There are three grades of seriousness. Fatalities are any persons who are killed outright or who die within 30 days as a result of the accident. Seriously or severely injured are persons who in the accident have sustained fracture, crash injury, severe cuts and lacerations, cerebral contusions or internal lesion or any other lesion entailing detention in hospital. The scale is not suitable for research purposes, but can sometimes be used in comparative studies between areas and time periods.

The injury scale used almost exclusively today is the Abbreviated Injury Scale (AIS)[1]. It is based on a more complicated scale—the Comprehensive Injury Scale. AIS is the result of collaboration between doctors in different specialities, engineers and traffic safety researchers and it is continuously revised. The parameters used to estimate severity of injury are energy dissipation, threat to life, permanent impairment, treatment period and incidence. It is however generally agreed that AIS mainly reflects "threat to life". The AIS grades are:

AIS	Severity Code (1980)
1	minor
2	moderate
3	serious
4	severe
5	critical
6	maximum, injury virtually unsurvivable
7	unknown

The revisions of AIS are compiled in a booklet where several examples of injuries and their coding are given.

In patients with multiple injuries the Injury Severity Score (ISS)[2, 3] is commonly used to judge the overall severity. ISS is the sum of the squares of the highest AIS for the three most severely injured body areas.

The six body regions used in ISS are:

1	skull/brain or neck
2	face
3	the extremities or pelvic girdle
4	chest
5	abdominal or pelvic content
6	external

AIS and ISS have not escaped criticism. The construction of ISS sometimes makes interpretation difficult. One fatal injury thus may have ISS 36 (6^2) while three severe, but not life threatening injuries have ISS 48 ($4^2 \times 3$). Recently the statistical treatment of AIS and ISS data has been criticized by Somers[5, 6]. He has constructed the Probability of Death Score (PODS). As compared to ISS PODS is based on a particular division of the body into regions, is not limited to just one AIS code per body region, includes a precise age factor, utilizes weighted rather than squared AIS codes and incorporates two rather than three AIS codes. Injury scales do not reflect permanent disability after injuries from traffic accidents as recently shown by Nygren[4].

References

1. Abbreviated Injury Scale. 1980 revision (1980) American Association for Automotive Medicine, Morton Grove, Ill.
2. Baker SP, O'Neill B, Haddon W, Long WB (1974) Injury severity score. A method for describing patients with multiple injuries and evaluating emergency care. J Trauma 14: 187–196
3. Baker SP, O'Neill B (1976) Injury severity score: An update. J Trauma 16: 882–897
4. Nygren Å (1984) Injuries to car occupants—some aspects of the interior safety of cars. Acta Otolaryngol (Stockh) [Suppl] 395
5. Somers RL (1983) The probability of death score: An improvement of the injury severity score. Accid Anal Prev 15: 247–257
6. Somers RL (1983) The probability of death score: A measure of injury severity for use in planning and evaluating accident prevention. Accid Anal Prev 15: 259–266

Author's address: P. G. Hansson, Department of Orthopedic Surgery, Länssjukhuset, S-30185 Halmstad, Sweden.

Acta Neurochirurgica, Suppl. 36, 23–24 (1986)

Time-Related Severity Scaling of Head Injuries—Discussion on the AIS-Severity Code—Early and Late

S. Lindgren

Department of Neurosurgery, Sahlgren's Hospital, Göteborg, Sweden

Summary

The deficiences of the present severity scaling of head injuries involve the absence of factors such as age, impact site etc. Moreover there is a terrible lack of agreement and of possibilities of translation between the AIS and the coma scales, presently more wellknown among neurosurgeons. The importance of noting the time after trauma for AIS-codifying must also be stressed, as well as of the presence of intoxication. A modified AIS-scale (EIS) is suggested to facilitate comparison with coma scales such as GCS, as well with the diagnostic terminology suggested for ICD 10 later in this supplement. An attempt to use the EIS as a late scaling after the "transition period" of the second to fourth week after injury is also suggested as a basis for a prediction of late residual disabilities.

Keywords: Head injury; modified severity scaling; coma scaling, diagnostic terminology.

It is nowadays a common knowledge that among the significant parameters influencing the evaluation of head injuries are not only the neurological and focal injuries themselves but also factors such as age, intoxication, impact site and impact severity and extracranial injuries and complications.

For the last factors the ISS or PODS have been commented upon by P. Hansson, but in Gothenburg we have also tried to consider the factors of age and impact site in a scale similar to the AIS. The AIS severity codes have themselves been subjects for modification with regard to discussion of coma scales, such as the Glasgow Coma Scale[1].

"Early Injury Scale"

As is shown in Table 1 the present scale temporarily called "*Early Injury Scale (EIS)*" only gives a rough indication of the prognostic importance of age below 20 years, between 20 and 50 years and above 50 years. At the same time consideration is also given to the impact site with frontal impacts regarded as less severe than temporal and occipital impacts.

Also simultaneously occurring cervical spine injuries in the lower and upper region are mentioned as prognostic factors. The severity scaling has been discussed previously particularly with regard to the patients "reaction levels" (AIS—Glasgow Coma Scale)[1]. Intoxication may be included as in group "2" or added from a separate coded group of intoxication diagnoses. The optimal number of factors is limited[3].

The scale was constructed to help the nurse or surgeon in the receiving emergency ward to get an opinion of the degree of threat to life of the injury as well as the emergency of management.

Table 1. *Early Injury Scale (EIS)*. (Gothenburg, 1979) (Degree of "threat to life") (> 30 min after accident). Impact sites, type. Age: < 20, 20–50, > 50 years

0. All ages: Head trauma. Alert. No immediate symptoms or signs.
1. All ages: Head trauma, slight (direct or indirect). Wounds. Slight non-localized pain in head or neck. Facial fractures. No unconsciousness. Dizzy. Confused. Slow answer.
2. All ages: Head trauma, moderate. Frontal impact. Wounds. Localized pain in head or neck. Facial displaced fracture. Eye ball damage.
   Unconsciousness < 30 min. PTA brief. Vomiting. Drowsy, eyes open, fixating; answers on request, confused and intoxicated.
   Spine: Dorsal and lumbar damage, no neurological symptoms.
3. All ages: Head trauma, moderate. Frontal or vertex impacts. Skull fracture (vault + temporal bone). Severe maxillar fractures. Unconscious < 6 hrs. Amnesia. If still unconscious: Localizing-warding off motor pattern with or without pain stimuli.
   Spine: Cervical damage, no neurological symptoms. Dorsal and lumbar damage with neurological symptoms.

4. < 50 years old (includes also no5 if < 20 years):
    ˙Head trauma: particularly temporal or occipital impacts. Skull fracture (open or base). Airway obstruction.
    Unconscious < 24 hrs. Stereotype flexor motor pattern. Hyperthermia.

    Intracranial expansive lesion ("secondary" complication) indicated by deeper unconsciousness, hemisymptoms, unequal pupils.
    Spine: Lower cervical damage with neurological symptoms.

5. > 50 years old—findings as in grade no 4—or
    All ages > 20 years: Head trauma, moderate to severe, all sites particularly occipital.
    Unconscious > 24 hrs. Respiratory abnormalities. Stereotype extensor motor pattern. Pupils fixed.
    Symptoms indicating intracranial expansive lesion.
    Spine: Upper cervical damage with neurological symptoms.

6. All ages: Head trauma, severe.
    Unconscious. Respiratory insufficiency—or lasting apnea. On pain no reaction or extensor motor pattern. Dilated fixed pupils. Anatomic lesions, related to this functional deficit.

    All head injury degrees may develop secondary complications indicating
    intracranial expansive lesion. Intrathoracic and intraabdominal injuries etc may add to the degree of injury. The "final" result may be graded according to neurological scales.

Main Factor considered

Age	Impact site, type
Fracture	Airway
Conscious impairment:	Respiration
defined conscious	Pupils
level	Paresis
intoxication	(add "extracranial inj"
	AIS-coded)

"Late Injury Scale (LIS)" (2–4 weeks after accident)

It is well-known that a certain serious sign after head trauma is becoming prognostically more severe after the initial, immediate and early, stage (see Fig. 6, Introduction).

It may then indicate a longstanding injury of less transient character or a superimposed complication.

However, two weeks after the head trauma the risk for such complications has become much less. The injuries sustained have stabilized and improvement rather than impairment may be expected. This seems also to be the finding of R. Braakman in his work on "prediction of outcome" in this supplement. He con-

siders the predictive power of some important posttraumatic indicators to change after one week and states that "it is only rarely possible to give a sharp prediction of the degree of final disability—even in two categories—within the first two weeks after onset of coma" (the separate phenomenon of vegetating states 3–4 weeks after the severe trauma has the same bad or even worse prognosis of survival as the prolonged posttraumatic coma).

After two weeks thus the same type of severity code could be used as in the presented EIS. In AIS-76 the grading was made with regard to "*threat to life*". The various degrees may empirically be shown as varying mortality percentages or "risk of death".

Braakman *et al.* (this supplement) have shown that four weeks after "comatose head injury" "sharp predictions" are possible using five outcome categories. They have also constructed a booklet "for bedside use" with probabilities of 6-months survival. The appropriate type and number of variables are discussed at powerful combinations.

With respect to the experience of Braakman *et al.* and the interest of predicting residual medical disability the LIS could be based on *threat to "normal" life* and then also include later morbidity. Neuropsychological and psychosocial deficit shown also after mild head injuries may be evident with more elaborate and behavioral testing[2] already 1 month after head injury.

The final outcome may not be evident until at least half a year to two years after the acute injury.

In special retrospective studies the power of the predictive tools mentioned above can be studied.

References

1. Lindgren S (1983) Coma scale—awareness of reaction levels as part of commonly used severity grading. Scott Med J 28: 203–204
2. McLean A, Jr, Dikman S, Temkin N, *et al* (1984) Psychosocial Functioning at one month after head injury. Neurosurgery 14: 393–399.
3. Miller GA (1956) The magical number 7 + or + 2: Some limits on our capacity for processing information. Psychol Rev 6: 81–97

Author's address: Prof. Dr. S. Lindgren, Department of Neurosurgery, Sahlgren's Hospital, University of Göteborg, S-413 45 Göteborg, Sweden.

Acta Neurochirurgica, Suppl. 36, 25–27 (1986)

Acute Injury Scaling Related to Residual Disability

Å. Nygren[1], P. G. Hansson[2], and **C. Tingvall[1]**

[1] Folksam Research and Development Division, Stockholm, Sweden
[2] Department of Orthopedic Surgery, County Hospital, Halmstad, Sweden

Summary

Injury scaling is an important issue in the traffic safety field. A comparison was made between the severity of injuries as graded according to the Abbreviated Injury Scale (AIS) and the severity 5 years after the accident. It was found that among persons with permanent medical disability $\geq 10\%$, 20% were given an AIS score of 1, i.e. they were initially judged as having a slight injury. This implies that the AIS scale needs to be re-evaluated to take into account possible long-term consequences.

Keywords: Injury scaling; head injury disability.

Background

Scaling of acute injuries has been a matter of concern regarding traffic accidents for the last three decades, since the mid-1950s, although division into killed and injured has been made since the 1930s. Injuries in surviving victims have been divided into slight and severe. In most countries this classification has been made by the police at the scene of the accident, thus leading to quality problems. There are two definitions of "severely injured", but most often the definition "spent at least one day in hospital" has been used. So far the term "slightly injured" has not been defined. This simple injury rating refers to the severity for the person as a whole, and not to the single diagnosis, although there are countries (e.g. Denmark) where the police also code the location of injuries.

Data from acute injury scaling are important as a source of information in traffic safety work, for example in identifying risks, establishing injury criteria, and in the construction and evaluation of traffic safety measures. Conventional police evaluations of the severity of injuries is very seldom sufficient in this work.

The Abbreviated Injury Scale (AIS)[1] has been accepted as a tool for assessing injuries in the acute phase. From the beginning it was intended for the evaluation of injuries from a variety of stand points. Today, the risk of death seems to be the only parameter that is judged with AIS. AIS is a scale with values from 1 to 6. Some examples of AIS values for skull/brain injuries are given below. AIS 1 represents very slight injuries, and AIS 6 unsurvivable injuries (AIS-80).

AIS 1 Head injury with no prior unconsciousness but the victim may have headache or dizziness.

AIS 2 Amnesia or trauma with no neurological deficit.

AIS 3 Cerebellar or cerebral contusion verified not only by clinical diagnosis.

AIS 4 Cerebellar or cerebral hematoma, epidural or subdural, $\geq 100\,cc$ or unspecified, not only verified by clinical diagnosis.

AIS 5 Brain stem compression.

AIS 6 Crush (or ring) fracture. ("6" certainly indicates accompanying fatal brain stem injury)

Great care must be taken when analysing the severity of an injury with AIS, as the values are not equidistant.

It is not enough to evaluate an injury in the acute phase solely in terms of the risk of death, but long-term consequences also have to be considered. Disability and handicap are costly to the society and unacceptable to those suffering from pain, mental disturbances and functional loss as a result of a trauma. Today there are no criteria that are accepted worldwide for the prediction of long-term consequences. Nygren[2] showed that AIS cannot be used for this purpose. In this report, long-term consequences of head injuries are described.

Material

During the period July 1, 1976 to December 12, 1980 all car occupants injured in cars involved in accidents reported to the Folksam Insurance company were studied and coded according to AIS and to their specific diagnoses. Hospital records and doctors' certificates were used to obtain adequate medical data. Four to five years after the accident all cases were collected a second time in order to study the long-term consequences, and all those subjects with residual problems over a certain limit were judged by a committee. The committee followed specific outcome criteria for evaluating the degree of objective disability based on objective loss of function and also on such factors as the patient's degree of pain. No attention is or was paid to handicap or to the patient's work and environment. The level of disability is or was set at 10 to 100%.

Examples of residual problems following head injury, and the corresponding disability levels, are given below:

Sensory disturbances	0–50%
Headache	5–10%
Epilepsy	
Mild-infrequent attacks with aura	15–25%
Severe-frequent attacks with aura	30–65%
Mild-infrequent attacks without aura	20–35%
Severe-frequent attacks without aura	35–100%
Mental complications (depressive, asthenic reactions, etc)	10–25%

Altogether 12,007 car occupants were injured during the period in question. Of these 563 (4.9%) had a residual medical disability of $\geq 10\%$.

Method

The number of injured persons with skull/brain injuries of different AIS levels were compared with the number with residual problems. Comparisons were also made for injuries of other locations.

Results

Table 1 shows the number of injuries to the skull/brain among the car occupants.

Table 1. *The Number of Injuries to the Skull/Brain of Different AIS Levels Among Surviving Patients*

AIS	Number of injuries	%
1	2,051	75.3
2	512	18.8
3	82	3.0
4	32	1.2
5	46	1.7
Total	2,723	

It is seen that the majority of the injuries were slight ones. The numbers of injuries of different AIS grades that led to $\geq 10\%$ medical disability are given in Table 2.

Table 2. *Number of Skull/Brain Injuries of Different AIS Levels Leading to Permanent Disability ($\geq 10\%$)*

AIS	Number of injuries	%
1	12	20.3
2	8	13.6
3	11	18.6
4	8	13.6
5	20	33.8
Total	59	

A total of 59 injuries led to permanent disability, i.e. 2.2% of all head injuries, which is lower than for all injuries (3.5%).

Table 3. *Ratio Between Injuries with Permanent Disability ($\geq 10\%$) and all Injuries to the Skull/Brain*

AIS	Ratio
1	0.6%
2	1.6%
3	13.4%
4	25.0%
5	43.5%

The disability risk, defined as the ratio between the number of permanently disabling injuries and all injuries to the skull/brain, increased rapidly with increasing AIS value, although the total number of AIS 1 injuries with permanent disability was 20% (12 out of 59).

Compared with injuries of other locations, skull/brain injuries carried a higher risk of leading to permanent medical disability, if the spine and lower extremities are excluded. It was concluded that AIS cannot be used as a tool for predicting long-term consequences unless the different body regions are separated.

Discussion

Acute injury scaling is the basis for epidemiological analyses in most traffic safety work. Simple scaling such as division into slight, severe and fatal injuries is seldom enough for deeper analysis. The AIS system and its outlines are considered to be a valuable tool for predicting a fatal outcome. For survivable injuries, however, it is important to have an idea of the long-term consequences, as it is considered that later impairment and handicap due to injuries should be avoided primarily.

To obtain an idea of the risks of having a disability as a result of injuries of different levels and types, patients must be followed up over a long period of time, and with clearly defined and consistent outcome criteria. Several authors have attempted to carry out such longitudinal studies with different criteria[3, 4, 5].

Death and permanent impairment are the most unacceptable consequences of road accident trauma. Better knowledge of the way in which these risks, especially long-term consequences, occur is essential both for reasons of protection and for biomechanical research. As the AIS scale is used all over the world, it is desirable to evaluate the possibility of predicting the long-term consequences by using this scale and ISS. Gustafsson *et al.* described a method of using the disability level applied by insurance companies in Sweden and compared it with AIS[7]. Further evaluation, taking into account both age and specific diagnoses, is required.

Conclusion

— It is important to have an injury scale whereby the long-term consequences can be predicted.

— For head injuries the AIS injury scale is inadequate for predicting long-term consequences among survivors.

— Further evaluation of the AIS scale is necessary.

References

1. Abbreviated injury scale 1980. Revision (1980) American Association for Automotive Medicine, Morton Grove Ill
2. Nygren Å (1984) Injuries to car occupants. Some aspects of the interior safety of cars. Acta Otolaryngol (Stockh) [Suppl] 395
3. Somers SL (1983) The probability of death score: A measure of injury severity for use in planning and evaluation accident prevention. Accid Anal Prev 4: 259–266
4. Bull JP (1975) The injury severity score of road traffic casualties in relation to mortality, time of death, hospital treatment time and disability. Accid Anal Prev 7: 249–255
5. Baker SP, O'Neill B (1976) The injury severity score: An update Journal of trauma 11: 882–885
6. Bull JP (1985) Disabilities caused by road traffic accidents and their relation to severity scores. Accid Anal Prev 17: 386–397
7. Gustafsson H, Nygren Å, Tingvall C (1985) Rating system for serious consequences (RSC) due to traffic accidents. Risk of death or permanent disability. Proceeding 10th Int Conf on Experimental Safety Vehicles, Oxford 1985

Authors' address: Å. Nygren, M.D., Ph.D., Folksam Research and Development Division, Stockholm, Sweden.

Acta Neurochirurgica, Suppl. 36, 28–30 (1986)

Biomechanics—Material Properties and "Tissue Damage"

P. Löwenhielm

Institute of Forensic Medicine, University of Lund, Sweden

Summary

Biomechanics is concerned with mechanical properties of tissues and their relation in living organisms. Material properties, of elements and specific tissues are discussed in relation to mechanical failure in terms of stress and strain. Some examples relevant to head injury are presented.

Keywords: Biomechanics; material properties; head injury.

Mechanics deals with the action and counteractions of forces. The mass of different tissue components acts by their weight and, in a dynamical situation by their inertia. The force actions are studied by means of the equilibrium laws of mechanics, *i.e.* equilibrium of forces and moments. However, the laws of equilibrium are seldom applicable in a biomechanical situation since tissue elements such as muscles are active components and a specific external force action does not imply that the body will assume a predicted position which would be the case if all the components were passive. Physiological terms such as "isometric" (maintained geometry) and "isotonic" (maintained force) have no counterparts in engineering. The skull, the cervical spine, and the brain can be regarded as "passive" while the muscles of the neck are "active".

Biomechanics is—in a broad sense—concerned with mechanical properties of tissues (*e.g.* stress-strain relationships, breaking strength) and their relations in living organisms. In the human being these tissues are bone, cartilage, ligament, muscles etc. In biomechanical analysis the anatomy is of crucial importance in the determination of how the different tissues and organs move in relation to each other, *e.g.* does slip constitute the movement in a knee joint or is it rolling or is it a combination of the two? How do the blood corpuscles deform and move in the narrow capillaries and how does the brain move within the skull when the head is subjected to acceleration?

Body tissues may have elastic or viscoelastic properties. A rubberband is elastic and resumes its original length when the force action ceases.—Most of the tissues of the human body regain their former size and shape after deformation, *i.e.* if tissue damage has not occurred. This return to size and shape occurs gradually, and is an example of the viscoelasticity of the tissues of the body. In order to deform a body a certain force is needed. If the body is viscoelastic the viscous component will oppose to the speed of force action, *i.e.* if the body is to be deformed rapidly a higher force is needed. This behaviour can be compared to an injection with a narrow needle. The syringe can easily be emptied slowly while a rapid injection requires considerable force. A deformation which is maintained when the force action is over is called a plastic deformation.

Muscles, bone, cartilage, and fibrous tissues such as tendons, ligaments and fascia are composed of different basic components of which collagen, elastine and apatite are the most important and exibit widely differing mechanical properties. Apatite is strong and brittle like glass, while elastine is not very strong but very elastic and resembles rubber (*cf.* Fig. 1). The yellow ligament of the neck at the back aspect of the spinal column is never unloaded even when the head is extremely extended. This pre-stretching prevents wrinkling of the ligament in order to avoid interference with the spinal cord.

Bone contains apatite and collagen. The apatite gives the bone its strength while the toughness of the collagen prevents the composite material to be brittle as pure apatite, *i.e.* the same construction method as in engineering composite materials such as fibre glass reinforced plastic (*cf.* Fig. 2).

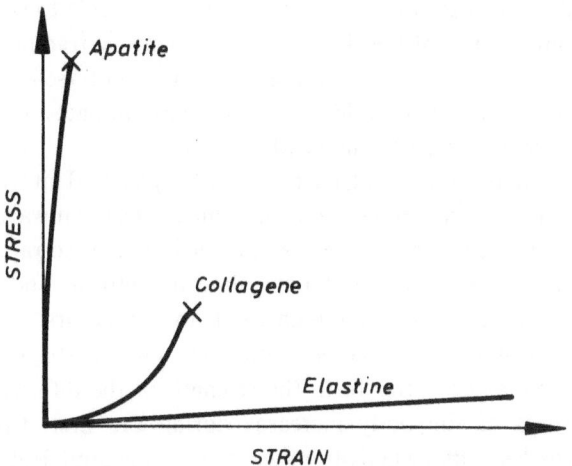

Fig. 1. Stress strain relationship for some mechanical elements of tissues of the body

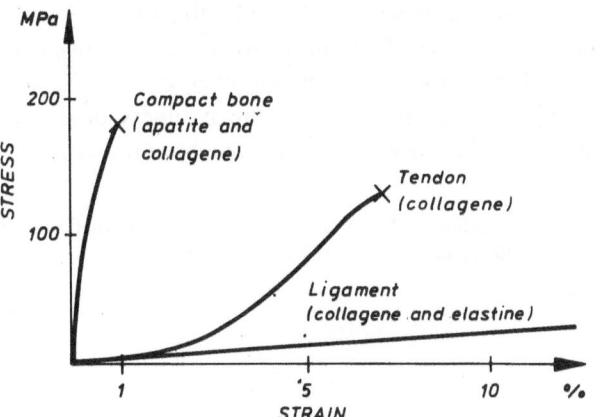

Fig. 2. Stress strain relationship for some tissues of the body

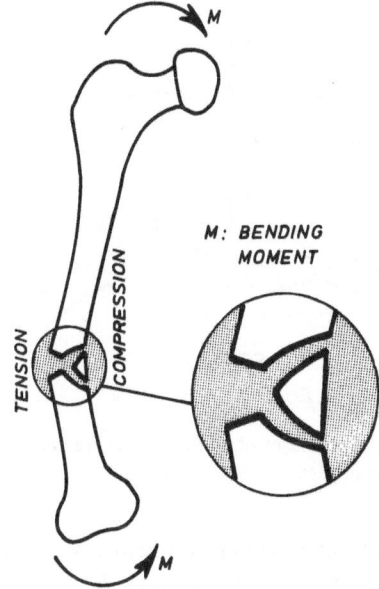

Fig. 3. Fracture mechanism of a tubular bone subjected to bending

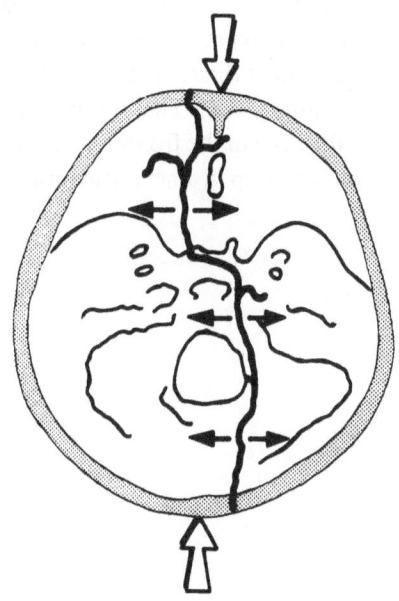

Fig. 4. Fracture mechanism of a fracture of the base of the skull. Bone is more resistant to compression than to tension

Mechanical damage to animate tissues are—at least on the microscopical level—mostly caused by tensile forces, which tear, anatomically, the structural elements apart. The counterpart at the macroscopical level may be shearing, bending etc.

The mechanical behaviour of the different tissues can be described in terms of a stress-strain curve. For biological tissues this relationship is quite linear for bone but not for soft tissues. The bladder can enlarge considerably before stresses in the wall develop, and an urge to urinate is felt, a design that is practical for normal living.

Mechanical failures occur when the stress (or strain) reaches a critical level for the tissue, *i.e.* the ultimate stress or ultimate strain. The ultimate strain for parenchymatous tissues is quite low compared with the values for bone and tendons. In viscoelastic tissues the critical levels are dependent on the strain rate also. When a parasagittal bridging vein is slowly strained it

can assume its double length before rupture occurs, while the maximal strain is about 15% when the strain rate is high.

As another example of a failure mechanism a long bone subjected to bending can be studied. When bent, there will be tensile stresses on the convex side of the bone and compressive stresses on the other (Fig. 3). The ultimate stress for bone differ in compression and in tension, the ultimate stress being somewhat lower in tension compared with compression. Therefore, the

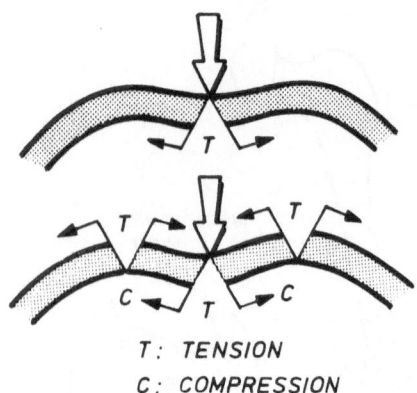

T : TENSION
C : COMPRESSION

Fig. 5. Fracture mechanism of an impression fracture of the skull after blunt head impact

fracture of a long bone in bending always begins at the convex side and at a right angle as the tensile stresses have the highest magnitude in this direction.

The same reasoning holds true for skull fracture: Let the skull be compressed in an anterior-posterior direction (Fig. 4). This will decrease the anterior-posterior diameter of the skull and at the same time increase the diameter in the frontal plane. The result is tensile stresses tangent to the skull in the frontal plane and the tensile stresses will open up a linear fracture in the anterior-posterior direction. Conversely, a side to side compression of the skull leads to transverse fractures. This is exactly how a nut breaks when compressed in a nutcracker. This holds true for blunt impacts with moderate speed to the head (Fig. 5).

On the other hand, if a bullet with high speed hits the skull, a conical bone fragment which enlarges inwards will be stamped out. In this case the impact is so rapid that the skull will not have time to deform, and a fracture caused by the high local stresses occurs.

Another factor that determines the ultimate stress or strain is age. After birth the strength of the different tissues of the body increases during the first two decades of life, whereafter there is a decline until death. Illness (osteoporosis, neoplasms etc) can steepen this decline. The following hypothetical experiment could be made: If the heart of the newborn is considered to be strong enough (mechanically) to be able to live outside the womb, when does the heart achieve its original strength after the maximum. In other words, which is the biomechanical length of life if illness does not intercept? The answer is: about one hundred years.

Author's address: P. Löwenhielm, M.D., Institute of Forensic Medicine, Sölvegatan 25, S-223 62 Lund, Sweden.

Acta Neurochirurgica, Suppl. 36, 31–32 (1986)

Head Injuries—Biomechanical Principles

P. Löwenhielm

Institute of Forensic Medicine, University of Lund, Sweden

Summary

The biomechanics of the head injuries is a most needed area of knowledge for the prevention of head injuries. Features of anatomy constituting natural protective parts as well as weak links in the injury process are discussed. Acceleration of the head can cause intracranial damage. The injury mechanisms associated with linear and angular acceleration of the head are presented. In addition comments are made on some injury criteria employed in the evaluation of head injury.

Keywords: Head injury biomechanics; physical injury criteria; traumatic head anatomy.

There is extensive literature on the possible mechanisms of head impact injury (*cf.* Viano[7]). When dealing with head injuries from a biomechanical standpoint, some special features of the anatomy of the head are worth attention:

One of the five layers of the scalp, the aponeurotic layer consists of dense fibrous tissue and is freely movable over the skull. This movability facilitates slip off of tangential blows to the head. On the other hand the looseness of the subaponeurotic layer allow the formation of enormous hematomas after tearing of connecting blood vessels between scalp and skull.

The cranial vault is a rigid container made up of several bones each with its own unique internal and external geometry. It encases the brain, and prevents local deformation of the brain at the impact site. The skull is in its turn protected by the scalp. It has been estimated that the scalp yields a forty fold increase of the skull fracture tolerance level (blunt trauma).

The cerebrospinal fluid has shock absorbing properties: a liquid applies uniform pressure without shearing stress to any surface it contacts (in this case the brain surface). Thus, the cerebrospinal fluid distributes any focally applied external pressure to a uniform stress which is also tolerated well by neural tissues. The density of the cerebrospinal fluid is slightly lower than that of the brain tissue why the brain will gradually sink. Pudenz and Shelden[5] observed a considerable increase in the amplitude of gliding movements of the brain surface after impact if cerebrospinal fluid was removed prior to impact. Thus, the cerebrospinal fluid seems to damp the brain movement after head impact, probably in combination with preserved elastance of the craniospinal compartment.

The falx cerebri and the tentorium cerebelli which support the brain and separate one neural part from another can serve as sharp instruments or space-limiting structures during traumatic episodes.

The brain, therefore, seems to be well protected within the cranial vault. However, the water content of the different intracranial tissues is high and makes them essentially incompressible. As the vault is rigid, any volume change of any one of the intracranial tissues, *i.e.* the brain matter, the cerebrospinal fluid volume and the blood volume, will necessarily influence the volume of the others and cause increased intracranial pressure; if a volume increase is focal brain deformation and dislocation will occur with tentorial herniation, brainstem compression etc.

Such intracranial volume shifts are the successors of trauma to the head. Then, which are the biomechanical prerequisites for such changes to occur? Impact to a freely moveable head causes acceleration of the head and destructive stresses may occur at the impact site as well as remote from the impact site.

Linear acceleration of the head does not produce any notable mass movement of the brain but produces negative pressure, which has been assumed to be able to exceed the cohesive strength of the brain tissue, thereby causing cavitation of the cerebral parenchyma (appearance of gas bubbles). Gross[2] was the first to outline the cavitation hypothesis from observations of bubble formation in waterfilled glass vessels. The negative pressure concept is an ingenious engineering solution of the contrecoup problem. Gross[2] also advocated that injuries at the impact site resulted from negative pressure generated by snap-back of the skull after initial skull indentation. The cavitation theory suggests that the damage is caused mainly by the forceful collapse of the tiny cavities. Using a head model subjected to impact, Lubock and Goldsmith[4] have shown evidence for bubble formation in the fluids in the cranial cavity but their results appear to negate any bubble formation in the brain tissue proper. Furthermore, medical observers have indicated that negative pressure theories do not provide a satisfactory explanation for the location of the traumatic injuries and the evidence for cavitation in biological systems is meager indeed.

Head impact generally imparts rotation—angular acceleration as well as linear motion. Because of its inertia, the brain resists simultaneous rotation with the skull, *i.e.* the brain lags behind. Pudenz and Shelden[5] viewed the motion of the brain surface using the lucite calvarium technique. They used living monkeys subjected to head angular acceleration. The rotational motion causes distortion of the brain tissue. The original work in this area was presented by Holbourn[3] who on theoretical grounds proposed that brain injury is caused by shear strains due to brain distortion following angular acceleration of the head. In a traumatic situation this distortion is of centimeter size which may be sufficient to produce mechanical failure, thereby providing a traumatic mechanism. The rotational theory gives fixed injury sites which are also found in practice, but fails to explain the predominance of contrecoup injury.

Head injury tolerance levels which correlate well with the injury severity and physical injury criteria (see Mellander this supplement) attempt to address the physiological failure level by relating a clinically (or pathologically) observable process, such as amnesia, coma or loss of reflex action. Tolerance levels are the most employed representations and are appropriate clinical correlations for many biomechanical descriptions. Here, component behaviour is described in terms of a stress-strain curve in a particular mode of loading (tension, compression, bending) and when fracture or failure occurs (ultimate stress).

The internationally accepted scale for classifying severity in terms of risk to life is the injury severity scale—AIS (see Hansson, this supplement). This has no direct correlation to the disability of the patient. A successfully treated subdural hematoma may disable a patient less compared with an open tibial fracture, although the subdural hematoma scores a higher injury severity.

The physical Mean Strain Criterion (MSC) was published by Stalnaker *et al.* in 1971[6]. Experiments with subhuman primates led to the establishment of the MSC and the results were extrapolated to humans. The MSC is a continuous criterion with respect to head injury and correlates well with the AIS. It is however valid for linear acceleration though. A criterion for head injury following angular motion of the head is needed and a tolerance level correlated with AIS has been proposed by Goldsmith and Ommaya[1].

Distinction should be made for the skull and the brain concerning injury criteria. While fracture characteristics of the skull can be quantified by a mean value, failure of the brain tissue cannot be so conveniently delineated because physiological dysfunction most likely occurs at levels well below that producing mechanical disruption of soft tissues and, furthermore, the tissues comprising the brain and the blood vessels are so complex that neither functional nor structural failure limits have been adequately established. In consequence, an injury level for the brain is normally specified in terms of the magnitude of some mechanical parameter considered to be a major indicator of cerebral trauma.

References

1. Goldsmith W, Ommaya AK (1984) Head and neck injury criteria and tolerance levels. In: Aldman B, Chapon A (eds) The biomechanics of impact trauma. Elsevier Science Publisher, pp 149–187
2. Gross AG (1958) A new theory on the dynamics of brain concussion and brain injury. J Neurosurg 15: 548–561
3. Holbourn AHS (1943) Mechanics of head injuries. Lancet 2: 438–441
4. Lubock P, Goldsmith W (1980) Experimental cavitation studies in a model head-neck system. J Biomechanics 13: 1041–1052
5. Pudenz RH, Shelden CH (1946) The lucite calvarium—a method for direct observation of the brain, II. Cranial trauma and brain movement. J Neurosurg 3: 487–505
6. Stalnaker RL *et al.* (1971) Driving point impedance characteristics of the head. J Biomechanics 4: 127–139
7. Viano DC (1985) Bibliography of head injury literature. General Motors Research Laboratories Report #GMR-4936

Author's address: P. Löwenhielm, M.D., Institute of Forensic Medicine, Sölvegatan 25, S-223 62 Lund, Sweden.

Acta Neurochirurgica, Suppl. 36, 33–46 (1986)

Experimental Models of Head Injury

D. Stålhammar

Department of Neurosurgery, Sahlgren's Hospital, University of Göteborg, Sweden

Summary

Experimental research in studies of head injury may be directed along theoretical, mechanical and experimental animal and clinical lines. The parameter of the results compared may thus be the mechanics of skull or the skull contents, pathophysiological changes or pathomorphological lesions. Due to the variation of the daily accidents and resulting injuries each series of problems must be studied with suitable technique.

Often the various types of studies determine the possibility of interpreting the results for clinical analysis and prevention. However, this is often possible if all experimental conditions and parameters studied are precisely defined.

Movements, deformations of skull and the intracranial contents, results from rotational and angular acceleration and velocities as well as the direction and the site of impact in the human being must always be considered.

Keywords: Head injury experimental models; experimental traumatic pathophysiology; posttraumatic pathomorphology; clinical traumatic analysis.

Introduction

Simulation of the events at head injury is a most important way to gain knowledge of the injury mechanisms and thereby produce a *rational basis for prevention and therapy* of these injuries. The efforts in this field, however, have not been restricted to mechanical trauma and its consequences, but has also included a variety of investigations of the circulatory, biochemical, bioelectrical, structural and other changes of various types of insults (temperature, hypoxia, ischemia, electrical current etc).

Therefore, for any neurosurgeon, even without a particular interest in experimental head injuries, it certainly is of great value not only to get an orientation among the abundance of various experimental models, but also to understand some of the principles and the difficulties involved in the development of such models because such understanding is a prerequisite for *critical interpretation* of experiments: to evaluate the validity of a model and the reliability of the measurements performed.

This paper will briefly discuss the mechanisms of head injury and orientate you about various models.

Basic Concepts of Tissue Injuring Mechanisms at Mechanical Trauma

General

The principal direct cause of dysfunction and structural *failure* as a result of external forces acting on the human body is the *relative displacement* of adjacent body tissues (deformation, strain).

In Fig. 1 this relative displacement is illustrated by a

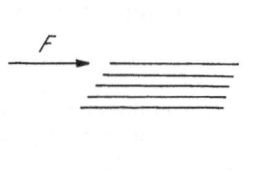

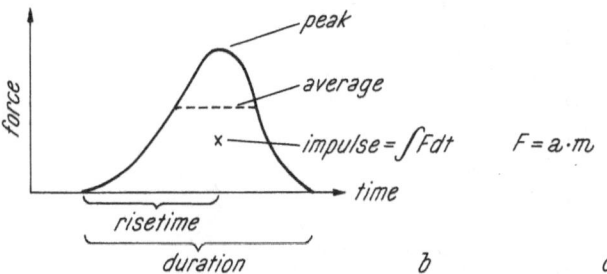

Fig. 1. a) A pack of cards deformed by a force that has a specific direction and point of action and which may vary in amplitude over time. b) The time course can be defined by rise, peak, duration, average value, impulse. c) Newton's second law: force and acceleration are directly related to each other

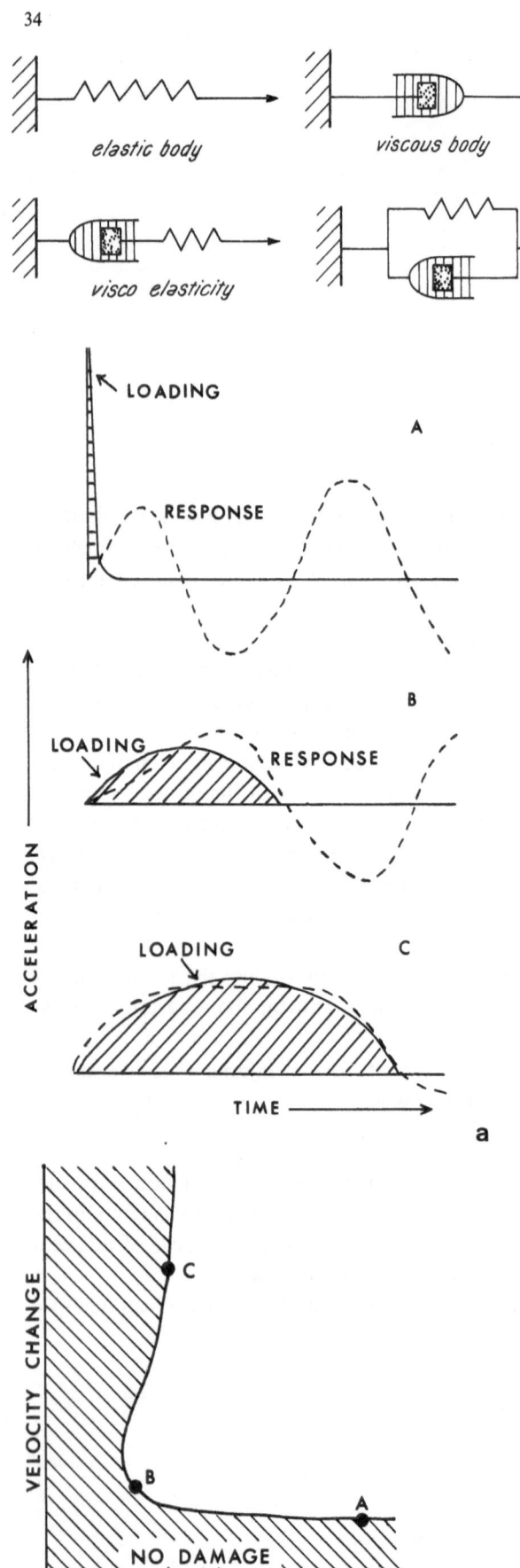

Fig. 2. Illustration of mechanical properties, elasticity, viscosity, plasticity and visco-elasticity

pack of cards deformed by a force. The *force* has a direction, a specific point where it acts and a magnitude varying over time. The *deformation* can be defined by the total distances of the displacement in three dimensions and the time courses of these. The deformations are denoted *strains* (compression, tension and shear) and the forces acting within a material are usually denoted *stresses*.

The relation between the external loading force and the resulting stresses and strains within a body is dependent upon the *mechanical properties* of the tissue (elasticity, viscosity etc) compare Fig. 2.

Data on properties of living tissue (elasticity, plasticity and viscosity) are known to some extent [12, 13, 16, 63, 67, 77] and are used in mathematical simulation [15, 39, 49, 58–60, 102].

The mechanical properties of a structure (and its geometrical characteristics) are decisive for which will be the lowest frequency at which free (natural) vibration will occur: the *natural frequency* of the material. The duration of one such oscillation is denoted the "natural period".

The *ratio* between the *duration of the loading* and the *natural period* is of direct importance for the magnitude of internal displacement and the degree of damage. Depending on this ratio different critical parameters can be identified: the average or peak magnitude of the force, the impulse or both. See Fig. 3.

— If this ratio is *small* compared to one: the same impulse will result in the same injury even if for instance the maximum force (and acceleration) will vary over a wide range.—The blow is over before the structure has started to move.

— if this ratio is *great* compared to one: the same maximum force (or acceleration) will produce the same

Fig. 3. a) Illustration of how the impact duration affects the peak acceleration necessary to induce a given amplitude level of response.—The shorter the duration of the loading the greater the acceleration required for the same velocity response. b) A sensitivity curve for a simple mass spring system subjected to half-sine pulses according to a. (From Kornhauser *et al.* 1962[48])

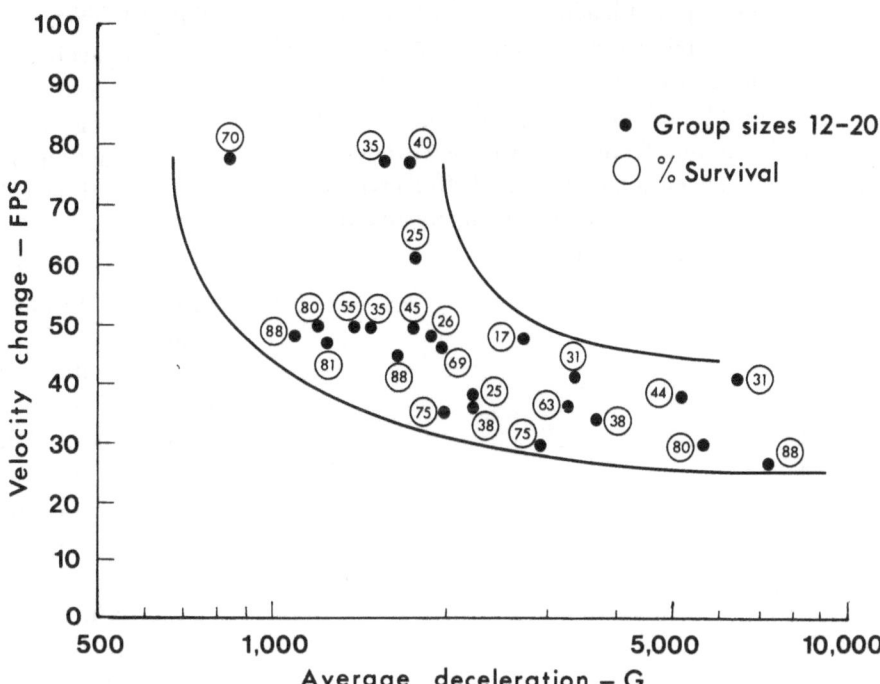

Fig. 4. Tolerance of restrained mice to transversely applied impact forces. (From Gold *et al.* 1962[24])

injury (even if the impulse and duration will vary over a wide range).

— If this ratio is *about one:* neither the impulse nor the maximum force alone can characterize the sensitivity. The complete force-time function must be considered.

In real head injury impacts and in experimental impacts the duration of the loading is in the same range as the natural periods of the structures involved. For the brain of an animal or man natural frequency is about 10–30 Hz (natural period 100–30 msec)[41, 93].

In Fig. 4 this is shown by a classical experiment from Aero Space Medicine in the beginning of the 60's. The impact tolerance of mice is a function of velocity change (corresponding to the impulse) and average acceleration. In these experiments death resulted primarily from "sudden displacement of the central nervous system"[24].

In Fig. 5 the same phenomenon is illustrated by another classical curve (5 a), the Wayne State University *Tolerance Curve.* Although this is extrapolated from very few and widespread experimental data (linear acceleration 3–5 msec) it shows the basic principle and also how these early data fits into later information (Fig. 5 b).

In Fig. 6 pathophysiological and pathomorphological changes are related to the duration of load and to the peak pressure amplitude in an head injury experiment; sudden volume load of the exposed rabbit brain[90, 91].

It is of interest to compare the development of experimental models for studying spinal injuries where for a long time only the potential energy of the impacts in gm-cm units were used and where it has been nicely shown by Dohrmann *et al.* that spinal cord injuries of different magnitudes can be obtained by the same gm-cm amount by various combinations of weight and height (velocity)[3, 10, 11] and *cf.*[97].

Mechanisms Specific for Head Injury

Head injuries can be divided into three categories on the basis of the *type of load application* and its *time history* (Fig. 7).

— *Impact load:* collision of the head and a solid object at an appreciable velocity. A "hard" impact (*i.e.* concrete floor, falling stone) will last about 1–3 msec. A less hard (*i.e.* interior vehicular structure) 5–15 msec. and a blow by a fist about 20–30 msec.

— *Impulsive load:* The head is set in sudden motion without direct physical contact. Such a load may in the range 50–200 msec. Ex. rear end car impact ca 200 msec with a whiplash trauma.

— *Compressive load:* A load lasting longer than 200 msec (*i.e.* crushing of a heavy object). Such a load may be denoted static or quasistatic and consequences due to speed of load application may be totally neglected.

These three types of mechanical loading will involve partly different physical phenomena. In daily life trauma these types of loading often occur at the same time and their relative importance for production of injury is difficult to distinguish. However, for understanding the physical processes producing head injuries it is helpful to consider these three main types of loading and their mechanical and biological effects separately. This is also the approach taken by many investigators of head injury mechanisms.

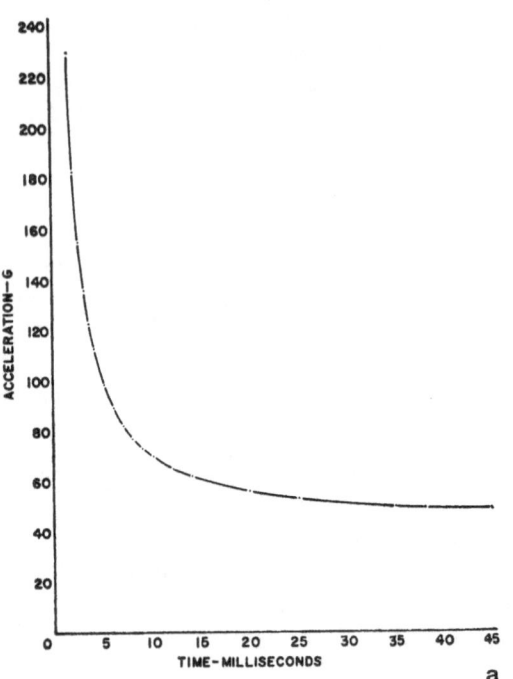

Impact Load

An impact is defined as a collision of the head with a solid object at an appreciable velocity. At an impact two types of effects occur (Fig. 8):

— Initiation and propagation of stress waves.

— Local disturbances at the impact site, "contact phenomena".

Stress waves initiated at the point of impact will propagate through the entire skull bone and the contents of the head. These stress waves are of several types, dilatational, shear, compressive, and their velocity of propagation (in human brain in the range of 2–2,500 m/sec) will depend on the physical properties of the tissues. At the boundaries between various media the stress waves are both transmitted and reflected. The transit time through the brain will be about 0.1 msec which is one order of magnitude less than the duration of shortlasting impacts. Although the injurious effect of the stress waves may not be very important (just because they exist for such a short time compared to the natural period of the brain *v.s*) some investigators have studied their effects[25]. Certainly these phenomena may contribute to dysfunction as well as structure failure, but experimental evidence has so far not appeared.

"Contact phenomena". In the bone, at the site of impact a temporary or permanent indentation will invariably occur: penetration, perforation, fracturing and fragmentation. For review of experiments related to these phenomena and especially the occurrence of skull fractures see[32, 33, 42].

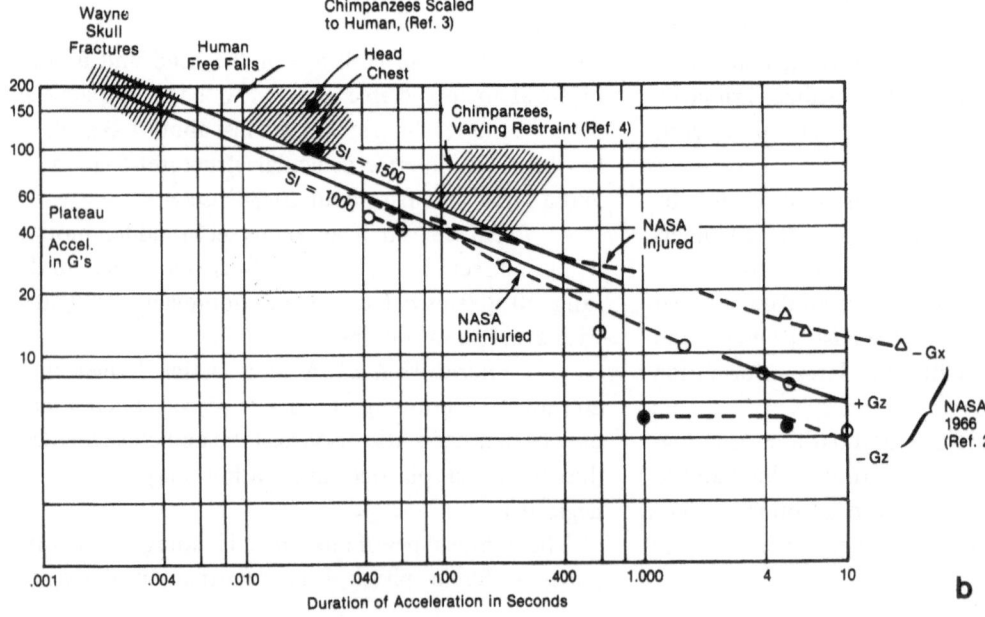

Fig. 5. a) The Wayne State University tolerance curve. At short duration of impact even very high acceleration may not cause injury.

b) Tolerance curves constructed from NASA 1959 and 1966 Literature Summaries for Tolerable Plateau Accelerations, Harnessed; with Other Data Superimposed. (From Gadd 1981[18])

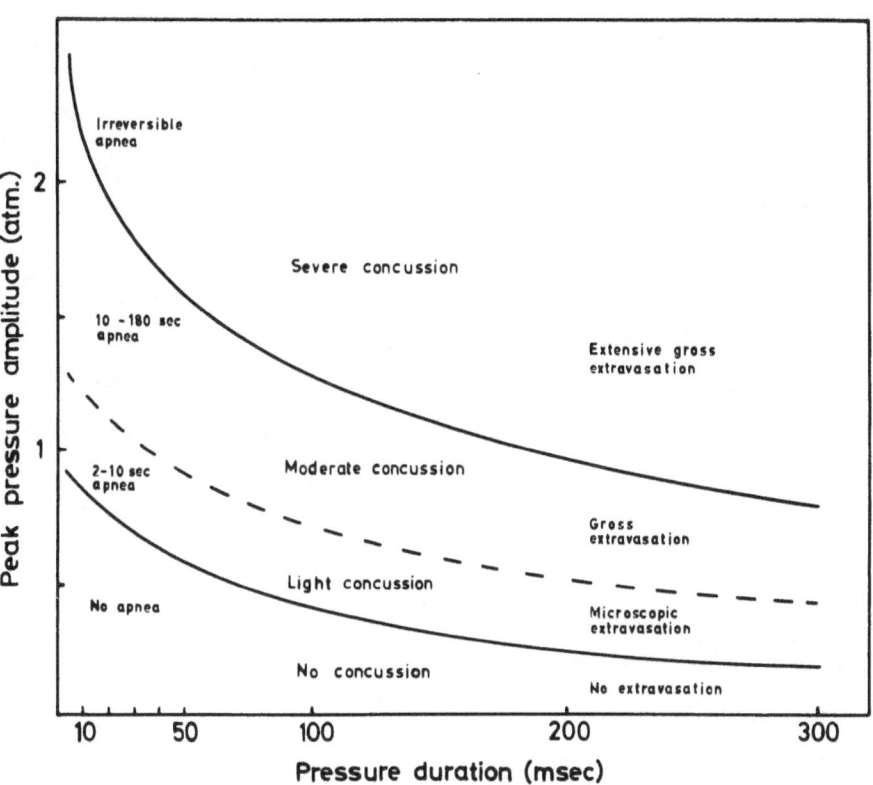

Fig. 6. Diagram showing approximate relations between peak amplitude of intracranial pressure increase at load input to the skull cavity, and "severity" of concussive response and extent of extravasation of labelled albumine at induction of pressure pulses of varying duration. Severe concussion: irreversible apnea, rise in blood pressure, tachy- or bradycardia. Moderate concussion: 10–180 sec apnea, rise in blood pressure, bradycardia. Light concussion: 2–10 sec apnea, fall in blood pressure, bradycardia. No concussion: No effects on recorded physiological parameters. (From Rinder 1969[90])

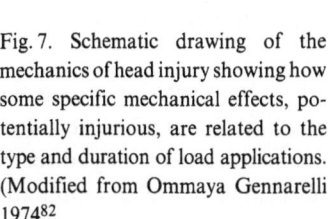

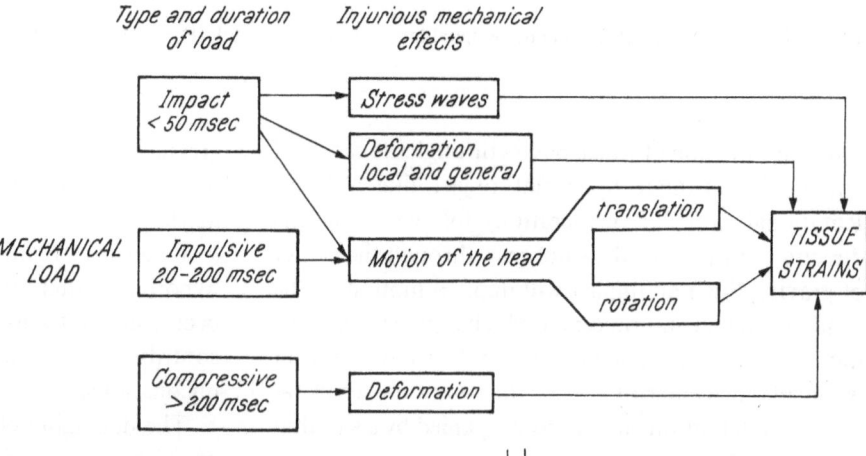

Fig. 7. Schematic drawing of the mechanics of head injury showing how some specific mechanical effects, potentially injurious, are related to the type and duration of load applications. (Modified from Ommaya Gennarelli 1974[82]

Impulse Load

In a pure impulsive loading (inertial loading, pure acceleration trauma) all effects are related to the sudden motion of the head and not to any effects due to direct impact. The movement of the head may be mainly *translational* or *angular* (rotation). See Fig. 9. In daily trauma situations the movement of the head will evidently be very complicated and include both types of motion. However, in attempts to understand the injury mechanisms it may be clarifying to study the effects of mainly translational or mainly angular acceleration separately.

Pure translational acceleration is produced by a

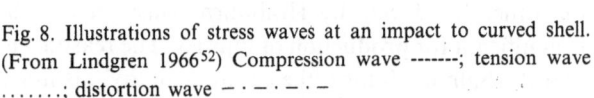

Fig. 8. Illustrations of stress waves at an impact to curved shell. (From Lindgren 1966[52]) Compression wave -------; tension wave ....; distortion wave — · — · —

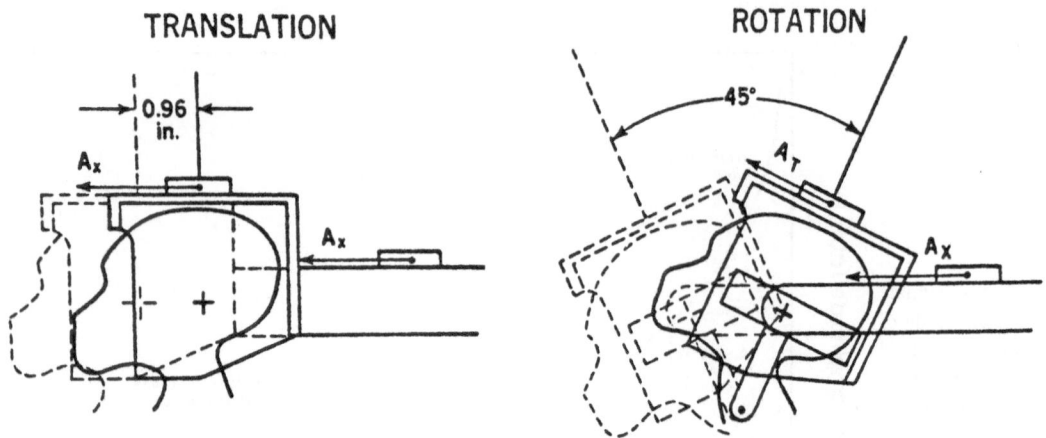

Fig. 9. Illustration of translational and rotational movement. (From Ommaya and Gennarelli 1974[82])

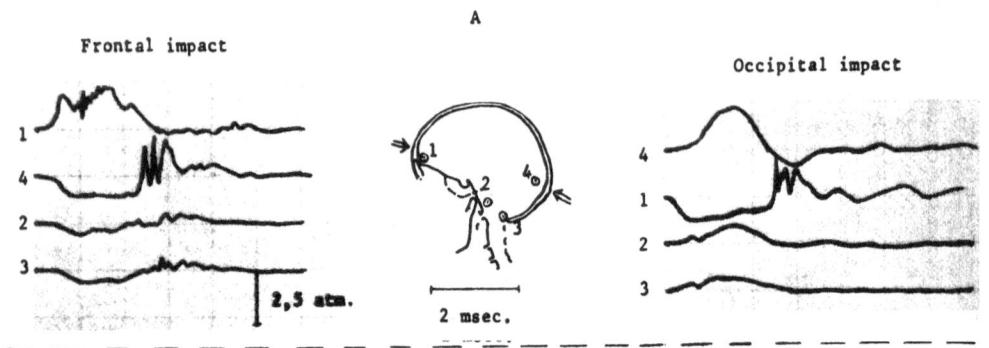

Fig. 10. Pressure changes at frontal and occipital impact to cadaver skull. (From Lindgren 1966[52])

force the direction of which passes through the center of gravity for instance by a flat object like a floor. Rotational (angular acceleration) follows when the direction of the force does not pass through the center of gravity. Such an impact will imply a motion of the head around a rotation center which in most cases will move. It should be noted that when the rotation center is outside the center of gravity the rotational acceleration is, by definition, always accompanied by a simultaneous translational movement.

A starting point for the development of a head loading device by which it should be possible to isolate the effects related to translational and rotational movement of the head respectively were some hypotheses by an Oxford physicist, Holbourn, at the beginning of the 40's[44, 45]. He claimed that rotational acceleration was the most important injurious factor because it should generate shear strain that could cause dysfunction as well as tissue damage. The translational acceleration on the other hand was by Holbourn considered to be insignificant for production of injuries. The reason was that the bulk modulus ("the compressibility") is much greater than the shear modulus ("rigidity") i.e. it is not possible to compress the brain but very easy to change its shape.

Other investigators[25, 35, 5], however, forwarded the hypothesis that the *intracranial pressure changes* occurring in translational acceleration may directly contribute to cerebral contusions as well as traumatic unconsciousness.

The damaging effects of translational acceleration have been proposed to depend on shear stresses at the brain stem and pressures and turbulence produced by the collapse of cavities near the contrecoup point. The support for this theory has been the large pressure differences recorded at translational acceleration[34, 35, 52].

Fig. 10 shows the pressure pattern at coup (occipital), at contrecoup (frontal) area and in foramen magnum region. The *pressure gradients* over posterior fossa-foramen magnum may indicate motion of the brain stem and concomitant shear stress.

The *subatmospheric pressure* ("negative pressure") in the frontal region may be accompanied by shortlast-

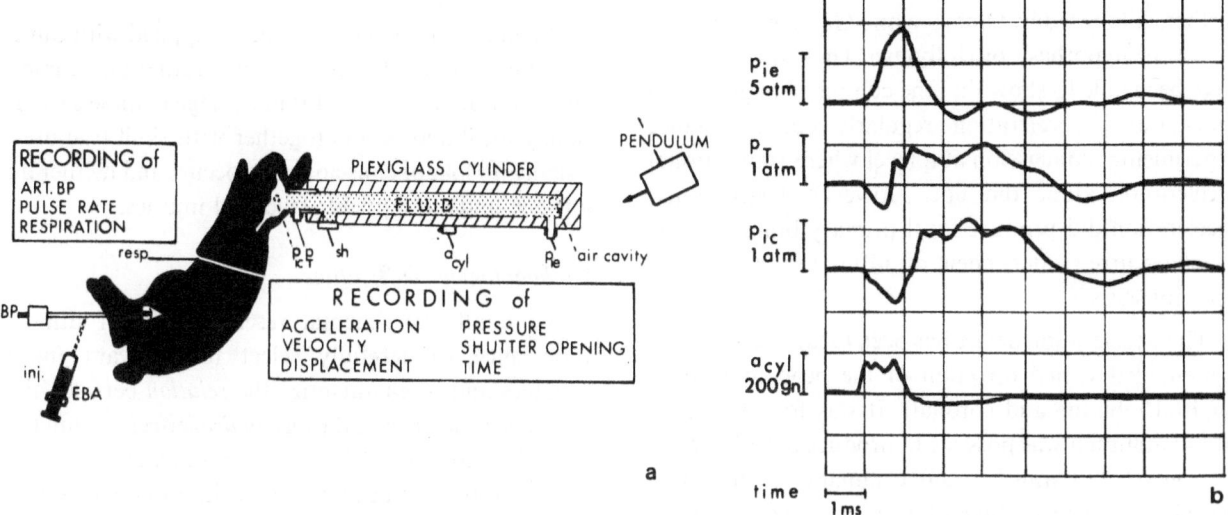

Fig. 11. a) Experimental arrangement for production of sub-atmospheric pressures in the skull cavity of the rabbit. b) Recordings of cylinder acceleration (*acyl*) and pressures at impact end (*pie*), in T-tube (*PT*) and in the skull (*pic*). (From Stålhammar 1974[98])

ing occurrence of cavities and the subsequent collapse of these. Similar subatmospheric pressures have been produced within the cranial cavity of a rabbit[98]. See Fig. 11.

No signs of tissue damage (tested by Evans blue albumin) were, however, produced unless "flow" of tissue was allowed[98].

The above mentioned findings of pressure gradients in the brain stem area at impact to the intact skull initiated elaboration of a device for direct loading of the exposed brain in order to produce a similar pressure pattern under experimental conditions more easily controlled. See[89–92]. See Fig. 12.

A clear and *reproducible relationship* was shown to exist between the magnitude of the *mechanical load* (in terms of peak of pressure amplitude as well as the duration) and quantifiable *pathophysiological*, (BP,

respiration, pulserate[91]) and *pathomorphological* (extent of EBA exsudation[89]) changes (*cf*. Fig. 6 and Table 3).

A modification of this model has been extensively used for investigations of a variety of effects, *cf*. Table 3 and also for trial of therapeutic measures[38, 95].

Fig. 13 shows a *head accelerating device* by which it is possible to produce either a translational or a combined translational-rotational movement[40, 78, 82]. The head is protected from any impact loading by a helmet closely

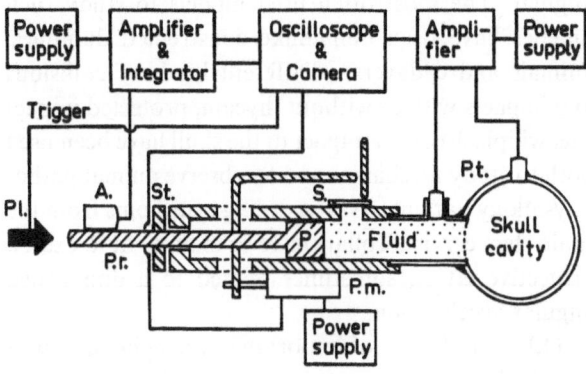

Fig. 12. Experimental arrangement for production of intracranial pressure changes in the rabbit. (From Rinder and Lindgren 1969[53])

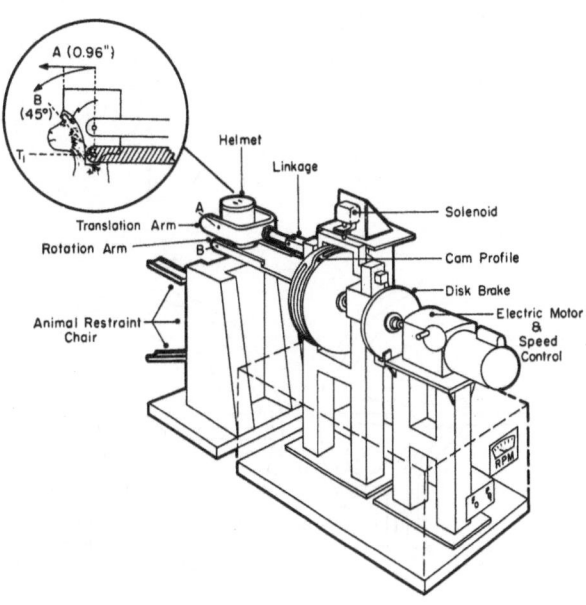

Fig. 13. Head accelerating device for application of impulse loading (head acceleration without direct impact). *Cf*. Fig. 9. (From Ommaya and Gennarelli 1974[82])

fitted to the head of the animal. This device has been further elaborated by Ommaya and Gennarelli in order to test the hypothesis of Holbourn. These investigators have been able to show that the combined angular and translational acceleration regularly could produce experimental concussion at a level where translational acceleration alone did not. However, translational acceleration did produce focal primary brain damage which occurred independent of diffuse lesion or loss of consciousness[82].

This acceleration device has been further refined and has enabled varied direction of the head movement (sagittal, oblique and coronal). It was found that by lateral motion it was possible to produce deep *longlasting coma*[19, 20]. Parallel to this traumatic unconsciousness characteristic findings of *diffuse axonal injury* were found[1]. This ist most remarkable because it is the first time that a "humanlike" prolonged unconsciousness has been simulated in animal experiments.

Fig. 14 shows two examples from recent experiments with physical models; a simplified head form of acrylic plastic with a transparent silicone gel in which photographic targets are introduced. The displacement of these targets during rotational motion of the model is recorded by high-speed cinematography. From Aldman *et al.*1981[2], *cf*[60].

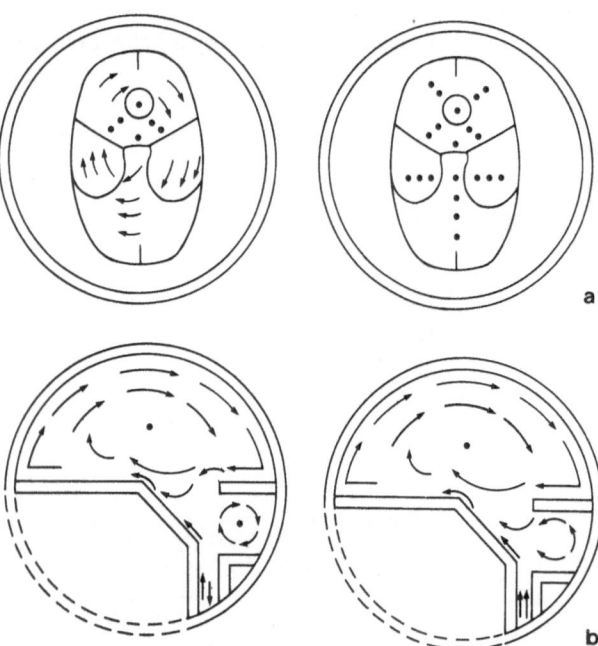

Fig. 14. Moulds of the skull with a gel in a soft bag and targets at different levels recorded by high-speed cinematography during rotational motion. a) sagittal plane, b) horizontal plane. (Aldman 1981[2])

Compressive Load

When the mechanical loading is applied with durations longer than 200 msec this is a rather uncommon cause of head injury. The brain damage in these cases is mainly focal and occurs together with skull fractures. Usually no loss of consciousness occurs and neither do amnesia and widespread structural injuries.

Methodological Difficulties

As in all experimental research it is of utmost importance to carefully select the relevant input variables and to characterize the *relation* between the *impact parameters* and the *mechanical* effects within the brain that are critical for injury production.

Therefore, in an experimental situation, where it is intended to relate a graded mechanical input to varied biological response it is required to perform *reliable recordings* of the movements of the head in terms of time course of acceleration, velocity and distance. Regarding these recordings of mechanical events under impact conditions it should be noted that several types of errors will easily be introduced[52, 55, 56]. Unfortunately, too often the description of the technical procedure and of control experiments are insufficient to make it possible to judge critically the reliability of the methods.

Survey of Head Injury Models

See Table 1.

Mechanics

The purpose of the study can be to record the mechanics with regard to *movement of the head* and neck in terms of displacement, velocity and acceleration after impact, or the type of response translational or angular. The most often used models to study such kinetics have been humanlike constructed dummies, animals and cadavers.—Different kinds of collisions and impacts with or without (hycam, protected impact site, whiplash) direct impact to the skull have been used both to study mechanics and to observe animal pathophysiology parameters. Regarding symptoms from the brain stem cervical collars have been thought to exert a protective effect, sometimes related to a diminished angular acceleration.

Other mechanics of importance are *deformations of the skull* sometimes causing impact site fracture or meridional fracture along the deformation transfer. The most frequently used models have been spherical

Table 1. *Models of Head Injury Studies*

Purpose of study	Models	Experimental variations	Parameters studied
I Mechanics			
Movements of	theoretical	collisions	velocities
head-neck	dummies	impacts	accelerations
Impulsive load	volunteers		HIC
Direct impact	animals	"Whiplash"	
Translat. response	cadavers	sled accel	
Angular response		Hycam	symptoms, sign
		cerv. collar	— brain stem
		direct impact	
		"Protected" impact	
		site	
Deformation	theoretical	shell properties	accelerations
Skull- shell	fluid filled	size	stress coat changes
Fracture	sphere	shape	holographic changes
	hemisphere	ground	intracran pressures
		hard- soft	
Intracran. contents	theoretical	compartments	movements
(Tissue properties)	physical	contents	pressure
Strain	sphere	properties	fluid displacement
Movements	hemisphere		
	cylinder		
	transparent shell		symptoms, signs,
	— also in animal		— brain stem
			tolerance level
	perc. concussion		
	(fluid input)		
	— animal		
II Pathophysiology:			
Changes	labor. animals		"Exper. animal brain concussion"
			brain contusions
	subhuman primates		long duration
			concussions
			tolerance levels
III Pathomorphology:			
Lesions	see above (animals) and		lesions severity
	cadavers, pressurized		location
Macroscopical			
Microscopical			
BBB studies			
Edema—axons—neurons			
IV *Clinical analysis:*			
Epidemiology	admission chart and		accident mechanics
Accidents and mechanics	observation recording		fall height, speed ground, sharp or
Injury types and severity	in each case		blunt object
			E-nr (WHO)
			age
			injury severity
			AIS
			Scales of impaired
			consciousness
			ICD (WHO)
			diagnostic severity

When animals are studied: mechanics, symptoms and morphology are correlated (usually brain stem signs).

When pressurized cadavers are studied: mechanics and hemorrages are correlated.

Table 2. *Survey of Animal (and Some Human Cadaver) Experimental Brain Injury Models by Mechanical Loading.* Basis for classification: type and size of contact surface and time course of loading. Figures refer to literature list

	Type and size of contact surface intact skull ("whole head")						exposed intracran tissues ("part of brain")	
	unprotected		protected				"macro"	"micro"
	"blunt"	"sharp"	for study of special phenomena					
			impact site	movements of head translat	rotat	cran-spin junction		
Time course Single load duration								
< 10 msec	9, 22, 29, 31 43, 51, 73–76, 79, 80, 81, 50	5	41	19, 20, 40, 41, 66	19, 20, 21, 40, 41, 100	43	37, 38, 53 84, 89–92 94, 95, 98, 99	7, 36
10–200 msec					63, 64, 78 87, 103	43	53, 88–92 65, 69, 97	63, 64, 68
> 200 msec							53, 88–92	8
min—hrs						43	6, 70, 101	28, 83
multiple repeated loads	22, 72						22, 47, 65, 88, 92	

based on material property knowledge, and with fluid filled spheres of varying experimental design.

Finally the mechanical *response of intracranial contents* has been studied theoretically or in physical transparent containers. A similar technique with high-speed photography has also been used through a transparent shell in the skull of animals.—Direct fluid input to imitate pressure differences at acceleration concussion has also been used as percussion concussion, usually with observation of brain stem signs. Transparent cylinders modified in compartments similar to the intracranial dural folds and with brainlike contents have also been used for studies of rotational movements.

Among the parameters studied HIC denotes *Head Injury Criteria*, which are functions of acceleration and duration of impact response and *tolerance levels* which is a grading of a mechanical disturbance and its duration causing severe brain stem signs such as interrupted respiration. A well known tolerance level curve is the Wayne State University Tolerance Curve, but a more reliable graded Tolerance Curve with more measurement points has been presented by Rinder 1969.

Pathophysiology

Pathophysiological studies in animals have mostly reported the occurrence of the degree of "experimental animal brain concussion" with graded severity within rather restricted time limit. Recently Gennarelli *et al.* have managed to obtain *long duration concussions* in subhuman primates more similar to the clinical human concussions.—Brain contusions have been studied by direct impact to the brain.

Morphology

Pathomorphology has also been studied in animals particularly with respect to findings in the brain stem and in the contrecoup region. During the last 10 years also human *cadavers* with artificially raised aortic blood pressure sometimes with respiratory ventilation have been used in collision studies during similar conditions as in daily traffic. The location and severity of hemorrhages within the brain have been studied to some extent.

Clinical Analysis

Every day we all have possibilities to study the *clinical* head injury model in our patients if we analyse

Table 3. *Survey of Animal Experimental Brain Injury Models.* Classification according to injury cause (input) and category of consequences (output), compare Table 2

Input	Type and size of contact surface intact skull ("whole head")						exposed intracran tissues ("part of brain")	
	unprotected		protected				"macro"	"micro"
	"blunt"	"sharp"	for study of special phenomena					
			impact site	movements of head translat	rotat	cran-spin junction		
Output								
Functional changes								
"Psychological"	79							
Reaction level	9, 29, 31, 73		41	19, 41, 66	19, 41, 78, 100		38, 69, 85, 91, 98, 99 101	
Cardio resp vasc	79, 81						97	
ICP					21		6, 99, 101	
CBF	22, 72, 75			19	19		22, 88	70, 7, 68
Structural changes								
contus, hemorr. swelling, edema BBB studies	9, 73, 80 51, 72, 97	5		1, 66	1, 87, 103 101	17	9, 97, 99 65, 85, 89, 92, 99	63, 64
neurons, diff axonal injury	29			1	1	17	84	28, 83
Biochemical changes							37	36
Electrical changes								
EEG				19, 66	19			
SER	50							7, 8
Metabolic *"Therapeutic"*	22, 74–76						22, 69, 94 6, 38, 47, 95	68

the accident, the mechanics and the injury types and severity. The parameters studied for the accident can be the E-numbers (WHO); for injury, injury severity scales (in general the AIS), or just scales of impaired consciousness (various scales among which the GCS is well known). It must be recognized that symptomatic scales are not conclusive regarding prognosis; there must also be a strong influence of the diagnosis of the condition. The diagnostic parameters have been listed in the ICD (WHO).

Classification of Animal Experimental Models by Mechanical Load

According to the description above of the injury mechanisms, a *classification* of animal experimental brain injury models by mechanical loading may be based on *type and size of the contact surface* and the *time course* of loading. For a rough and rapsodic orientation in the field Table 2 presents some of the literature and in Table 3 these experiments are grouped according to the type of output.

Acknowledgement

This study is supported by Swedish Medical Research Council proj no B86-27X-6613-03B and the Folksam Insurance Company.

References

1. Adams JH, Graham DI, Gennarelli TA (1983) Head injury in man and experimental animals: Neuropathology. Acta Neurochir (Wien) [Suppl] 32, 15–30
2. Aldman B, Thorngren L, Ljung C (1981) Patterns of deformation in the brain models under rotational motion. Proceedings of a Workshop on Head and Neck Injury Criteria. U.S. Department of Transportation. National Highway Traffic Safety Administration. Washington, pp 163–168

3. Allen AR (1911) Surgery of experimental lesion of spinal cord equivalent to crush injury of fracture dislocation of spinal column. JAMA 57: 11: 878–880

4. Caveness WF, Walker AE (eds) (1966) Proceedings of head injury conference. University of Chicago, Lippincott

5. Clemedson CJ, Falconer B, Frankenberg L, Jönsson A, Wennerstrand J (1973) Head injuries caused by small-calibre, high velocity bullets. An experimental study. Z Rechtsmedizin 73: 103–114

6. Clubb R, Maxwell R, Chou S (1980) Experimental brain injury in the dog. The pharmacological effects of pentobarbital and sodium nitroprusside. J Neurosurg 52: 189–196

7. Crockard HA, Brown FD, Trimble J, Mullan JF (1977) Somatosensory evoked potentials, cerebral blood flow and metabolism following cerebral missile trauma in monkeys. Surg Neurol 7: 281–287

8. Crockard A, Iannotti F, Kang J (1982) Posttraumatic Edema in the Gerbill. In: Grossman R, Gildenberg P (eds) Seminars in neurological surgery. Head injury: Basic and clinical aspects. New York, pp 159–168

9. Denny-Brown D, Russel WR (1941) Experimental cerebral concussion. Brain 64: 93–164

10. Dohrmann GJ, Panjabi MM (1976) Standardized spinal cord trauma: Biomechanical parameters and lesion volume. Surg Neurol 6: 263–267

11. Dohrmann GJ, Panjabi MM, Banks D (1978) Biomechanics of experimental spinal cord trauma. J Neurosurg 48: 993–1001

12. McElhaney JH, Fogle JL, Melvin JW, et al. (1970) Mechanical properties of cranial bone. J Biomech 3: 495–512

13. McElhaney JH, Melvin JW, Roberts VL, Portnoy HD (1973) Dynamic characteristics of the tissues of the head. Perspectives in Biomedical Engineering: Kenedi RM (ed). Macmillan Press Ltd, London, pp 215–222

14. McElhaney J, Stalnaker R, Roberts V (1973) Biomechanical aspects of head injury. Human impact response. Plenum Press, pp 85–112

15. Engin AE (1969) Axisymmetric response of a fluid-filled spherical shell to a local radial impulse—a model for head injury. J Biomech 2: 325–341

16. Fallenstein GT, Hulce VD, Melvin JW (1969) Dynamic mechanical properties of human brain tissue. J Biomech 2: 217–226

17. Friede R (1958) Biophysics of concussion (Neurohistopathological studies). WADC Tech Rep 58–193, Wright-Patterson Air Force Base, Ohio

18. Gadd C (1981) Head injury discussion paper. Proceedings of a Workshop on Head and Neck Injury Criteria. U.S. Department of Transportation. National Highway Traffic Safety Administration, Washington, pp. 177–182

19. Gennarelli T, Segawa H, Wald U, et al. (1982) Physiological response to angular acceleration of the head. In: Grossman R, Gildenberg P (eds) Seminars in neurological surgery. Head injury: Basic and clinical aspects. New York, pp 129–140

20. Gennarelli TA (1983) Head injury in man and experimental animals: clinical aspects. Acta Neurochir (Wien) [Suppl] 32: 1–13

21. Gennarelli T, Marcincin R, Thibault L, Thompson C (1983) Effect of direction of head movement on ICP in experimental head injury. In: Ishii S, Nagai H, Brock M (eds) Intracranial pressure. Springer, Berlin Heidelberg New York, pp 483–486

22. German W, Page W, Nims L (1947) Cerebral blood flow and cerebral oxygen consumption in experimental intracranial injury. Trans Am Neurol Ass 72: 86–88

23. von Gierke HE (1966) On the dynamics of some head injury mechanisms. In: Caveness WF, Walker AE (eds) Head Injury Conf Proc. Lippincott, Philadelphia, pp 383–396

24. Gold A, Hance H, Kornhauser M, Lawton R (1962) Impact tolerance of restrained mice as a function of velocity change and average deceleration. Aerospace Med 33: 204–208

25. Goldsmith W (1966) The physical processes producing head injuries. In head injury Conf Proc Caveness WF, Walker AE (eds) pp 350–382

26. Goldsmith W (1972) Biomechanics of head injury. In: Fung YC, Anliker M, Perrone N (eds) Biomechanics. Its foundation and objectives. Prentice-Hall, New Jersey, pp 585–634

27. Gosch HH, Gooding E, Schneider RC (1970) The lexan calvarium for the study of cerebral response of acute trauma. J Trauma 10: 370–376

28. Gray J, Ritchie JM (1954) The effects of stretch on single myelinated nerve fibers. J Physiol 124: 84–99

29. Groat RA, Windle WF, Magoun HW (1945) Functional and structural changes in the monkey's brain during and after concussion. J Neurosurg 2: 26–35

30. Gross AG (1958) A new theory on the dynamics of brain concussion and brain injury. J Neurosurg 15: 548–561

31. Grubb R, Naumann R, Ommaya A (1970) Respiration and the cerebrospinal fluid in experimental cerebral concussion. J Neurosurg 32: 320–329

32. Gurdjian ES, Lissner HR, Webster JE (1947) The mechanism of production of linear skull fracture. Further studies on deformation of the skull by the "stresscoat" technique. Surg Gynecol Obstet 85: 195–210

33. Gurdjian ES, Webster JE, Lissner HR (1949) The mechanism of skull fracture. J Neurosurg 7: 106–114

34. Gurdjian ES, Lange WA, Patrick LM, Thomas LM (eds) (1970) Impact injury and crash protection. Ch C Thomas, Springfield

35. Gurdjian ES (1975) Re-evaluation of the biomechanics of blunt impact injury of the head. Surg Gynecol Obstet 140: 845–850

36. Hamberger A, Rinder L (1966) Experimental brain concussion. J Neuropathol and Exp Neurol 25: 68–75

37. Hayes R, Kulkarni P, Galinat B, Becker D (1982) Evidence for the release of endogenous opiate substances after experimental closed head injury in the cat. In: Grossman R, Gildenberg P (eds) Seminars in neurological surgery. Head injury: Basic and clinical aspects. New York, pp 179–188

38. Hayes R, Galinat B, Stålhammar D, Becker D (1983) Effects of Naloxone on ICP and systemic cardiovascular responses after experimental closed head injury in the cat. In: Ishii S, Nagai H, Brock M (eds) Intracranial pressure V. Springer, Berlin Heidelberg New York, pp 572–576

39. Hickling R, Wenner ML (1973) Mathematical model of a head subjected to an axisymmetric impact. J Biomech 6: 115–132

40. Higgins LS, Schmall RA (1967) A device for the investigation of head injury effected by non-deforming head acceleration. Proc 11th Stapp Car Crash Conf, Soc Auto Engg, New York, 57–72

41. Hirsch A, Ommaya A, Mahone R (1970) Tolerance of subhuman primate brain to cerebral concussion. In: Gurdjian, Lange, Patrick, Thomas (eds) Impact injury and crash protection. Ch C Thomas, Springfield, pp 352–369

42. Hodgson V (1967) Tolerance of the facial bones to impact. Am J Anat 120: 113–122

43. Hollister NR, Jolley WP, Horne RG (1958) Biophysics of concussion. WADC Tech Rep 58–193, Wright-Patterson Air Force Base, Ohio

44. Holbourn AH (1943) Mechanics of head injuries. Lancet 438–441

45. Holbourn AH (1945) The mechanics of brain injuries. Br Med Bull 3: 147–148

46. Joseph PH, Crist JDC (1972) On the evaluation of mechanical stresses in the human brain while in motion. Brain Res 26: 15–35

47. Karvounis P, Smith M, Piccone V, *et al.* (1968) Effect of proteolytic enzymes in brain contusion after controlled head injury. Surg Forum 19: 416–417

48. Kornhauser M, Gold, A (1962) Application of the impact sensitivity method to animate structures. Proceedings of a Symposium: Impact Acceleration Stress. National Academy of Sciences, National Research Council, Washington, pp 333–344

49. Lee YC, Advani SH (1970) Transient response of a sphere to symmetrical torsional loading—a head injury model. Math Biosci 6: 473–483

50. Letcher F, Carrao PG, Ommaya AK (1973) Head injury in the chimpanzee: Part II. Spontaneous and evoked epidural potentials as indices of injury severity. J Neurosurg 39: 167–177

51. Lewis P, Ramirez R, McLaurin L (1968) Intracranial blood volume after head injury. Forum 19: 433–435

52. Lindgren SO (1966) Experimental studies of mechanical effects in head injury. Acta Chir Scand [Suppl] 360

53. Lindgren S, Rinder L (1969) Production and distribution of intracranial and intraspinal pressure changes at sudden extradural fluid volume input in rabbits. Acta Physiol Scand 76: 340–351

54. Lindgren S, Rinder L, Stålhammar D, Åsberg Å (1973) Correlation between brain injuries and mechanical response of the head at impact. Injury 5: 31–34

55. Lindgren S, Rinder L (1965) Experimental studies in head injury. I. Some factors influencing results of model experiments. Biophysik 2: 320

56. Lindgren S, Rinder L (1966) Experimental studies in head injury. II. Pressure propagation in "percussion-concussion". Biophysik 3: 174

57. Lindgren S (1983) Interaction between the skull base and the skull contents at impact to the skull. In: Samii M, Brihaye J (eds) Traumatology of the skull base. Springer, Berlin Heidelberg New York, pp 44–49

58. Liu YK, Chandran KB (1975) The exact solution to the translational acceleration of inviscid compressible fluid in rigid spherical shells. Math Biosci 24: 1–16

59. Liu YK, Chandran KB, von Rosenberg DU (1975) Angular acceleration of viscoelastic (Kelvin) material in a rigid spherical shell—a rotational head injury model. J Biomech 8: 285–292

60. Ljung C (1975) A model for brain deformation due to rotation of the skull. J Biomech 8: 263–274

61. Ljung C, Lindgren S, Aldman B (1981) On the analytical approach to head injury criteria. Proceedings of a Workshop on Head and Neck Injury Criteria. U.S. Department of Transportation. National Highway Traffic Safety Administration. Washington, pp 194–197

62. Lombard, C, Ames S, Roth H, Rosenfeld S (1951) Voluntary tolerance of the human to impact accelerations of the head. J Aviation Med 22: 109–116

63. Löwenhielm P (1974) Dynamic Properties of the parasagittal bridging veins. Z Rechtsmedizin 74: 55–62

64. Löwenhielm P (1974) Strain Tolerance of the vv. cerebri sup. (bridging veins) calculated from head-on collision test with cadavers. Z Rechtsmedizin 75: 131–144

65. Marshall J, Jackson L, Langfitt T (1969) Brain swelling caused by trauma and arterial hypertension. Arch Neurol 21: 545–553

66. Masuzawa H, Nakamura N, Hirakawa K, *et al.* (1976) Experimental head injury and concussion in monkey using pure linear acceleration impact. Neurologica medico-chirurgica 16: 77–90

67. Melvin JW, McElhaney JH, Roberts VL (1970) Development of a Mechanical Model of the human head—determination of tissue properties and synthetic substitute materials. Proc of 14th Stapp Car Crash Conference, pp 221–227.

68. Meyer J, Kondo A, Nomura F, *et al.* (1969) Cerebral hemodynamics and metabolism following brain trauma. Demonstration of luxury perfusion following brain-stem laceration. In: Brock M, Fieschi C, Ingvar DH, Lassen NH, Schurmann K (eds) Cerebral blood flow, clinical and experimental results. Springer, Berlin Heidelberg New York, pp 199–201

69. Meyer J, Kondo A, Nomura F, *et al.* (1970) Cerebral hemodynamics and metabolism following experimental head injury. J Neurosurg 32: 304–319

70. Miller J, Stanek A, Langfitt T (1971 b) Effect of expanding intracranial lesions on cerebral blood flow. Surg Forum 22: 422–423

71. Nakatani S, Ommaya AK (1973) A critical rate of cerebral compression. In: Brock M (ed) Intracranial pressure. Springer, Berlin Heidelberg New York

72. Nelson L, Auen E, Bourke R, *et al.* (1982) A comparison of animal head injury models developed for treatment modality evaluation. In: Grossman R, Gildenberg P (eds) Seminars in neurological surgery. Head injury: Basic and clinical aspects. New York, pp 117–128

73. Nilsson B, Pontén U, Voigt G (1977) Experimental head injury in the rat. Part I: Mechanics, pathophysiology, and morphology in an impact acceleration trauma model. J Neurosurg 47: 241–251

74. Nilsson B, Pontén U (1977) Experimental head injury in the rat. Part 2: Regional brain energy metabolism in concussive trauma. J Neurosurg 47: 252–261

75. Nilsson B, Nordström CH (1977) Experimental head injury in the rat. Part 3: Cerebral blood flow and oxygen consumption after concussive impact acceleration. J Neurosurg 47: 262–273

76. Nilsson B, Nordström CH (1977) Rate of cerebral energy consumption in concussive head injury in the rat. J Neurosurg 47: 274–281

77. Ommaya AK (1968) The mechanical properties of tissues of the nervous system. J Biomech 2: 1–2

78. Ommaya AK, Faas F, Yarnell PR (1968) Whiplash injury and brain damage: An experimental study. J Am Med Assoc 204: 285–289

79. Ommaya AK, Geller A, Parsons LC (1971) The effect of experimental head injury on one-trial learning in rats. Int J Neurosc 1: 371–378

80. Ommaya AK, Grubb Jr RL, Naumann RA (1971) Coup and contre-coup. Observations on the mechanics of visible brain injuries in the rhesus monkey. J Neurosurg 35: 503–517

81. Ommaya AK, Corrao P, Letcher FS (1973) Head injury in the chimpanzee. 1. Biodynamics of traumatic unconsciousness. J Neurosurg 39: 152–166

82. Ommaya AK, Gennarelli TA (1974) Cerebral concussion and traumatic unconsciousness: Correlation of experimental and clinical observations on blunt head injuries. Brain 97: 633–654

83. Persson L (1976) Experimental brain injury. Thesis. University of Göteborg

84. Povlishock JT, Becker DP, Miller LW, Dietrich WD (1979) The morphopathologic substrates of concussion? Acta Neuropathol (Berl) 47: 1–11

85. Povlishock J, Kontos H (1982) The pathophysiology of pial and intraparenchymal vascular dysfunction. In: Grossman R, Gildenberg P (eds) Seminars in neurological surgery. Head injury: Basic and clinical aspects. New York, pp 15–29

86. Proceedings of a Workshop on Head and Neck Injury Criteria. U.S. Department of Transportation. National Highway Traffic Safety Administration, Washington, 1981

87. Pudenz RH, Shelden HC (1946) The lucite calvarium. A method for direct observation of the brain. II. Cranial trauma brain movement. J Neurosurg 3: 487–505

88. Reivich M, Marshall J, Kassell N (1969) Loss of autoregulation produced by cerebral trauma. In: Brock M, Fieschi C, Ingvar DH, Lassen NH, Schurmann K (eds) Cerebral blood flow, clinical and experimental results. Springer, Berlin Heidelberg New York, pp 205–208

89. Rinder L, Olsson Y (1968) Vascular permeability changes in experimental brain concussion. Acta Path Microbiol 72: 350–352

90. Rinder L (1969 a) Experimental brain concussion by sudden intracranial input of fluid. Göteborg, Sweden: Dept. of Hygiene, Univ. of Göteborg. Dissertation

91. Rinder L (1969 b) Concussive response and intracranial pressure changes at sudden extradural fluid volume input in rabbits. Acta Physiol Scand 76: 352–360

92. Rinder L, Olsson Y, Lindgren S, Stålhammar C (1972) Comparison of effects from single and repeated trauma to the animal brain. Scand J Rehab Med 4: 97–99

93. Ripperger EA (1975) The mechanics of brain injuries. In: Vinken PJ, Bruyn GW (eds) Injuries of the brain and skull. Handbook of clinical neurology. Am Elsevier Publ Co, New York, pp 91–109

94. Rosenthal M, Duckrow B, LaManna J, et al. (1982) Consequences of cerebral injury on oxidative energy metabolism measured in situ. In: Grossmann R, Gildenberg P (eds) Seminars in neurological surgery. Head injury: Basic and clinical aspects. New York, pp 69–78

95. Rosner M, Becker D (1984) Experimental brain injury: successful therapy with the weak base, tromethamine. With an overview of CNS acidosis. J Neurosurg 60: 961–971

96. Sato K, Massing W, Zulch KJ (1971) Experimental concussion in the cat. Clinical and morphological findings. Z Neurol 200: 201–212

97. Smith D, Ducker T, Kempe L (1969) Experimental in vivo microcirculatory dynamics in brain trauma. J. Neurosurg 30: 664–672

98. Stålhammar D (1974) Experimental brain damage from fluid pressure due to impact acceleration. Göteborg, Sweden: Dept of Neurosurg Univ of Göteborg Dissertation

99. Sullivan HG, et al. (1976) Fluid-percussion model of mechanical brain injury in the cat. J Neurosurg 45: 520–534

100. Unterharnscheidt F, Higgins LS (1969 b) Traumatic lesions of brain and spinal cord due to non-deforming angular acceleration of the head. Texas Reports on Biol and Med 27: 127–166

101. Weinstein J, Langfitt T, Bruno L, et al. (1968) Experimental study of patterns of brain distortion and ischemia produced by an intracranial mass. J Neurosurg 28: 513–521

102. Ward C (1981) Status of head injury modeling. Proceedings of a Workshop on Head and Neck Injury Criteria. U.S. Department of Transportation. National Highway Traffic Safety Administration, pp 157–162

103. Voigt G, Löwenhielm P, Ljung C (1977) Rotational cerebral injuries near the superior margin of the brain. Acta Neuropathol (Berl) 39: 201–209

Author's address: Prof. D. Stålhammar, Department of Neurosurgery, Sahlgren's Hospital, University of Göteborg, S-413 45 Göteborg, Sweden.

Acta Neurochirurgica, Suppl. 36, 47–50 (1986)

Head and Neck Injuries

K. P. G. Krantz and **C. G. P. Löwenhielm**

Department of Forensic Medicine, University of Lund, Sweden

Summary

A survey of cranial, intracranial and neck injuries caused by blunt trauma to the head is presented. The different types of fractures to the skull (impression fractures, linear fractures and ring fractures) are discussed as well as the injury mechanisms. Brain injuries are discussed under the heading of focal brain injury (*i.e.* brain laceration, cortical contusion, hemorrhages of the meninges and traumatic intracerebral hemorrhages).

The different types of neck injuries, including atlanto-occipital dislocation, are listed and the stability of the different fractures are discussed. Facial injury is not included.

Keywords: Skull fracture; brain injury; neck injury; injury mechanisms.

Introduction

Impact against the head can give rise to external and/or internal (cranial and intracranial) injuries as well as injuries to the neck. This communication deals with the internal injuries which could be divided into fractures, hemorrhages and injuries to the neural tissue. Facial injuries are not discussed.

Head Injuries

Fractures

Skull fractures by themselves are very seldom life-threatening. Nevertheless they are of importance in the determination of the characteristics of the impact. Certain kinds of fractures as well as the direction of trauma often indicate the intracranial injuries to expect.

The neurocranium is mechanically a complicated construction, which is composed of thin and thick elements of bone tissue. The numerous foramina, sutures and fissures of the base of the skull constitute the weak parts of the structure.

Direct impact can lead to impression fractures or to linear fractures of the skull. If the violence is transferred to the vault of the skull two different kinds of impression fractures could be distinguished. When a flat object with a large surface area impacts against a convex surface of the skull, a globus fracture (pond fracture) can be produced. Such a fracture is characterized by circular fracture lines crossed by radially directed fractures running from the impact centre to often far outside the impact zone. In other cases when the impacting object is smaller the fracture will correspond to the form and size of the impacting object. These fractures are often enlarged conically into the skull (stamp-fracture). The above mentioned fractures (direct fractures) are mostly seen as the result of an impact of considerable magnitude. In cases with less impact magnitude different kinds of linear fractures may appear. These fractures may also affect other parts of the skull and are often proceeding into the base of the skull.

Vault fractures can be accompanied by dural injuries, intracranial hemorrhages or neural tissue injuries which depend of the magnitude and the direction of the impact.

Fractures of the base of the skull can be linear or ring shaped and they always arise indirectly. The linear fractures may have a sagittal, oblique or transverse direction. They correspond to impact from anterior-posterior, from oblique anterior-posterior or from the side, respectively. These fractures are often ramified.

Ring fractures of the base of the skull are annular and mostly involve the sella turcica or the junction between the dorsum sellae and the corpus ossis occipitale, run in front of the pyramides and through the squama ossis occipitale [10]. The ring fractures arise from different trauma mechanisms: *e.g.*

- Traction (hyperextension), often associated with angular acceleration of the head (Fig. 1 a).
- Torsion of the upper part of the head in relation to

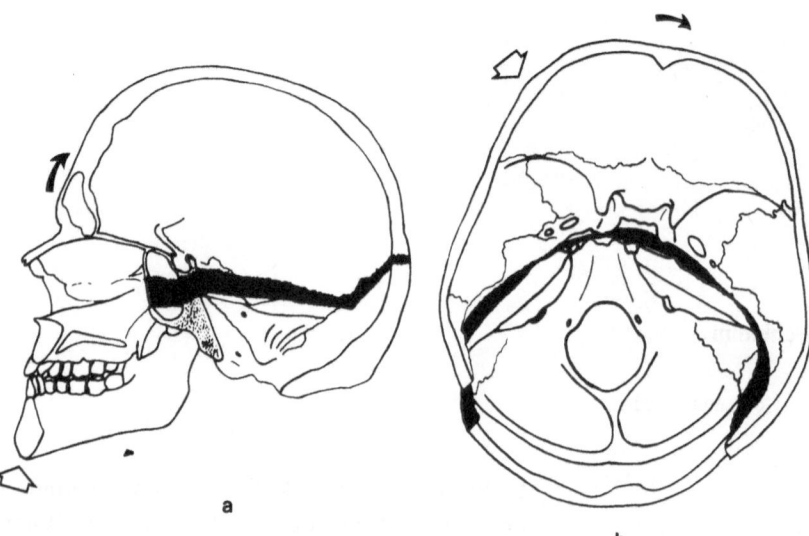

Fig. 1. The two most common types of ring fracture of the base of the skull according to Voigt and Sköld (1974). a) Classical ringfracture due to traction. b) Ringfracture due to torsion

the base of the skull, mainly seen as a result of oblique impact against the temporal or posterior part of the side of the head. This ring fracture is then often asymmetric (Fig. 1 b).

● Impact against the frontal bone cleaving the anterior part of the skull base right back to the pituitary fossa where the fracture divides and runs laterally in front of the pyramides towards the temporal bones (wedge-effect).

● Impact against the top of the head causing displacement of the atlas and thereby the bone around the foramen magnum into the cranial cavity.

Fractures of the base of the skull are often accompanied by focal brain damage and dura lacerations which open up the cerebrospinal fluid spaces outward.

Fractures of the frontal fossa and of the corpus ossis occipitale can lead to laceration of the mucosa of the nose or the throat. Aspiration of blood is then a big hazard when blood vessels are disrupted. The ring fractures almost always have a fatal outcome due to the concomitant injuries to the brain stem.

Brain Injuries

Brain injuries include two distinct varieties:

● Focal injuries result from primary localized tissue damage. The brain laceration, cortical contusion, epidural-, subdural-, subarachnoidal- and traumatic intracerebral hematomas comprise the focal injuries. They can cause coma if they are sufficiently large so that the focal damage leads to brain shifts, herniation and brain stem compression.

● The diffuse brain injuries are fundamentally different and are associated with widespread primary brain damage. This damage may be principally functional or structural—diffuse axonal injury[2]—(see Boström et al., this supplement) from primary injury to the cerebral hemispheres or the brainstem. The diffuse brain injuries are most often associated with disruption of several or all parasagittal bridging veins and with a malignant brain edema, with a brain weight 200–300 grams above normal.

These intracranial injuries could also be related to the point of impact or remote from this point. With exception for those cases with widespread fractures of the skull epidural hematomas, local brain laceration and cortical contusions are examples of injuries at the point of impact.

Injuries located remote from the point of impact can be exemplified by subdural hematomas originating from a disrupted parasagittal bridging vein, presumably caused by angular acceleration of the head due to impact against the chin or frontal bone. This may also cause cortical and/or subcortical hemorrhages, designated as gliding contusions[6]. These injuries and the disruption of the parasagittal bridging veins were also designated rotational cerebral injuries[11].

Cortical contusions are often located both at the point of impact (coup injuries) and at the contra-lateral side of the brain (contrecoup injuries). The latter occur particularly in the frontal and temporal lobes. Contusions at these sites are perhaps more confined to the lower brain surfaces in posterior impacts than at impacts to the front of the head. Geometric configuration of the brain and skull at these sites is probably a significant factor in the injury process. Frontal impact does not give rise to contusion of the posterior part of the brain.

Skull fracture can occur with or without substantial or fatal brain damage; conversely, serious or lethal brain trauma can occur without skull fracture. In about 20% of cases with bridging vein disruption there are no skull fractures[11].

Disruption of one or a few of the veins may lead to a subdural hematoma; on the other hand in acute cases, dying very early after the trauma, many or all of the parasagittal bridging veins may be torn without a noteworthy subdural hematoma[12]. This can be found also when life has been maintained by respirator treatment (brain death?). As part of the accompanying diffuse brain injury often microscopical brain stem lesions are found[7].

Neck Injuries

Following head impact, the axial and/or transverse loading of the neck and subsequent hyperflexion or extension are the probable mechanisms for severe neck injuries causing death or quadriplegia. Without head impact, flexion/extension caused by inertial loading (whiplash) is the injury mechanism observed. Whiplash seldom causes lethal injuries.

The outcome of fractures of the upper cervical spine depends highly on the stability of the fractures[8]. In the list of injuries of the upper cervical spine presented below, reference is also made to the direction of the impact trauma to the head (cf. Sköld, 1978)[9].

● Atlanto-occipital dislocation. Survival is rare and the injury is in our material sometimes encountered in helmet wearing MC or moped riders (increased head weight?)[5]. The impact direction is frontal or oblique frontal.
● Fracture of the posterior arch of the atlas or comminuted fracture of the ring are mostly due to axial loading (the so-called Jefferson fracture). The fractures are as a rule stable and heal without surgery.
● Fracture of the odontoid process of the axis:
   A) Fracture involving the tip of the odontoid process is asymptomatic and rare.
   B) Fracture at the junction of the odontoid process and the C 2 body is dangerous and often associated with spinal cord injury due to dislocation.
   C) Fracture of the odontoid process and part of the body is usually stable with good outcome. Impact direction is often frontal causing compression and hyperextension.
● Sagittal atlanto-axial dislocations are commonly associated with fractures of the odontoid process and as they are unstable they often cause spinal cord injury. Dislocations may also appear without fractures. A

dislocation of the odontoid process of the axis both anterior and posterior towards the atlas is reported in several cases. The posterior luxation of the odontoid process of the axis is accompanied with disruption of the transverse ligament of the atlas. These dislocations are often caused by anterior or posterior sometimes somewhat oblique impact against the face or the occiput[4].
● Rotational atlanto-axial dislocations are caused by axial rotation and has generally good outcome.
● Fractures of the neural arch of the axis (Hangman's fracture) can be caused by an extension-distraction mechanism and this injury seldom involves neurologic deficit[9].
● Fractures in the parts of the cervical spine below the level of atlas and axis mostly occur in the level of C 5–C 7. Different kinds of fractures in this region appears as the result of a hyperextension of the head. These injuries are often seen among young male mc-riders and in swimmers jumping into shallow water. They often survive the initial trauma but remain tetraplegic cripples.

Concerning the fractures of the odontoid process of the axis it could be mentioned that in a comparative study (Ersmark and Löwenhielm[1]) between a clinical and a forensic autopsy material of cases suffering such fractures it was shown that while among the surviving cases neurologic deficit was seldom at hand, there were as a rule injuries to the spinal cord in the forensic cases. Concomitant injuries to other body regions also contributed to the fatal outcome in the forensic cases and although the selection of cases was not primarily based on the injuries to the cervical spinal cord the anterior-posterior diameter of the uninjured spinal canal at the C 1 level was significantly lower in the forensic cases compared with the clinical material.

Epidemiological Considerations

The different causes of head injury, traffic accident, falls etc may indicate the type of head injury. The frequency of different kinds of injuries occuring in victims from various kinds of accidents is well known from numerous investigations. Such knowledge can sometimes be of guidance for diagnostic considerations. E.g. according to Gennarelli, Spielman and Langfitt[3], the less severe focal and diffuse injuries (contusion and concussion respectively) occur with equal frequency in vehicular and non-vehicular trauma. The more severe focal injuries (subdural hematoma, epidural hematoma and intracerebral hematoma) are two to four times more common in non-vehicular injury while the more severe diffuse brain injuries (moderate and severe diffuse axonal injury) are seventeen times more frequent in vehicular trauma.

References

1. Ersmark H, Löwenhielm CGP (1986) Factors influencing the outcome of cervical spine injuries. Submitted to J Trauma
2. Gennarelli TA *et al.* (1982) Diffuse axonal injury and traumatic coma in primate. Ann Neurol 12: 564–574
3. Gennarelli TA, Spielman GM, Langfitt TW (1982) Influence of the type of intracranial lesion on outcome from severe head injury: a multicenter study using a new classification system. J Neurosurg 56: 26–32
4. Krantz KPG (1980) Isolated disruption of the transverse ligament of the atlas; an injury easily overlooked at postmortem examination. Injury 12: 168–170
5. Krantz KPG (1985) Head and neck injuries to motorcycle and moped riders—with special regard to the effect of protective helmets. Injury 16: 253–258
6. Lindenberg R, Freytag E (1960) The mechanism of cerebral contusions. Arch Path 69: 440–469
7. Löwenhielm CGP (1975) Mathematical simulation of gliding contusions. J Biomech 8: 351–356
8. Paradis GR, Janes JM (1973) Posttraumatic atlantoaxial instability: the fate of the odontoid process fracture in 46 cases. J Trauma 13: 359–367
9. Sköld BG (1978) Fractures of the axis caused by hanging. Z Rechtsmed 80: 329–331
10. Voigt GE, Sköld BG (1974) Ring fractures of the base of the skull. J Trauma 14: 494–505
11. Voigt GE, Löwenhielm CGP, Ljung CBA (1977) Rotational cerebral injuries near the superior margin of the brain. Acta Neuropathol (Berl) 39: 201–209
12. Voigt GE, Saldeen T (1968) Über den Abriß zahlreicher oder sämtlicher Vv. cerebri sup. mit geringem Subduralhaematom und Hirnstammläsion. Dtsch Z ges gerichtl Med 64: 9–20

Author's address: P. Krantz, M.D., Department of Forensic Medicine, University of Lund, Sölvegatan 25, S-223 62 Lund, Sweden.

Acta Neurochirurgica, Suppl. 36, 51–55 (1986)

Aspects on Pathology and Neuropathology in Head Injury

K. Boström and **C. G. Helander**

Institution of Forensic Medicine, University of Göteborg, Göteborg, Sweden

Summary

Some principal differences of the head injury materal available to clinicians, hospital pathologists and forensic pathologists are discussed with reference to the primary and secondary findings at focal and diffuse brain injury and intracranial injuries after trauma. The importance of cooperative understanding between the different disciplines is stressed in order to cover the whole head injury pattern. Examples are given.

The importance of intracranial arterial hemorrhages is stressed and may also be the cause of a particular group of acute subdural hematomas; it may be of special prognostic importance because of their probable availability to successful surgery in the acute stage. The cause may be a tearing of arterial connections between the peripheral branches of the middle cerebral artery and the dura.

The diagnosis of different types of primary diffuse brain injury is discussed with particular reference to the non-satisfactory common histological methods of investigation early after trauma.

Diffuse brain injury due to hypoxia at the trauma can be serious but give few macroscopical findings; disseminated intravasal coagulation can appear isolated in the brain or be part of a systemic manifestation.

Keywords: Fatal head injury; acute subdural hematoma; diffuse brain damage.

Injuries of the brain after trauma have been classified in injuries caused directly as a consequence of mechanical events at the trauma and injuries subsequent to and caused by the primary injury. Today clinicians and pathologists often at first classify the brain injuries as focal or diffuse and then determine if they are primary or secondary.

However, it has become quite evident to us, that there are some differences in aspects on the victims not only those available to clinicians and pathologists but also those investigated by hospital pathologists and by forensic pathologists because of the different types of injuries from the accidents they investigate. In this paper we will try to elucidate some features of the knowledge apparent for each group of investigator but less known to the other disciplines. The experience is founded on autopsies during a 15-year period. About 30 thousand autopsies were performed. Death was caused by blunt trauma in about 15%.

Focal Intracranial Injuries

Among primary focal head injuries are brain contusions and intracranial hematomas.

Primary Brain Contusions

Cortical brain surface contusions are characterized by hemorrhages in the cortex and a focal subarachnoid hemorrhage. If the contusion is restricted to the surface the hemorrhages in the cortex are limited to the convexity of the gyri. At more severe injuries the hemorrhages may continue through the cortex into the white matter. The cortical contusions are caused by mechanical violence to the head and their location is due to the impact site on the head. If this is located frontally the contusions are limited mainly to the frontal and temporal lobes and mainly at their basal surfaces. This may be caused by the movement of the skull base in relation to the brain surface at trauma.

Cortical-subcortical contusions: If the impact is directed to the temporal or occipital region of the head contusions will appear both inside the site of contact of the trauma (coup) as well as in the diametrically opposite part of the brain (contrecoup). It is remarkable that the coup injury can be much less apparent macroscopically than the contrecoup injury. The latter may be extensive and in serious cases combined with contusion-laceration of the brain surface with subsequent subdural hematoma.

Parasagittal contusions: This special type of contusions are located parasagittaly in the frontal, parietal and occipital lobes. Hemorrhages are seen subarachnoidally, cortically and subcortically; they can appear in one of the tissues or together[7].

These contusions will be produced at acceleration of the head of an impulsive loading type without direct impact. The contusional changes are often bilateral and symmetrical and are often revealed only after special attention to an investigation of the parasagittal region. Thus, the location and appearance of the contusions can indicate the site of the trauma to the head and the kind of violence occurred.

Intracranial Hematomas

These can be intracerebral, subdural and extradural. The causes of the hematomas are injuries of vessels, arteries or veins or both.

Extradural hematomas are often caused by injuries of meningeal arteries. They may sometimes also occur inside the location of a linear fracture in continuity with hemorrhage from the spongiosa of the bone, filling the space between the bone and the perhaps immediately disconnected dura. (At severe impact site fractures and simultaneous tearing of the dura the epidural hemorrhage may extend subdurally.)

Intracerebral and subdural hematomas may result from injuries of arteries as well as of veins after contusion—laceration of the cortex. For radiologists and clinicians it is also well known that a less severe course of intracerebral contusion may be followed by CT scanning from the contusional salt-pepper pictures to the confluent more homogenous intracerebral hematoma a few days later.

Acute subdural hematomas of arterial or venous origin: According to general opinion the acute subdural hematomas are usually of venous origin and due to rupture of parasagittal bridging veins. It seems to us that subdural hematoma also can be produced by injuries of small arteries from the peripheral branches of the middle cerebral artery to the arachnoidal and dural tissue. These small arteries are located on the convexities of the temporal lobe, frontal lobe and parietal lobe in the vicinity of the Sylvian fissure. It seems to be well known for surgeons that sometimes when carefully removing a rather limited and coagulated subdural hematoma a torn and pulsating bleeding proximal stump of a small artery can be revealed in this collection of clots. Such vessels are easily overlooked at routine autopsies because they are small and are hurt at

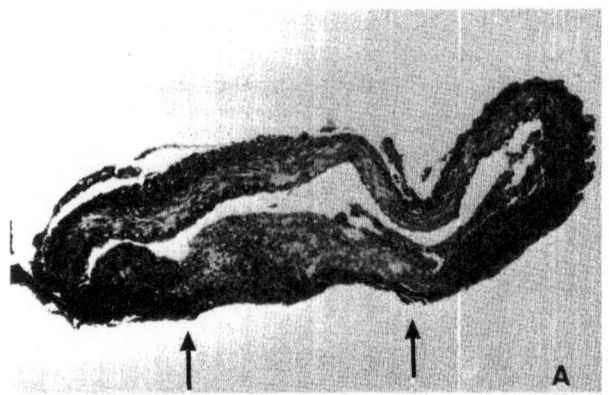

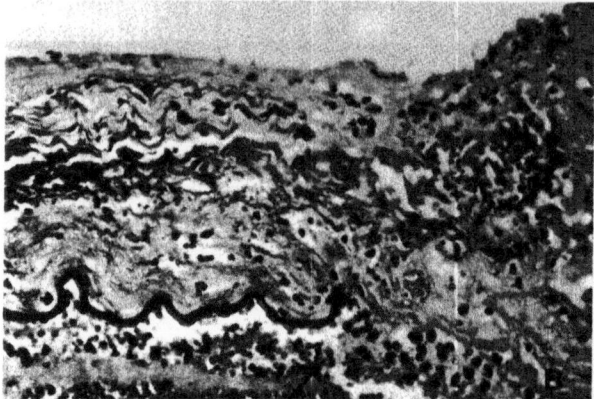

Fig. 1. Basal intracranial subarachnoidal hemorrhage in a 20-year-old man (alcohol-intoxicated) after trauma to the skull base. "Survived" one day with respirator-ventilation. A) Rupture, between arrows, of ordinary vessel wall—left p.i.c.a. (posterior-inferior-cerebellar artery). B) Vessel wall in detail with clot (arrow) at the site of rupture. Staining: Elastica and Van Gieson

the autopsy exposure of the brain. A special technique is required to reveal these vessels[3].

Traumatic *basal subarachnoidal hemorrhage* of arterial origin seems on the other hand more frequently observed by the forensic pathologists[5]. They are found in persons with alcohol intoxication and with a trauma to the head at the level of the skull base. These persons die often immediately after the trauma. The cause of the subarachnoidal bleeding is a rupture in the wall of the vertebral or basilar artery or of one of their branches with extensive hemorrhage underneath the base of the pons, cerebellum and medulla oblongata. There is often a fracture in the first vertebra (atlas). The vessel rupture causing the bleeding is usually very small, of pinpoint size, and therefore difficult to reveal. To find the rupture in the arterial wall a very careful dissection must be performed on a formalinfixed brain (Fig. 1).

"Secondary brain damage" from intracranial focal injuries occurs because of their often expansive nature

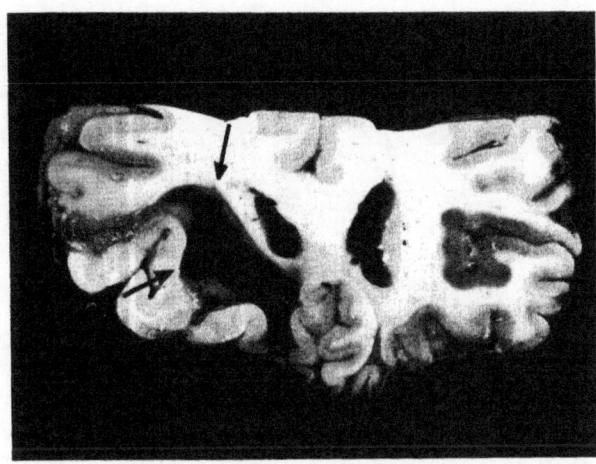

Fig. 2. Old "healed" contusion basally in left frontal lobe with cyst formation (between arrows). Occasional finding at autopsy. (Necrotic cortex of orbital frontal lobe—downward)

(edema, hemorrhages); if they result in the patient's death this is usually caused by compression and deformation effects to the brain stem.

If the evolution of an intracranial hematoma is very rapid, the patient can succumb in a brainstem injury without evidence of hemorrhages or infarctions at the autopsy. If the hematoma is more slowly developed hemorrhages and infarctions can be seen and be due to herniation effects through the tentorium opening, underneath the falx or through the foramen magnum.

Patients with the extensive and multiple focal brain injuries can survive. In patients who have died from other causes it is possible at autopsy to find healed focal brain injuries of large extension (Fig. 2).

Diffuse Brain Injury

"Primary diffuse brain injury" may cause deep unconsciousness of the person from the moment of trauma and he will never wake up from his comatous condition. CT scanning of the brain can show normal pictures in the acute stage.

From a pathoanatomical view the primary diffuse brain injury can be divided in two types:

1. Patients who die immediately at the time of trauma, and

2. patients who survive some day or somewhat longer.

Type 1: In patients with primary diffuse brain injury after trauma dying immediately or within the first 24 hours there are few findings at the autopsy. The macroscopical examination may show petechial hemorrhages in the white matter of the cerebral hem-

ispheres, most often in frontal and temporal lobes between the cortex and the ventricular walls. Petechial hemorrhages may be found also centrally in the basal ganglia, in the mesencephalon and in the pontine region, mostly in its rostral part; they also occur around the aqueduct and in the peduncles. The hemorrhages may be numerous or sparse. At examination only hemorrhages are found in the tissue. Many more hemorrhages may be seen microscopically than macroscopically.

Isolated petechial hemorrhages in the brainstem have not been evident in the persons in our autopsy material. If hemorrhages have been evident in the brainstem also small bleedings have been seen in other parts of the brain.

Type 2: May appear in patients unconscious but surviving more than a day or up to some weeks, and be more often recognized also by hospital pathologists. The macroscopical examination of the brain reveals few hemorrhages characteristically located to corpus callosum and the rostral part of the pons. However, hemorrhages can be found also in other parts of the cerebral white matter and the brainstem. They are usually small and vary in diameter from a few millimeters to one centimeter. Parasagittal contusions with hemorrhages are often revealed while cerebral cortical contusions on the convexity or base may be very few or may be missing. Some brain swelling with flattened gyri may be seen (Fig. 3).

This type of primary diffuse brain injury has been called "diffuse axonal injury" because of the findings at the microscopical investigation. With silverstaining it is possible to find ruptures of axones in the cerebral white matter, in the brainstem and in cerebellum often located to certain tracts and projections[1, 2, 6].

If the patient survives some months the macroscopical and microscopical picture will be different. The brain surface can be without pathological changes. The brain cortex seems intact but a reduction of the volume of the white matter will be found with a corresponding dilation of the cerebral ventricles. As a remaining evidence of earlier hemorrhages small cysts in the tissue will be seen. The microscopical investigation in these cases will reveal demyelination of the white matter in the cerebrum, brainstem and cerebellum. The location of the demyelinated areas correspond to the areas[1, 2, 6] where ruptured axones have been found in silverstained preparations of patients who died some days after the trauma.

Thus, in our material there are two groups of patients with primary diffuse brain injury: type 1—

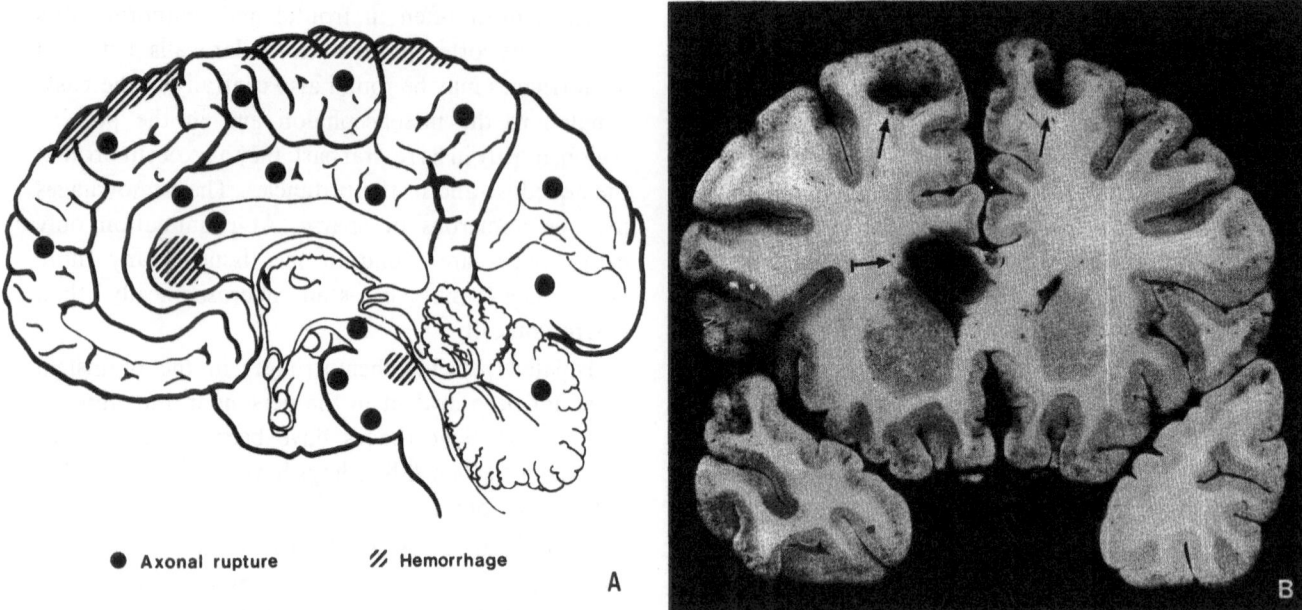

Fig. 3. Diffuse axonal injury. Location of axonal injuries and hemorrhages. A) Drawing illustrating common localization of hemorrhages and ruptures of axones. B) Hemorrhage in corpus callosum (———>). Bilateral parasagittal contusions (arrows directed upward)

patients who died within the first day and type 2—the patients who survived some days or longer. Both groups of patients have been victims of the same type of violence (usually traffic accidents) and have a similar clinical picture with deep unconsciousness after the trauma. The macroscopical findings at the investigation of the brain in this early posttraumatic phase are surprisingly few in relation to the reported very serious clinical picture. In both groups of patients parasagittal contusions are revealed as well as hemorrhages in the cerebral white matter and in the rostral part of the brainstem.

At the microscopical investigation of the group of patients surviving some day or longer silverstaining will help to reveal axonal injuries.

In patients surviving months it is also possible to see demyelination of the axonal tracts. Thus, in these cases it seems evident that a diffuse axonal injury has occurred. The histological examination is the basis for the diagnosis. However, the silverstaining technique cannot help in defining axonal injuries in patients dying within one day.

Probably the difference between these two groups of patients of primary diffuse brain injury is a difference of degree rather than of type of injury. This is also supported by the similarity in clinical picture and macroscopical findings in the brain.

Intracranial Effects of Acute Extracranial Injuries

In patients with brain injuries caused by trauma there are often also other and multiple extracranial injuries. These will severely influence the patients' general condition: blood pressure fall may result because of hemorrhages or respiratory obstruction occur due to thoracic injuries. The result can be ischemia and hypoxia for which the brain is particularly vulnerable.

It is well known that hypoxic injuries of the brain are common in patients dying after head injury. The hypoxic damages may be pathophysiologically serious but the resulting pathomorphological changes difficult or impossible to reveal macroscopically in patients with short survival after the trauma. The microscopical investigation will be more clarifying. It is well known that the areas most vulnerable for hypoxia are hippocampi and basal ganglia. Hypoxic damage is also often seen in the cortex in cerebellum and in the cerebrum.

In the cerebral cortex hypoxic damage is most common in the borderline between the nutritional areas of two arteries and most often between the anterior and the middle cerebral arteries (compare "watershed infarction"). Diffuse damage in the cerebral cortex is also common.

Within the frame of the diffuse secondary brain damage are also effects of "disseminated intravasal coagulation" (DIC). This can be elicited in two ways: at the s.c. "extrinsic pathway" tissue damage will deliver thromboplastin and thromboplastic products; at the s.c. intrinsic pathway disseminated intravasal coagulation can follow damage to the endothelial cells of the vascular walls. DIC in the brain can be part of the systemic manifestation or be located only to the brain.

This last "isolated" location has been reported to be elicited by hypoxemia and subsequent endothelial damage[4]. DIC will be evident in two ways: the appearance of microthrombi or hemorrhages. Microthrombi can result in microinfarctions, perivascular demyelination, focal edema and petechies. In similarity with hypoxic brain injury the macroscopical findings may be very few at disseminated intravasal coagulation in the brain. Also in these cases the microscopical examination elucidates the diagnosis.

Discussion

It is evident from this report that both at primary as well as at secondary diffuse brain injury in spite of serious clinical symptoms the macroscopic pathoanatomical changes are not impressive, particularly not in the forensic cases usually dying early after trauma. A macroscopical observation only of a nonfixed brain may in these cases give no contribution to the diagnosis or the cause of death. This stresses the importance of thoroughful examination of the brain particularly in the cases where the clinical cause of death has not been revealed by the surgeon or anesthesiologist.

References

1. Adams JH, Gennarelli TA, Graham DI (1982) Brain damage in non-missile head injury: observations in man and subhuman primates. In: Smith WT, Cavanagh JB (eds) Recent advances in neuropathology. Churchill Livingstone, Edinburgh London Melbourne New York, pp 165–290
2. Adams HJ (1985) Cerebral trauma. In: Blackwood W, Corselis JAN (eds) Greenfield's Neuropathology, 4th edn. E Arnold, London, pp 85–124
3. Boström K, Helander CG, Lindgren SO (1986) Bridging arteries between the middle cerebral artery and the dura. To be published
4. Kaufman HJ, Mattson J-C (1985) Coagulopathy in head injury. In: Becker DP, Povlishock JT (ed) Central nervous system trauma. Status report, pp 87–206. National Institutes of Health, London
5. Lindenberg R (1971) Trauma of meninges and brain. In: Minckler J (ed) Pathology of the nervous system, vol 2. McGraw Hill, New York, pp 1705–1765
6. Strich SJ (1976) Cerebral trauma. In: Blackwood W, Corselis JAN (eds) Greenfield's Neuropathology, 3rd edn. Ed Arnold, London, pp 327–360
7. Voigt GE, Löwenhielm P, Ljung CBA (1977) Rotational cerebral injuries near the superior margin of the brain. Acta Neuropathol (Berl) 39: 201–209

Authors' address: K. Boström, M.D., Institution of Forensic Medicine, University of Göteborg, S-413 45 Göteborg, Sweden.

Acta Neurochirurgica, Suppl. 36, 56–57 (1986)

Care at Accident Site and During Transport

E. Gordon

Karolinska Hospital, Stockholm

Summary

The immediately performed measures at the site of accident including adequate ventilation of an unconscious person with head injuries may be lifesaving. As a matter of fact, these measures are far more important than a rapid transport to the nearest hospital.

Keywords: Head injury; first aid; acute management; accident site.

Comments

There are many reports in the relevant literature[2–4], which show that between 15 and 20% of head injured patients die after road accidents not because of the severity of their brain injury, but because of cerebral hypoxia due to aspiration of blood, vomit, minor chest injuries, and cardiac arrest. These complications are potentially reversible and if handled within 10 min the patients would have a much greater chance of survival and probably complete recovery. Therefore, patients with head injuries have to be assessed and treated within 10 min of the accident by qualified personnel to avoid or minimize secondary brain damage which develops with extreme rapidity, if untreated (Fig. 1).

Brain injury in the initial stages is a dynamic process, and therefore the time factor is one of the most important factors in this period of the trauma. Treatment in the "therapeutic vacuum"—the time period between injury and admission to hospital—cannot only interrupt the development of vicious circles, but also provide the surgeon more time available to perform the evacuation of an acute hematoma.

Head injured patients without gross multiple injuries have most often an intact cardiovascular function. Therefore, the most crucial among vital functions must be provided by the *restoration of free airways and adequate ventilation*. These have to be secured with the most simple method that is effective—as soon as possible: that is at the site of accident[1].

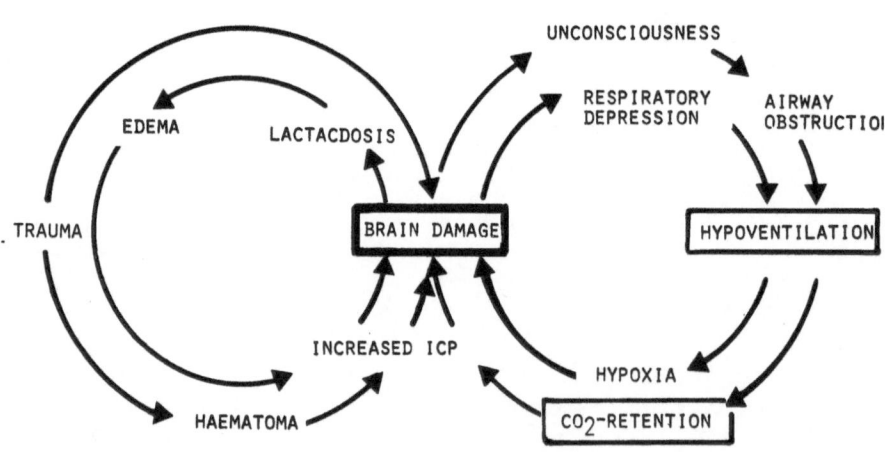

Fig. 1. Some of the vicious circles facing the head-injured patient

References

1. Andreasson R, Baker ME, Halldin M (1976) Report from First International Workshop on First AID at the Scene of an accident. Discussion. Opuscula Medica 21: 12–18
2. Frey C, Huelke DF, Gikas PW (1969) Resuscitation and survival in motor vehicle accidents. J Trauma 9: 292–310
3. Maloney AF (1970) The fatal head injury and some neuropatho-logical observations. Head Injury Symposium, Churchill-Livingstone, Edinburgh London Madrid, pp 28–32
4. Ringkjøb R (1970) Care at the roadside-prevention of second accident. Head Injury Symposium, Edinburgh London Madrid, pp 23–36

Author's address: E. Gordon, M.D., Karolinska Hospital, Stockholm, Sweden.

Acta Neurochirurgica, Suppl. 36, 58–59 (1986)

Guidelines for Care in the Acute Phase in Hospitals Without Neurosurgical Specialists

Introduction

U. Pontén

Department of Neurosurgery, University Hospital, Uppsala, Sweden

In 1984 the Swedish neurosurgical and anaesthesiological societies agreed upon a priority list on admission to hospitals without neurosurgical unit of patients with acute traumatic cranio-cerebral injuries. This list was published in Läkartidningen in a series of papers on the care of head injured patients [1–5]. The main points in this priority list is shown in the paper by E. Gordon (see below).

This first priority list is recommended for all Swedish hospitals without a neurosurgical service.

For the continued management, however, it was realized that special recommendations have to be decided for each hospital according to the available resources and competence, the distance to the regional neurosurgical unit and similar factors. Appropriate admission charts and observation charts have to be standardized for cooperation between the different links in the chain of management (see chapter of "Management charts" in this supplement).

The priority list for acute management should be modified and regularly revised by the surgeons and anaesthetists of the local hospital together with the neurosurgical department. An example of this type of recommendations was also published [1] (see also Gordon).

References

1. Gordon E, Pontén U, Stånge K, Wiklund L (1984) Principles of treatment in acute head injured patients at hospitals without neurosurgical services (in Swedish) Läkartidningen 81: 1521–1523.
2. Messeter K, Nordström C-H, Pontén U, Sundbärg G (1984) Guidelines for management of patients with acute head injuries in the south region (in Swedish) Läkartidningen 81: 1529–1530.

Author's address: U. Pontén, M. D., Department of Neurosurgery, University Hospital, S-75185 Uppsala, Sweden.

Guidelines for Management

E. Gordon

Karolinska Hospital, Stockholm, Sweden

As material and personnel resources vary in different hospitals, a very detailed program of treatment is neither possible nor is it necessary. Routines of care should be worked out by the respective units, with the cooperation of the regional neurosurgical clinic.

Nevertheless, it is reasonable to put forward general guidelines for the acute care and management of these patients in the very early phase after the trauma, e.g. before a possible contact with the neurosurgical clinic can be established. The goal is to stress the necessity of the early judgement of the neurological state, particularly the grade or level of impairment of consciousness, and then to point to the extreme importance of free airways and adequate ventilation; the principles behind these recommendations are now well established and basically not controversial.

Thus control and management has to be guided by the grade of consciousness and neurological findings. The primary goal is to hinder the development of secondary lesions. In this stage the care of the head injured patient has to be conducted through a close cooperation between surgeon and anaesthetist, with the responsibilities for the various diagnostic and therapeutical procedures (care of vital functions, lowering of ICP, operations etc.). All the involved specialists should know the necessary techniques for neurological examinations, and be well aware of basic neurological pathophysiology.

Table 1. *Priority List at Admission of Patients with Acute Cranio-cerebral Traumatic Injuries*

1. Assess the reaction level	(Reaction level scale 1–8)
2. Assess and secure the airways and the ventilation	Oxygen for all unconscious patients (RLS 4–8) Tracheal intubation for airway obstruction or unconsciousness > ½ hour
3. Assess and secure the systemic circulation	Shock usually indicates multiple injuries
4. Second assessment of the reaction level within 10 min + neurological examination	Use special watch sheet
5. Blood sampling	Blood gases Glucose/s Screening for intoxication when necessary
6. Consult neurosurgeon	If the patient has/is A. Deteriorating reaction level B. Still unconscious (RLS 4–8) > 2 hrs C. Open brain injury or depressed skull fracture D. Severe complicating disease (*e.g.* pulmonary or cardiovascular insufficiency) E. Difficult to assess or treat for other reasons.

Intubation should be performed by an anaesthetist or other personnel with sufficient knowledge not only of technical details, but also of effects of pain stimuli and anaesthetic drugs on cerebral blood flow and intracranial pressure.

In case of transfer to another hospital all records containing the case history and findings should follow the patient.

A simple list of priorities can be followed according to the list in Table 1.

It is obvious that immediately after admission to hospital the most urgent task of the anaesthetist is to secure the patient free airways and adequate ventilation, if not cared for previously. It is equally important to assess the patient's neurological state, especially the level of consciousness. It is important to assess if the patient has some other or multiple injuries and focal or diffuse brain lesion. If neurological symptoms are observed and recorded continuously, a trend will be noticed very soon indicating an improvement or deterioration of the patient.

After the preliminary acute assessment and treatment, further diagnostic measures can be taken (skull X-ray, CT-scan) followed, if necessary, by surgical intervention.

Reference

1. Gordon E, Pontén U, Stånge K, Wiklund L (1984) Principles of treatment in acute head injured patients at hospitals without neurosurgical services (in Swedish) Läkartidningen 81: 1521–1523.

Author's address: E. Gordon, M.D., Department of Neuro-anesthesiology, Karolinska Hospital, S-10401 Stockholm, Sweden.

Acta Neurochirurgica, Suppl. 36, 60–61 (1986)

Resources for Head Injury Patients at Different Hospital Levels

U. Pontén

Department of Neurosurgery, University Hospital, Uppsala, Sweden

By law (Hälso- och Sjukvårdslagen 1983) all patients in Sweden are granted a good and equal care irrespective of where they live and what their financial status is. For specialized care like neurosurgery Sweden is divided into 6 regions with catchment populations varying from 0.9 to 1.8 million inhabitants. In our Uppsala-Örebro region (1.6 million inhabitants) 50% of the referring hospitals are situated at a distance between 200 and 390 km from the neurosurgical department in Uppsala. Nevertheless the neurosurgical unit in Uppsala has the responsiblity of organizing good and equal care all over the region for all the inhabitants.

In this region some 5,000–8,000 head injuries should occur per year, 300–500 of these patients should benefit from neurosurgical care or evaluation.

Referral of all these cases to a neurosurgical unit which is possible in a city like Stockholm (1.5 million) is not practical in the Uppsala-Örebro region due to available resources and to the large distances.

To improve, *e.g.* the often poor results with acute subdural hematomas the patient has to be on the operating table within one or two hours in many cases. Thus it is often impossible to reach the neurosurgical unit in time. It is well known from studies in Scotland and also in Sweden that delay in the treatment of expanding hematomas is the most frequent "avoidable factor" in the treatment chain causing poor result in traumatic brain injuries.

The problem has to be solved by

1. Optimal competence and resource allocation to peripheral hospitals with a definition of the type of patients which should be observed and treated in the different hospitals.

2. Close collaboration between the neurosurgical unit and the local hospitals with educational programs and uniform principles for management of the patients.

Standardized acute head injury and supervision sheets. For each hospital specially prepared guidelines for the management according to available resources and geographical situation.

3. Frequent consultations, with use of modern techniques for communication (*e.g.,* of CT records).

4. A safe and fast transport system.

The object is to arrange a safe continuous supervision and care of the patient from the site of the accident through all the different levels of medical resources needed, and to rapidly determine the competence level which is accurate for the patient. The neurosurgical unit

Table 1. *Minimum Competence and Resources Required for Observation and Treatment of Traumatic Brain Injuries*

Type of hospital	Surgical	Anesthesiological ICU	Neuro-radiological
I	Evacuation of extradural hematoma. Dural incision (for subdural hematomas?)	Supervisions by specially trained personnel. Anesthesia with controlled ventilation. Intensive care for transport.	Skull and spine X-ray (angiography)
II	Simple depressed skull-fractures. Evacuation of all extracerebral and simple intracerebral hematomas.	ICU, conventional non-surgical treatment of raised ICP (in some hospitals monitoring of ICP and EEG, EVR, Barbiturate coma)	CT (head-scanner), a–y, myelography.
III	Full neurosurgical competence	Specialized cerebral ICU. Full neuroanesthesiological competence	Full competence

furthermore has a responsibility of improving the treatment of severe traumatic brain injuries by own research and by evaluating new methods and principles in the field and finally to transfer those principles through the whole organization as soon as possible.

Three main levels of competence are recognizable for hospitals in which head injured patients are to be observed and treated in the acute stage.

I Local hospital (länsdelssjukhus)

II Central hospitals (länssjukhus och regionsjukhus) without neurosurgical unit

III Hospitals with neurosurgical unit

The competence and resource allocation needed for these different types of hospitals are given by table 1.

Modern clinical and laboratory research facilites are required at least in the type III hospitals.

The management is also governed by the well-known principles that a deterioration indicates an operable expansive process until proven otherwise.

However, the safety margins for the patients will definitely differ in various hospitals human to available personnel and material resources.

Author's address: U. Pontén, M.D., Department of Neurosurgery, University Hospital, S-751 85 Uppsala, Sweden.

Acta Neurochirurgica, Suppl. 36, 62 (1986)

Resources for Mild, Moderate and Severe Head Injury Patients

Introduction

B. Jennett

Department of Neurosurgery, The Southern General Hospital, University of Glasgow, Scotland

The overall objective of head injury care is to minimize the occurrence of avoidable mortality and morbidity. Most avoidable mortality is due to delayed diagnosis and management of intracranial hematoma or the overlooking of systemic extracranial events. Most avoidable morbidity is in mild and moderately disabled patients. Overall too much attention has probably been paid to very severely injured patients both in the acute stage and during rehabilitation.

In most countries only a minority of injuries have been considered to need neurosurgical care (in the UK in 1974 5% of admitted patients were transferred on average, but in many places it was only 1 or 2%). The effect of the advent of CT scanning on this policy depends on the number and location of scanners and of neurosurgical units. In most of UK head scanners have so far been largely located in neurosurgical units and there has been an increased referral rate of patients in order to secure a scan; many such patients have been returned to primary surgical wards once the scan had excluded an intracranial hematoma. With the increased availability of scanners in general hospitals it has been proposed that there might be fewer patients transferred to neurosurgical units as scanners are used for screening patients for surgical complications. It is estimated that about 10% of head injuries admitted in the UK justify a scan. How wise it is to depend on scanning without skilled neurosurgical assessment or continued monitoring is a matter of controversy.

It is believed that in Britain too many mild head injuries are admitted to primary surgical wards and that better assessment in accident and emergency departments, with proper use of plain skull X-ray could reduce this number substantially. Where scanning facilities are readily available they are sometimes used for patients in accident and emergency departments— but it is difficult to see this as a sensible policy[1, 2].

Guidelines have been evolved by a national panel of neurosurgeons and estimates made of the neurosurgical bed requirements to operate these guidelines. The basis of these guidelines is statistical evaluation of the risk factors predicting the likelihood that an intracranial hematoma will develop, as well as on identifying patients who for other reasons require various levels of investigation or treatment[3-5].

References

1. Bryden JS, Jennett B (1983) Neurosurgical resources and transfer policies for head injuries. Br Med J 286: 1791–1793
2. Jennett B *et al.* (1984) Guidelines for initial management after head injury in adults. Br Med J 288: 983–985
3. Mendelow AD, Campbell DA, Jeffrey RR, Miller JD, Hessett C, Bryden J, Jennett B (1982) Admission after mild head injury: benefits and costs. Br Med J 285: 1530–1532
4. Mendelow AD, Teasdale G, Jennett B, Bryden J, Hessett C, Murray G (1983) Risks of intracranial haematoma in head injured adults. Br Med J 287: 1173–1176
5. Teasdale G, Galbraith S, Murray L, Ward P, Gentleman G, McKean M (1982) Management of traumatic intracranial haematoma. Br Med J 285: 1695–1697

Author's address: B. Jennett, M.D., Department of Neurosurgery, Institute of Neurological Sciences, Glasgow G51 4TF, Scotland.

Acta Neurochirurgica, Suppl. 36, 63–66 (1986)

Resources, Distribution and Management Levels of Head Injury Patients; Place of CT-Scanning

D. Stålhammar

Department of Neurosurgery, Sahlgren's Hospital, Göteborg, Sweden

Summary

The task for the medical profession is to diagnose, to treat, to evaluate results of the management and to deliver information about the management to those who are responsible for the regional planning of head injury care and preventive work.

The impact of CT scanning on diagnoses and distribution on different levels of managements is discussed. These considerations are related to the degree of severity of the patient's symptoms early after the accident. The strategy of priority with more restrained economical resources will make the above mentioned considerations even more important.

Keywords: Head injury management; levels of resources; the place of CT scanning.

The overall objective is an allocation of resources that optimize the outcome for all categories of head injury patients. The resources concerned are not only hospital care but also prevention and post primary care. Information about the various aspects of management is required to accomplish such an allocation.

The task for the medical profession is
— to diagnose
— to treat
— to evaluate the results of the management
— to deliver information about the management to those who are responsible for the regional planning of head injury care and preventive work.

Diagnosing and treating have been the doctors' primary responsibilities. Evaluation of the results of the medical interventions has also been part of the care, but is performed only occasionally and only for a very small proportion of all head injury patients. Although continuous, valid and reliable information is a prerequisite for large scale planning it is a fact that the information currently delivered about the process of head injury management in terms of hospital statistics is insufficient in these respects.

The question of resources for the head injured patients may be considered in a short and a long time perspective. The most urgent current problems relate to avoidable morbidity and mortality by referring the patients in time to units with adequate resources; the CT-scanner, general surgery ICU, neurosurgery, ICP-monitoring etc.

For the future it is most important to establish continuous feed-back regarding the quality of and the costs for the care. This will require a system for classification of type and severity of lesions and also an accounting system that relates the costs to the individual patients.

In the last decade there has been an increasing interest to identify deficiences in the current management; delays in evacuation of intracranial hematoma[5, 7, 13, 15, 16], undetected airway complications and hypotension[12], transportation of patients without proper precautions etc[3, 10].

One action taken to minimize these "avoidable" causes of bad management is the publication of national and regional recommendations regarding the early management of head injuries[6, 4, 9]. In these guidelines the patients are classified according to the time course of responsiveness after the accident. Fig. 1 shows the patient categories used in the recommendations from the South Region of Sweden[9].

Fig. 2 presents the situation the doctor faces on the first admission of the patient. The influence of time delay on outcome has been clearly demonstrated. Selig *et al.* have showed a significant increase in mortality for subdural hematomas when the delay exceeded four hours[15]. Mendelow *et al.* have shown similar results for epidural hematomas[7].

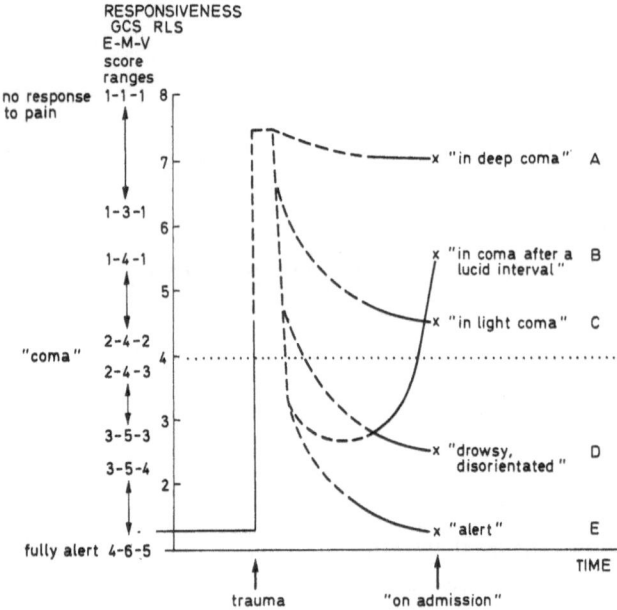

Fig. 1. Head injury patients grouped in five categories according to the level of responsiveness, and its early time course, as recorded on admission to the first hospital. *GCS* = Glasgow Coma Scale, *E—M—V* score = eye—motor—verbal aspects of the GCS, *RLS* = Reaction Level Scale in eight steps

In order to reveal a unilateral complication earlier Salem and Price[14] have argued for measurement of the midline shift in primary hospital because such measurements adequately performed add important information regarding the assessment of the risk of hematoma.

Fig. 3 shows the current guidelines in the Western Region of Sweden. These are based upon the experience of inappropriate management during the last few years[16] and stress that decisive and rapid action is a prerequisite to achieving good results. Thus they em-

phasize the basic principle forwarded by the Glasgow group and others[8, 15, 18] to consider, early and rationally, the risk of development of an intracranial hematoma and not wait until the signs of deterioration appear.

Those criteria for secondary referral are similar to the recommendations published by the Swedish Societies of Neurosurgeons and Anesthesists[4] and to those by the British neurosurgeons[6]. However, there are some discrepancies which it may be fruitful to discuss, particularly when compared with the practice in the Western Region of Sweden in 1977[17] which is presented in Table 1. That situation may partly still exist and perhaps also reflect the policies in other regions and countries.

As further background information for an analysis regarding resources and distribution of head injured patients Table 2 shows the approximate number of patients in different categories and the estimated risks of intracranial hematoma.

Finally Table 3 presents the alternative costs for primary hospital care for head injury patients of various degrees of severity. When considering which is the most efficient strategy of management of these patients it is important to realize the total costs for society. What really repays is adequate prevention and the highest possible quality of care.

In Western Scotland a change to a more liberal admission policy at the neurosurgical unit clearly improved the outcome for patients with intracranial hematoma[18]. Probably this improvement was related to an earlier diagnosis and better treatment. Neurosurgical skill is certainly required for successful evacuation of intracranial hematomas. For head injury patients

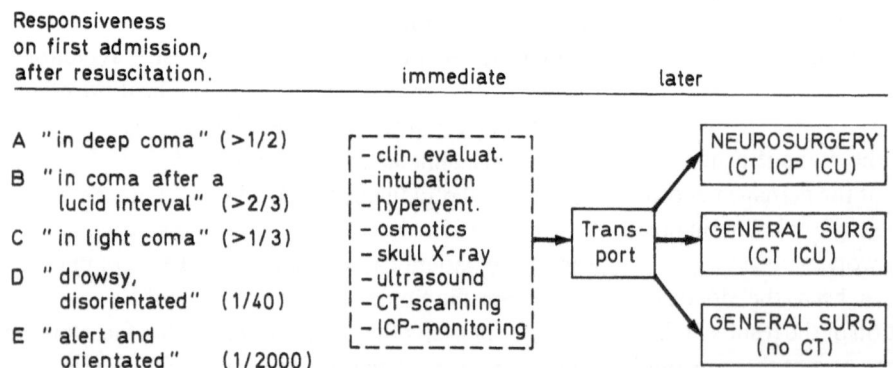

Fig. 2. An overview of alternatives in acute management of head injury patients. These are categorized according to their responsiveness after resuscitation on the first admission to hospital, *cf.* Fig. 1. An approximate statistical risk of development of an intracranial hematoma that needs operation is given within brackets. The resources are available at three different types of hospitals. The outcome will strongly depend on, undelayed, correctly performed diagnostic and therapeutic procedures. The influence of time delay and the occurrence of a midline shift are illustrated in Figs. 3 and 4. The doctor has to consider: Which are the immedaite most appropriate measures? Should the patient be kept or referred to a unit with better facilities? Guidelines for initial management are presented in Fig. 3

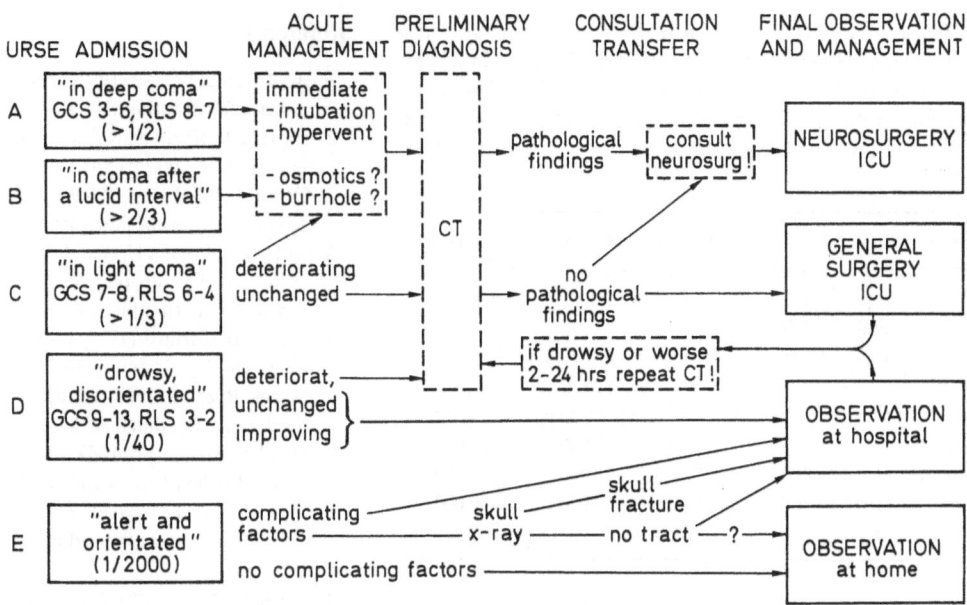

Fig. 3. In these guidelines the head injury patients are classified according to the time course of responsiveness early after the impact *A–E* (*cf.* Fig. 2). Figures within parentheses give a rough statistical estimate of the risk of developing hematoma in an adult patient[8, 17]. "Complicating factors" may be: Nontraumatic: intoxic., resp/cardiac disturbances, anticoagul. Traumatic: amnesia, unconsciousn., neurol deficit, EP fits, headache, vomit, blood/CSF nose, ear, multiple inj.

Table 1. *Recommendations for referral of Patients to Neurosurgery Published for Great Britain (GB)*[6], *for Sweden (Sw)*[4]. As comparision is shown the actual management in the West Region of Sweden 1977. (G = Goteborg)[17]. * = always, + = sometimes, 0 = not recommended or performed

Patient categories		GB	Sw	G
"deep coma"	with hematoma	*	*	+
	without hemat.	*	*	0
"in coma after lucid interv"	with hematoma	*	*	+
	without hemat.	*	*	0
"light coma"	with hematoma	*	*	+
	without hemat.	*	+	0
"drowsy, disoriented"	skull fract	*	0	0
	no sk fract	0	0	0
"alert"	skull fract	+	0	0
	no sk fract	0	0	0

Table 2. *Number of Head Injury Patients of Various Categories per 100,000 Population a Year and Risk of Development of a Surgically Significant Intracranial Hematoma.* Modified after Mendelow *et al.* 1983[8] and Stålhammar *et al.*[8]

		Number of patients	Risk of hematoma
"deep coma"		3	> 1/2
"in coma after lucid interv"		5?	> 2/3
"light coma"		5?	> 1/3
"drowsy disoriented"	skull fract	9	1/4
	no fract	43	1/100
"alert"	skull fract	10	1/30
	no fract	160	1/5,000

for 1977 there is no evidence for a better outcome at a neurosurgical clinic for those patients[17].

Resources will always differ between hospitals and regions and also over time. Therefore, in order to approach an optimal balance in the distribution of head injury patients, we must elaborate a system of continuous information regarding the quality of and the costs for the management. One important step toward a better feed-back is a classification system taking into

without any significant mass lesions however, it may well be that those treated in the ICU at a well equipped (CT-scanner, ICP-monitoring?) and adequately staffed (general surgeons with neurosurgical training) district hospital will show the same outcome as similar patients managed at a neurosurgical unit. In our investigation

Table 3. *Costs for Primary Hospital Care at Neurosurgical and General Surgical Clinic Respectively and Total Costs for Society for Patient with Head Injuries of Varying Degree of Severity.* The figures on hospital costs are calculated in our study from the western region of Sweden. The costs for society are deduced from a study by Persson 1982[11]

| Type of patient | Stay in hospital days | Number of patients per 100,000 a year | Costs for primary hospital care per patient at | | Total costs for society per patient |
			neurosurg SEK	gen surg SEK	SEK
Slight	2	175	5,000	2,000	10,000
Moderate	11	30	30,000	21,000	75,000
Severe	21	6	80,000	50,000	1,400,000
Fatal	3	14	12,000	9,000	700,000

account the type and the severity of the injuries. Such an improvement of the ICD system is presented by Lindgren in this volume.

Moreover it is mandatory that our efforts include the slightly and moderately injured patients. Slight head injuries are 20–30 times more frequent than severe head injuries. In a study of slight head injuries Fritzson et al.[2] illustrate the importance of early and adequate rehabilitation. They have shown that the total costs for the patients directly rehabilitated were half (SEK 7,500) of that for those not adequately taken care of (SEK 15,000).

In a situation with more restricted economic resources it will be even more important to consider the costs and benefits of the entire process of head injury care for optimal allocation of the resources to the various types of injuries and to different phases of the management.

Acknowledgement

This study is supported by Swedish Medical Research Council proj no B86-27X-6613-03B and the Folksam Insurance Company.

References

1. Bryden JS, Jennett B (1983) Neurosurgical resources and transfer policies for head injuries. Br Med J 286: 1791–1793
2. Fritzson L, Karlsson R, Lund L (1982) Lätta skallskador — stor utslagning. Folksam, Stockholm
3. Gentleman D, Jennett B (1981) Hazards of inter-hospital transfer of comatose head injured patients. Lancet ii: 853–855
4. Gordon E, Pontén U, et al. (1984) Behandlingsprinciper för akut skall-hjärnskadade patienter vid sjukhus utan neuokirurgisk expertis. Läkartidningen 81: 1521–1523
5. Jennett B, Carlin J (1978) Preventable mortality and morbidity after head injury. Injury 10: 31–39
6. Jennett B, et al. (1984) Guidelines for initial management after head injury in adults. Br Med J 288: 983–985
7. Mendelow AD, Karmi MZ, et al. (1979) Extradural haematoma: effect of delayed treatment. Br Med J i: 1240–1242
8. Mendelow AD, Teasdale G, Jennett B (1983) Risks of intracranial haematoma in head injured adults. Br Med J 287: 1173–1176
9. Messeter K, Nordström CH, et al. (1984) Riktlinjer för handläggning av patienter med akuta skallskador i södra sjukvårdsregionen. Läkartidningen 81: 1529–1530
10. Messeter K, Nordström CH, et al. (1984) Mortalitet och morbiditet vid svåra skallskador. Läkartidningen 81: 1523–1527
11. Persson U (1982) Vägtrafikolyckornas samhällsekonomiska kostnader. Institutet för Hälso- och sjukvårdsekonomi, Lund
12. Price JE, Murray A (1972) The influence of hypoxia and hypotension on recovery from head injury. Injury 3: 218–224
13. Rose J, Valtonen S, Jennett B (1977) Avoidable factors contributing to death after head injury. Br Med J ii: 615–618
14. Salem FA, Price DJ (1982) Monitoring of head injuries. In: Brock M (ed) Modern Neurosurgery I. Springer, Berlin Heidelberg New York
15. Seelig JM, Becker, Miller JD, et al. (1981) Traumatic acute subdural hematoma. Major mortality reduction in comatose patients treated within four hours. N Engl J Med 304: 1511–1618
16. Stålhammar D (1979) Akuta skallskador — bristfälligt omhändertagna. Läkartidnigen 76: 2234–2238
17. Stålhammar D, Holmgren E, et al.: The management of head injuries in the south and west regions of Sweden during one year. In preparation.
18. Teasdale G, Galbraith S, et al. (1982) Management of traumatic intracranial hematoma. Br Med J 285: 1695–1697

Author's address: Prof. D. Stålhammar, Department of Neurosurgery, Sahlgren's Hospital, University of Göteborg, Sweden.

Acta Neurochirurgica, Suppl. 36, 67–69 (1986)

Is Diagnostic Severity Grading for Head Injuries Possible?

D. J. Price

Department of Neurosurgery, The General Infirmary, Leeds, Great Britain

Summary

The classification of head injured patients is more difficult than that for most other disease processes. The quantum of data to be embedded into each patient's grading code depends on the purpose to which that grading is used.

If the information is merely required for broad epidemiological surveys, it may be confined to a double rubric which represents the most significant diagnostic component and an arbitrary index of associated severity. For this purpose, diagnostic severity grading is possible provided the task is delegated to experienced members of the neurosurgical team. If the grading is to be used in attempts to compare one patient group with another or for predictions of complications or outcome, a more detailed data-set is required. This may be accomplished with the use of multiple ICD diagnostic codes but assignations of severity to each diagnostic component requires very subjective judgement. Such an approach is unlikely to be successful and the only alternative is to define a data-set of "pure" information which includes all the relevant clinical, radiological, and operative findings without resorting to artificial data compression by using potentially misinterpretable deduced codes.

Keywords: Head injury; diagnostic codes; severity scores; database.

Introduction

Diagnostic severity grading infers that for each patient, diagnostic components can be qualified by severity scores. Unlike many other disease processes in medicine, the effect of a head injury is virtually unique for every individual patient and this may well explain why most earlier attempts at simple classification have failed. This problem has also beset many workers who have tried to compare groups of patients with differing treatment regimes. To allocate patients into two therapeutic groups by simple pairing with the aim of comparing "like with like", only 3 or 4 features can usually be used as otherwise the numbers of patients in each group becomes too small to achieve statistical significance. More complex statistical techniques which overcome this problem seem less acceptable as neurosurgeons are always suspicious of conclusions which cannot be confirmed from published raw data with a simple calculator!

The Need for Diagnostic Severity Grading

The ranking of head injuries by severity is necessary for practical management, for prognosis, for estimation of subsequent risks of epilepsy, for assessing the relative value of alternative methods of management and for assessing personal damages for legal compensation. In the past, we have relied on one or two arbitrary parameters for measuring the overall severity of brain insult such as the durations of coma and of post traumatic amnesia but they only allude to parts of the usually complex clinical picture.

From the moment of impact, a dynamic pathological process begins and this may lead to immediate or delayed brain damage. The eventual disability will depend on both the total global organic brain insult and the brain's capacity to compensate to that partial disruption of function. The complex sequence of events may be captured as a series of "snapshots" but unless the minimal information required to describe the clinical, radiological and operative findings is carefully recorded at the time it happens, the cases notes are incomplete and subsequent retrospective retrieval is limited. What information there is, is often disseminated amongst the verbiage of the medical notes and the "number jumble" of the nurses' records[5].

Diagnostic severity coding implies a method of recording total global cranio-cerebral insult sustained at or after impact with the hope of making ranking possible. The reason for such coding is threefold:

1. To monitor the effects of preventative measures and allow resource allocation.

2. To evaluate the effectiveness of interventional therapy in a search for better alternative methods of treatment.

3. To allow more accurate prediction of both complications and eventual outcome.

Diagnostic Severity Coding

Diagnostic Components

It would be naive to even contemplate the concept of assigning each head injury with a single diagnostic code. The components of the impact injury to scalp, cranium and brain alone often require several codes and any complications require others.

As an alternative, combinations of ICD codes may be considered but guidelines for the selection of these codes for each patient would need to be very strict to ensure compatibility between one physician's choice and anothers. To given an example, 12 codes are required to describe a patient with multiple skull fractures, cranial nerve injuries and complications.

Bony Injuries
800.1	Open fracture of vault
801.1	Fractured base with CSF leak
804	Facial fractures

Cranial Nerve Injuries
950.0	Optic nerve injury
951.4	Facial weakness
951.5	Auditory nerve damage
781.1	Anosmia

Complications
345.1	Generalized seizure
852	Extradural hematoma
851	Intracerebral contusion
320.2	Streptococcal meningitis
324.0	Cerebral abscess

Even with this extended use of ICD coding, there are no indications of the relative severity of each component and this rather complex example illustrates the need for additional severity indices to generate a more comprehensive summary of individual patients. The use of multiple diagnostic codes alone does not solve the problem and British neurosurgeons use ICD coding and the only recorded indication of severity (the length of stay in hospital) for the crudest of regional head injury statistics and epidemiological studies[2].

Severity Components

The dataset for measurement of severity must include all the initial features, the severity of subsequent complications, the rate at which these complications arise, the duration of impairment of consciousness, and amnesia and the eventual sequelae in terms of both mental and physical disabilities. For international comparative studies, any improvements in coding would have to be agreed by each country and any one patient may require as many as 20 diagnostic and severity coded features to allow inclusion of the minimum of the relevant information necessary for serious studies. In recent years, some of us have diverted our attention away from prediction of eventual outcome towards predicting the complications as in this way, we are more likely to actively influence the outcome by early anticipation and reversal of threatening secondary events. Whatever our aim in either prediction or comparison of management regimes, a detailed dataset which includes all the relevant diagnostic and severity information is essential.

As it took some 30 years to develop the current ICD system, it is unlikely that a sufficiently comprehensive system will become internationally accepted by the end of this century. Many of the failings of the current ICD code are related to the way it is applied (often by untrained "coding clerks"). This information does however supply crude epidemiological data for intranational and international comparison and allows the observation of broad trend with time. It has been shown that the response to accident preventative measures such as drink and drive legislation and seat belt regulation is of significance and there is almost sufficient detail to allow for resource allocation planning[2].

Limitations of Even Extended Applications of Diagnostic and Severity Coding

Although improved coding would provide better opportunities for more accurate and useful epidemiological studies, I consider that for other data applications, a much higher number of items of information is required.

If any serious study of the effectiveness of various interventional therapies of severe head injuries or of management criteria for the apparently minor head injury is needed, a far more detailed dataset is necessary.

Alternative Data Collection Systems

Neurosurgeons in Glasgow and Rotterdam were pioneers in developing such a comprehensive dataset for severe head injuries enabling them to collect arrays of separate items of information about each patient. This provided valuable statistical data and a means of predicting outcome[3].

The data were necessarily obtained by the extraction of information by a research team from records of patients during their stay in hospital. For routine clinical use however, this duplication of effort is an unacceptable chore for the junior staff and most of us have found it difficult to achieve within a normal clinical programme. As it may take up to an hour to write the initial case record of each head injured patient on admission, we are attempting to replace that record with a structured proforma which ensures that with 80 coded features, all the diagnostic and severity information can be collected during the time of the patient's admission. Completed proformas can be difficult to read but if the data is then transferred to a computer in the ward, automatic text generation of typed case records, case summaries, correspondence and ICD coding is possible.

This relieves some of the more tedious aspects of our work and it has the additional advantage of providing data for both clinical and financial audit for prediction of complications and outcome and as a tool for future comparative studies of therapeutic regimes without duplication of effort.

Figure 1 shows a flow chart which attempts to summarize the main components of the overall dynamic process following head injury which must be included within the diagnostic severity dataset. Time plays a vital part in determining the degree of brain damage and must be included. The longer hypoxia

continues, the less of a chance of a good recovery[4]. The more rapidly an intracerebral hematoma expands and the longer the delay in evacuating it, the worse is the outcome[1, 6].

The planning of our own project has involved the careful selection of information and in particular the choice of pupil and coma scales. Calculations of the time intervals, pupil trends, coma scale trends and the referral to physiological tables for normal ranges are tasks well suited to a computer. When the problems of adequate data collection are overcome, it is tempting to contrive scoring systems to "measure" the global severity of injuries to the cranium and brain. Mathematical addition of non-parametric data is however renowned for generating misleading results. We consider it preferable to concentrate our efforts towards developing a mutually accepted dataset containing each contributory component of information rather than to attempt to merge them into an artificial composite code or score.

Conclusion

I consider that artificially contrived diagnostic severity grading is desirable and may be useful provided the limited information it contains is used only for epidemiological surveys. The inclusion of severity grading is in theory useful but in practice may prove difficult to define in numeric terms.

A more comprehensive dataset is required for any attempts to compare the influence on outcome of one management policy with another or to predict complications or outcome.

References

1. Bricolo A, Pascut LM (1984) Extradural haematoma: toward zero mortality. Neurosurgery 14: 8–12
2. Field JH (1976) Epidemiology of head injuries in England and Wales. Her Majesty's Stationery Office, London
3. Jennett B, Teasdale G, Braakman et al. (1976) Predicting outcome in individual patients after severe head injury. Lancet 1: 1031–1034
4. Kohi YM, Mendelow AD, Teasdale GM et al. (1984) Extracranial insults and outcome in patients with acute head injury—relationship to the Glasgow Coma Scale. Injury 16: 25–29
5. Price DJ, Mason J (1986) Attempts to resolve the numerical chaos at the bedside. In: Bryant J (ed) Current perspectives in health computing. Br J Healthcare Computing pp 147–157
6. Seelig JM, Becker, DP, Miller JD et al. (1981) Traumatic acute subdural haematoma. N Engl J Med 304: 1511–1518

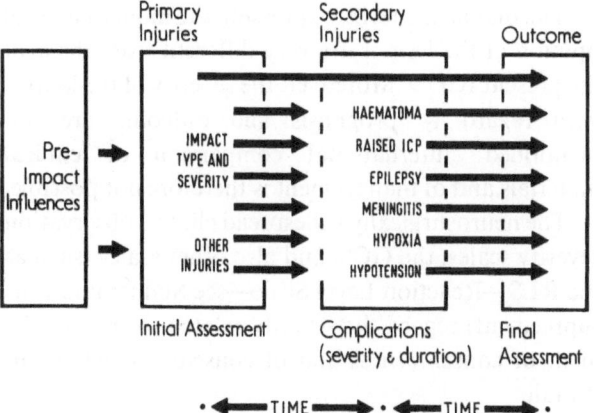

Fig. 1. A flow chart to summarize the main components of the dynamic process which follows head injuries. Most of them contribute to the global brain insult and subsequent outcome

Author's address: D. J. Price, F.R.C.S., Department of Neurosurgery, The General Infirmary, Leeds, Great Britain.

Acta Neurochirurgica, Suppl. 36, 70–80 (1986)

Diagnostic Terminology of Head Injuries—Related to Severity

S. Lindgren

Department of Neurosurgery, Sahlgren's Hospital, University of Göteborg, Sweden

Summary

The 10th revision of ICD (International Classification of Diseases and Injuries, WHO) is now being prepared. Before its codifying starts the contents must be revised to fulfil the requirements of modern clinical medicine. A modified diagnostic severity graded classification on the part of head injuries Chapter XVII is suggested here.

More attention is now being paid to the intracranial injuries. An attempt to classify the severity of conscious disturbances is also made. The severity grading of AIS-76, -80, and -85 is discussed and partly used.

In view of the worldwide medical importance of ICD for facilitating clinical comparisons and improved management it is urgent to extend the basis of knowledge in an accurate diagnostic terminology. This will facilitate and shorten the time necessary for the daily differential diagnostic and prognostic work.

Keywords: Terminology head injuries; diagnostic severity—head injuries; ICD—AIS.

Introduction

The importance of recognition of the severity of impairment of consciousness or of other neurological functions resulting after head injuries as well as of its cause (nature) has been observed and noted during the management of these patients for a very long time. Several reasons for this have been mentioned by David Price in this supplement.

However, in the stage of final clinical evaluation of the individual case (at discharge) within a diagnostic frame this importance has very often been forgotten; only the patho-anatomical name of a later occurring posttraumatic complication (such as an "intracranial hematoma") has been mentioned.

If such a complication has not occurred, there have been different terms for the traumatic unconsciousness of brief or of long duration. The diagnostic term of unconsciousness elsewhere in the medical disciplines "coma" has been rarely used as a posttraumatic diagnosis.—It seems as the general terminology and not only the specific clinical contents for classification must be discussed.

Some time ago (1960)[18] a plea was made for recording all the head injury lesions within the diagnostic frame to be able to compare clinical materials and results of treatment.

This policy was also recently supported (1982)[11]:

"The type of lesion is thus as important a factor in determining outcome as is" the level of the patients conscious impairment; this is notified in coma scales (including the GCS Glasgow Coma Scales-score) "and both types of recording must be considered when describing severely head-injured patients".

The present official diagnostic terminology of WHO (International Classification of Diseases and Injuries—ICD, 9th revision, 1977, HMSO) is clinically unsatisfactory within large fields of neurosurgery (such as tumors) and particularly in neurotraumatology, Chapter XVII; also ICD 9 CM will be discussed.

The diagnostic terms expressing the modern clinical opinion of the lesions are very different from those of the present ICD 9. Moreover, the severity of the lesions with regard to prognosis and outcome are not mentioned: international comparison of clinical materials and of management is therefore not possible.

The neurosurgically widespread clinical observation severity scales, the GCS, and also other scales (such as the RLS—Reaction Level Scale—see Stålhammar this supplement) regard the severity related to the impairment of consciousness and of conscious reactions to stimuli.

However, there is a general severity scale related to the various types of head injuries and based on their "threat to life"—the Abbreviated Injury Scale (AIS) of the American Medical Association and the American Association for Automotive Medicine (AAAM) (see P.

Hansson, this supplement). Its general principles are flexible and adaptable also to the above mentioned coma scales. The AIS is more well known in other surgical specialities than in neurosurgery.

In the Sixth International Conference of the International Association for Accident and Traffic Medicine in Melbourne 1977, (§ 5), the AIS was recommended for worldwide use[19].

The aim of this paper is to discuss the diagnostic terminology, review deficiencies and suggest an improvement of the ICD 9 for "Head Injuries" (ICD 9: N 800-804, 850–854), as well as some additional code numbers of interest. In this connection there is a hope that the four first digits in ICD 10 (in preparation) will be international and the fifth digit can be used for specification for special purposes in each region or country.

An additional, combined use of the AIS for severity grading of the diagnosed conditions is also suggested.—The E-code (external causes) will not be discussed.

General Clinical Considerations in the Acute Stage

The importance in detecting and observing the possibility of injury to the intracranial tissues makes it perhaps desirable to point out in the acute stage the occurrence of a "*head trauma*" ("trauma capitis"). Later there may be more obvious signs indicating a previous head trauma.—Due to the serious and often different consequences of the indirect impulsive traumas to the head (see Fig. 1, Introduction this Suppl.), perhaps also the terms "direct" and "indirect" may be added to the diagnostic term.—This, "head trauma", may by itself be severity graded and of value for the clinical analysis if the course of the accident is not clear: "head trauma + epilepsy" will mean that an epileptic fit has occurred as a result of head trauma, while "epilepsy + head trauma" will call for a diagnosis of the original cause of epilepsy.—Patients with very slight head traumas with no acute effect have attended hospital but been sent home without any note. Subsequent complications, such as subacute or chronic subdural hematoma, have occasionally been the first note that there has been a head trauma.

In some cases with symptom of vertigo, impaired hearing etc it may be difficult to decide if the cause is due to intracranial or to skullbase injury: diagnoses will then be: "Head trauma + Vertigo" etc or "Posttraumatic vertigo" if it is clear that the eliciting cause was a trauma. A similar diagnostic policy will also be of help in cases of dizziness and in some disturbances of attention, particularly in old people.

Other arguments with respect to appropriate codifying are that posttraumatic symptoms such as "drowsiness, somnolence, coma, amnesia" etc (780 ICD 9) are referred to another chapter, XVI, "General symptoms—Illdefined conditions", where also another frequent posttraumatic condition, "anosmia", is coded. Moreover, "posttraumatic confusion" will be found in chapter V, mental disorders (293.0 acute confusional state—posttraumatic organic psychosis). This makes the possibility of an addition of the diagnosis and code of "Head trauma" even more important.

The detecting and recording of injury to the intracranial tissues should perhaps also be facilitated by referring contusions (910, 920 ICD 9) or wounds of the skin of the head (873) closer to the cranial and intracranial injuries in a "*body regional division concept*", but only for the injury chapter (XVII).—Note in each case which region of the head is impacted is important also for the acute injury scaling (see this supplement—EIS).

Administrative Use

Chapter XVII uses a three-digit code for describing injury and poisoning (800–999); this code is an integration of type of injury with site of injury.—Langley[17] reports on suggestions to replace the system with a modular system with a unique code for types of injuries and a unique code for each body site. At present there is lack of a similar pattern and differentiation. In some cases the fourth digit allows for a specific site description, while in other examples the provision of a fourth digit is not satisfactory.—In Scandinavian countries the Committee of "Nomesco" has allowed a fifth digit to be used in each country to provide an accurate and more specific description.

Clinical Deficiencies in ICD 9 (1977, HMSO), and ICD 9 (1979, CM).—Suggested Improvements

These classifications are here called "ICD 9" resp. "ICD 9 CM" and if both are involved only "ICD".

General Objection

The discussion by Langley[17] of the ICD construction, mentioned above, is of interest also for the structure of clinical contents. The importance of detecting and recording of an intracranial injury recognizing the external signs of *site of* impact, *skin contusions* and wounds was stressed.—Regarding the arrangement of such a combined *head injury concept* the superficial skin injuries (910 ICD 9), the contusions with intact skin (920 ICD 9) and with open wounds (873 ICD 9) could be combined and differentiation recorded with fourth digits. These skin injuries could also be referred to the same part of the Chapter XVII as the fractures of the head and the intracranial injuries.—The term "crushing injury" (925 ICD 9) perhaps refers both to external causes and mechanics as well as to contusions. The injury part of that term could perhaps be called "contusions".

However, the location recorded for these injuries to the skin in ICD 9 should also be described and specified for an impact site of the anterior (frontal and facial) part of the head as well as of the occipital, temporal, and vertex regions. Each of these impact regions (see "Injury scaling" this supplement) has its corresponding cranial and intracranial injuries and the anterior and vertex impacts may also be combined with cervical spine fractures.—These facts make such a differentiation of location important (head regions).

Not only the skin injuries but also the skull fractures may indicate the accurate diagnostic specification and probable complications provided that the intracranial injuries also are differentiated!

In the introduction to ICD 9, Chapter XVII, it is noted:—"The principle of multiple coding of injuries should be followed wherever possible".—However, in practice this is not always followed.

Specific Objections

Fractures (ICD—N 800—N 804) and intracranial injury *excluding* those with skull-fracture: ICD N 850–N 854.

1. Additions to Coded Skull Fractures

a) It is not at all satisfactory that an addition (to a codified fracture) such as a "fourth-digit subdivision" "1" or "3" should cover the vast area of "with intracranial injury" (see ICD 9 800–801, 803–804).—This has been improved in ICD 9 CM, with addition of seven specified and two unspecified intracranial injuries as a fourth digit (800.0–800.9, 801.0–801.9, 803.0–803.9, and 804.0–804.7). (Compare below: 6 d.)

Both modes of procedures seem unnecessary as the *intracranial injuries* mentioned have their *own code numbers*. (Example: Fracture of vault with focal cerebral contusion: 800 + 851—the last number can be more specified in ICD 9 CM).

b) Moreover, a fourth digit (ICD 9) and fourth and fifth digits (ICD 9 CM) cannot be used for intracranial injuries with category 802. Such additions are there only for extracranial facial skeletal injuries.

The intracranial injury (such as a brief coma or concussion) at a knock-out from an impact to a boxer's closed or open mandible (802.2–802.3—ICD) seems anyhow possible to cover with addition of its own code number (850). Thus both types of injury must be mentioned, in this case with the impact site injury before the more distant effect.

c) In the same way the code for "leak of CSF" in a rhinorrhoea or otorrhoea should be combined with a code for "fracture of the base of the skull" 801 ICD 9 801.9 ICD 9 CM. It is probable that there must be a fracture of the skull and probably a tear of the meninges, but so far the "CSF leak" has no diagnostic code in ICD.—Air found at X-ray of the skull in subarachnoidal or ventricular spaces may also be coded here and also indicate danger of later infection ("open"). Intracerebral "pneumocephalus" is a similar lesion, but also characterized by its focal expansive nature (see 851) (see below 6c).—Posttraumatic carotid-cavernous fistulas may also be considered.

d) A depressed skull fracture, with intact skin surface or an open wound, and with tear of the dura and a focal brain contusion could be coded in the same way provided the focal brain contusions are coded. This type of injury is very common and must be easily identified when computerized.

2. Intracranial Injuries—General Late Effects

A rare type of inaccuracy is seen in code 853 ICD 9 and 853.0 ICD 9 CM where "cerebral compression due to injury" is mentioned. The term "cerebral compression" as a diagnosis is not used in modern neurotraumatology as it does not specify the cause or pathogenesis of the condition.

3. Initial and Late Intracranial Injuries

often called primary and secondary injuries, should be diagnosed and coded. The common course at head injury with initial severe conscious impairment and later complications (see below) requires a more differentiated diagnostic code. This may be a measure to analyse and decrease avoidable morbidity and mortality.

4. Intracranial Hematomas

Subarachnoid, subdural and extradural hemorrhage following a head injury have the same code number 852 in ICD 9 in spite of their quite different pathogenesis, prognosis and management. It is urgent also for general surgeons to have these conditions separated in a diagnostic code.

However, in ICD 9 CM the different conditions have been separated with the use of a fourth digit (852.0–852.5). On the other hand only one code, 852.2, is for subdural hemorrhages but clinical differentiation is still common in acute, subacute and chronic subdural hematomas when operated as they have different prognosis, pathogenesis, additional injuries and management.

Thus, it is most important that different hemorrhages in 852 ICD 9 are separated, if possible with a three-digit code.

5. *Focal Brain Injuries*

These are commonly called "focal" as a diagnostic term, nowadays, to differentiate such injuries and their sometimes serious consequences with brain tissue displacement from so-called "diffuse" brain injuries. This differentiation has become even more important with a more frequent use of CT scanning.—The clinical symptoms may appear within a few hours after a mild trauma as visual defects (Gjerris, see this supplement), paresis of one arm etc; when these symptoms are transient they have also been called "focal cerebral commotions"[18]. Also focal epileptic fits may occur in the early stage with a usually good prognosis.

If the clinical symptoms occur later, within some days, they may be revealed as focal lesions of expansive nature and should be diagnosed and treated accordingly.

6. *"Cerebral Laceration and Contusion"*

code 851 in ICD 9 and the more specified—with regard to location—code 851 in ICD 9 CM.

a) The codes do not differentiate the nature (focal *nonexpansive* or *expansive*) of the types of focal brain lesion; the later occurring "expansive lesion" and its recognition may make surgical treatment necessary. Use of fourth digit in ICD 9 CM for locations such as 851.4–851.7 seem sometimes less necessary to differentiate clinically.

Regarding the terms cerebral "laceration" and "contusion" the pathogenesis and pathoanatomical picture may be similar and both may later result in CT diagnosed intracerebral hematomas. It seems as one term: "focal cerebral contusion" may be satisfactory; presence of meningeal laceration may appear from the descriptive terms "open wound" or "fracture" "with focal brain contusion".

b) On the other hand there may be use for codes for "multiple focal injuries" and "cerebral edema".—When injury to blood vessels of head and neck (900 ICD 9) is coded, the effect of this injury with brain ischemia, often focal edema, may also be pointed out.

c) Intracerebral pneumocephalus is also a focal intracerebral lesion, often expansive.

d) "Intracranial injury" with "fourth-digit subdivisions for use with 850–854:—with open intracranial wound" (ICD 9):

If this should occur, there are certainly several other diagnostic and coded findings to be mentioned in such a case and the focal brain lesions can be diagnosed with code 851 in ICD 9.

Diagnostic Severity Scaling

General Features

Before discussion of the terminology and grading of the conscious disturbances after head injury, it must be stated that also the above mentioned injuries can clinically be severity graded in each case.

However, *ICD 9* has only occasionally applied severity grading: regarding burns code 941–946 and 949 the severity degree of burns is graded 0–4 and regarding the extent 0–9 in 948 with fourth digit subdivisions. (See also Langley[17].)

The *Abbreviated Injury Scale—AIS—*applies a worldwide known severity scaling to all types of injuries and is graded according to the principle "threat to life". It has six different levels (see Hansson, this supplement) and is therefore not only concerned with survival or death in the acute stage.

Can this scale be used as additional severity numbers after the ICD code number?

(Example: Skull-fracture + Extradural hematoma—*Fractura cranii (800.00-2) + Hematoma extradurale (852.00-4)*.

The *AIS code (second number within brackets)* varies somewhat with the severity judged by the observer.—If initial disturbance of consciousness it should be recorded first, before "Fractura cranii".

Garthe[10] found 1982 that out of 2,099 ICD 9 CM—injury descriptions 1,487 were not compatible with the AIS 80 descriptions, most of them because of denominations such as "unspecified injuries" and ICD rubrics combined injuries of different severity.

Moreover, AIS is specified to body regions—except

for "external" (skin) while this is not always the case in ICD Chapter XVII. AIS-76 was based on morphological findings and even if AIS-80 covers more functional neurological deficits, morphological aspects are still better described.—It seems as AIS "anatomic lesion" corresponds to the structural part of prolonged "focal brain injury".—In AIS-85 the addition of 1.1 for *"neurological deficit"* to impairment (level or length) of consciousness is open to the same criticism as "the additions to coded skull fractures" in ICD 9.—A minor question is the same code number for skull base fracture both "with or without CSF leak".

Intracranial hematomas are partly graded with regard to size (more or less than 100 cc) but the patients secondarily impaired condition must also be considered. Such severity grading of serious intracranial "complications" has been performed by Stålhammar *et al.* 1981[25] (*cf.* Löfgren, this supplement).

With regard to scaling of *multiple injuries* and the ISS (Injury Severity Score) in the recently published AIS-85 there is a note that the use of PODS (Probability of Death Score) (see "Injury scaling", this supplement) will be an improvement; moreover it is also related to the same body regions as AIS.

If some of the above mentioned deficits in ICD are removed and AIS is better modified to clinical situations along the adaptable principles of "threat to life" expressed in AIS-76, the situation will certainly be improved.

An improvement of such a clinical situation is a clinical consideration of the classification of the important conscious disturbances after head injury.

Conscious Disturbances

A. *Noncomatous* Posttraumatic *Disturbances*

of attention, of memory—such as traumatic amnesia, whether retrograde (RA) or anterograde (PTA)—and confusion (incoherence of thoughts[12]) belong to this group. However, alterations of attention and memory as well as of cognitive efficiency, behaviour, emotional and autonomic symptoms may appear as transitional states or be so subtle that they will not be revealed in the ordinary examination[24]. Amnesia has been specially studied in this respect (memory islands); regarding PTA also its duration as a severity measure was studied as well as its relation to duration of posttraumatic unconsciousness and rehabilitation outcome[5, 9, 15, 26].

Courville[8] with his seven degrees of "concussion" did not discuss confusion and amnesia.—Ommaya[21] is one of the few neurosurgeons who has attempted a

"concussive brain injury grading correlation" with AIS levels. Of the six levels the two first deal with "confusion without amnesia" and "amnesia without coma": the amnesia was graded in slow onset and rapid onset.

Present state: In ICD 9 Chapter V acute confusional state of posttraumatic origin, code 293.0 is differentiated from excitative (298.1) and reactive (298.2) states.—Retrograde amnesia may be found in Chapter XVI code 780.9 of "Ill-defined conditions".

Amnesia may occur after trauma not directed to the head but it would be of value to code *posttraumatic confusion* and *traumatic amnesia* among the "intracranial injuries" in Chapter XVII; otherwise the term and code for "Head trauma" can be added. However, 850.0 ICD 9 CM means mental confusion or disorientation.—In AIS-85 amnesia has only one code: 206-04.2; dizziness and headache are two alternatives at admission under one code (206-01.1) but not "confusion".

B.1. *Impairment of Consciousness*

This has been extensively discussed in the present supplement together with clinical reaction level scales. Their symptomatological instantaneously used terminology is, however, less suitable for diagnostic synthesis as the head injuries may result in various clinical pictures due to which neuronal subsystem is injured (see Lindström, this supplement).

The terminology, partly based on animal experiments, is often less precise, defined and differentiated with respect to other related conditions in the posttraumatic course in humans.

Moreover, there may be a *lack of terminology* describing both the remaining *and* the involved mental functions; this may be particularly evident in the relationship between the constructs of the widely used "states" of "remaining functions":

a) *"wakefulness"* (see Norrsell, this supplement "up to" alertness).

b) *"Mental accessibility"* may be evident from any reaction, also autonomic or emotional, on strong request.—Plum & Brennan[22] further discussed such accessibility in syndromes such as "locked in" syndrome—see also Cabezudo[6]—and "akinetic mutism".

c) *"Specific mental responsiveness"*: more complicated responses with involvement of mental, complex, integrated functions may be elicited at action such as "obey command". This type of activity may perhaps be called: "more specific mental responsiveness"—as it is not a simple verbal or a simple motor reaction.

d) *"Awareness"*, a well known term, is usually related to environment or to one-self but this "state" may be assumed by an observer to be present from some responses usually occurring on uniform stimulations (auditive request with the subjects name, gives verbal response, pain gives warding off movement).

e)*"Alertness"* is a common term for "normal" mental, associative general responsiveness and attentional behaviour.

Plum & Brennan[22] further discuss the differential diagnoses of altered states of consciousness and try to differ between deranged and depressed consciousness.

Courville's[8] second degree of "concussion" describes the patients as dazed or stunned (while his first degree comprises "paralytic cortical phenomena").— Ommaya[21] does not consider these symptoms and their denominations in his six level scale.

The influence of "damage or depression of the brain at nearly every level"[22] on respiration and also on "sleep-like cycles" is sometimes considered; Price in his admission chart also estimates respiration.

However, it is still not possible to refer the components of the first mentioned "reaction level scales" or of the above mentioned different expressions of accessibility and of other remaining reactions observed as part of different functional neuronal subsystems.

Therefore general terms describing general defects in behaviour are used.

Under "General symptoms" in ICD 9, Chapter XVI, drowsiness, somnolence and semicoma are denominated before "unconsciousness" and under the heading "Coma and Stupor" (780.0).

In the introduction of "Glossary of Neurotraumatology"[12] it was mentioned that terms such as "clouding of the conscious state after trauma" were "left for consideration in the future". Obnubilation and obtundation are other terms. In "Stupor" the subject can still be aroused by vigourous external stimulation[22].—*"Posttraumatic lethargy"*, *of varying degrees*, seems therefore to be a term which can cover most of these states; it is also used in AIS-terminology (AIS-85 206-08.2). Degrees and length of lethargy can be coded as described later for symptomatic and/or duration severity for unconsciousness.

It is also important that more *diagnostic attention* is paid to the state of *intoxication* as this influences the traumatic picture of impaired consciousness.

B.2. *AIS and Impairment of Consciousness*

AIS-76, AIS-80, and the recently published AIS-85 show some variations of AIS severity code, see Fig. 1.—

Code number	-76	-80	-85
0	no injury		
1	minor	minor	minor
2	moderate	moderate	moderate
3	severe (not life-threatening)	serious	serious
4	serious (life-threatening, survival probable)	severe	severe
5	critical (survival uncertain)	critical	critical
6	maximum (currently untreatable)	maximum injury virtually unsurvivable in AIS-80	maximum injury virtually unsurvivable in AIS-85
9	unknown	unknown	unknown

Further necessary information is available in the separate revisions.

Fig. 1. AIS. Severity code

That severity code is in AIS-85 referred to a sixth digit, to the right of a decimal point. Thus, the first three digits refer to body region, organ or specific area while the next two refer to severity level "within each organ or body part entry".

To me the AIS-76 terms related to "life threatening" seem to be of practical value in estimating the AIS-severity code, related to any clinical diagnostic system.

In AIS-85 "Head" (skull, brain) the first three digits comprises 201–207 while the face has 301–328.

Unconsciousness is involved in the code numbers 206-06.2—206-37.2; the first part (206-01.1—206-07.3) is called "level of consciousness" while the later part (206-30.2—206-37.2) is called "length of unconsciousness".—Addition of 1.1. if "neurological deficit" is present.

However, the length of unconsciousness is described in both parts.—The *level of consciousness* is not appropriately described except in patients unconscious more than 24 hours in two groups: "appropriate movements, but only upon painful stimuli" (206-27.4) and "inappropriate movements" decerebrate, decorticate, flaccid, no response to pain" (206-29.5);—Stereotype flexion movements are among serious signs not mentioned.

Length of Unconsciousness: Borderlines
(Severity code before/after time limit given—*within brackets*.)

AIS-76: *15 minutes* (2-3—ICD No), *less than 12 hours* (4—ICD No) (other neurol. signs added—n.s.)(5-); *more than 12 hours* (severe n.s.) and *more than 24 hours*—other n.s.: all(5-).

AIS-80: *15 minutes*(2-3-), *1 hour*(3-4-), *more than 24 hours*(5-). Addition of 1 if neurologic deficit.

AIS-85: (First three digits 206):—when conscious level initially or at admission unknown—*less than 1 hour* (-30.2); *1-6 hours* (-32.3); *6-24 hours* (-34.4); *more than 24 hours* (-36.5)—with neurol. deficit add 1.1.

Similar lengths of unconsciousness are differently coded but similarly graded if the patient was awake, lethargic, or unconscious at admission.

A modified AIS severity grading, more similar to the neurosurgical reaction level scales or coma scales has also been presented elsewhere[19]. It might be seriously considered as an adaptable help for comparison of different scales.

C. *Unconsciousness—Diagnosis of Severity—Duration*

Type of Terminology

Immediately occurring unconsciousness after trauma to the head shows a similar symptomatology irrespective of its further duration. It may therefore be appropriate to use the same basic term "Coma". It seems, however, less adequate to use the common two-degree classification: brain concussion or commotio cerebri for short durations of the coma and for the more prolonged posttraumatic coma, varying types of terms: clinical, pathological, or patho-mechanical types.

Also the term "concussion" has been interpreted differently, such as defining the trauma of the head or transient impairment of neurological functions other than consciousness. (See Courville, above.)

Such misunderstandings can be avoided by use of the term *"Posttraumatic coma"*. It must be possible to recognize the diagnoses clinically.

Its *symptomatic severity* can be scaled with the AIS, the modified AIS[19], GCS or RLS scales discussed in the supplement and instantaneously coded (time after trauma noted) and added to the diagnosis. Its *duration* can also be included in the diagnostic term and coded, thereby giving an indication of the *severity* also of the *nature* of the disturbance.—The "duration"—term is more easily understood verbally, but is here also coded by Roman numerals (see below).—*Combinations* of serious or light symptomatic severity and brief or long durations can thus be coded (II–VI: 2–6). A similar combination of codes may be possible with the fifth (duration-nature) and sixth (AIS-severity) digit in AIS-85.

With regard to severity coding in ICD 9 CM for brief posttraumatic coma, 850 ("concussion") the fourth digit in 850.0 describes mental confusion or disorientation without loss of consciousness, which, however, occurs in 850.1 for less than one hour.

For the purpose of simplifying and transferring scaling numbers such as in AIS and the coma scales of various kinds we have suggested a similar symptomatic and diagnostic severity grading, which also can be verbally presented.

I: The "severity grade 1" is assigned to confusion, amnesia and lethargic conditions, which are specified in their diagnostic terms. In Fig. 6 "Introduction" we have included those noncomatous symptoms under I.

Differentiated Diagnostic Duration of Unconsciousness

Provided that unconsciousness as defined in this supplement as "Coma" is present, the following time differentiation may be practical (see Fig. 6, Introduction).

II. Brief posttraumatic coma ("coma breve posttraumaticum" ICD). Severity grade -2 with unconsciousness *less than 30 minutes*. There are several reasons for this "borderline" (see pp 22–23[18], *cf.*[11a]). It often corresponds to the time for transportation from the place of accident until reliable information can be obtained. Moreover, secondary clinical impairment, for instance elicited from an intracranial hemorrhage, and discernible from the primary brain injury, is usually not evident earlier.—"Coma breve posttr. 850,00-2".

III. Intermediate posttraumatic coma (coma intermedium posttraumaticum) (ICD) (-3) may be assigned to a duration of coma of *30 minutes to 6 hours*. The last mentioned borderline, 6 hours, is a practical limit to be able to include all clinical materials scaled according to the widespread Glasgow Coma Scale (GCS) where a time limit of estimation is fixed at 6 hours. In this way comparison between this diagnostic severity "scale" and the GCS-"severity scored"-material will be facilitated.—Moreover, the direction of acute management of head injuries is often dependent upon the result of acute examinations during these first 6 hours after trauma usually contributing to diagnosis and prediction of prognosis.

IV. Long posttraumatic coma (coma longum posttraumaticum) (ICD no-4) *6 hours–24 hours*. The last-mentioned time is often used to delineate clinical materials in the acute stage.

V. Prolonged posttraumatic coma (coma prolongatum posttraumaticum) (ICD no-5). *24 hours to 2 weeks*.—After the last mentioned limit of duration usually the posttraumatic condition is more stable and "new acute" extra- and intracerebral hemorrhagic complications do not occur.

VI. a) Protracted or persistent posttraumatic coma (ICD no 5-6). b) Persistent posttraumatic vegetating states (status posttraumat. veget.) (ICD no 5-6) *more than 2 weeks,* ("locked-in" syndrome, akinetic mutism etc may be referred to this group of rare conditions, specified by name).

The posttraumatic course may particularly in children be somewhat different with prolonged lethargic or comatous conditions with a better ultimate prognosis.—However, many of the adult head injuries of this type may often die from extracranial causes.

Other Posttraumatic Consequences

Among the most severe acute head injuries are those where the brain is the site of *multiple contusions* or "malignant edema", even with the so-called lucid interval[18] with a very high mortality. Posttraumatic *thrombosis* of one or more of the dural *sinuses;* fat *embolism* to the brain and "DIC" may require special coding.

Conditions of less acute serious character but important cause of disability: *posttraumatic hydrocephalus* (hydrocephalus posttraumatica ICD) is usually believed to be a result of posttraumatic subarachnoid hemorrhage—and is nowadays readily diagnosed after a few months with CT scanning and CSF-absorption studies.

Posttraumatic syndrome, syndrome after "Head trauma", is a well known neuropsychological-neuropsychiatric syndrome which deserves an own ICD number. Lishman[20] (p 241) concludes that "while often initially founded in physiogenic disturbance, readily thereafter becomes prolonged, nonetheless disabling, by virtue of purely psychogenic factors".

Discussion

It is quite obvious that the developing ICD has a long tradition and can still be improved with better precision for helping the daily clinical routine and the coders. The change between the above mentioned ICD 9 HMSO and the later ICD 9 CM shows a development in the right direction. In a personal communication T. Kruse and P. A. Frandsen in Odense, Denmark, mention that a new 3- and 4-digit version of Chapter XVII for ICD 10 is re-codified and should "lend itself to linkage with injury severity scoring instrument".

Removal of the "clinical" deficiencies shown here

and the improvements suggested may further improve the use of ICD.—This seems also of value as the economic consequences of diseases and injuries as in the DRG-system ("Diagnose-related-groups")[4, 23] must be considered in the future.—Individual variations within the range of costs is considerable in each "DRG"-group; there may be better sensitivity with improved contents of a severity-related ICD.

During the first 2–4 weeks after trauma there is a continuous flow of instantaneously revealed, diagnosed and often classified information. The time appropriate for observations of diagnosis and severity of injury as well as for prediction and treatment of complications (worsening the patient's condition) is of continuous importance. However, the observations are of value also in prospective studies and for indication of prognosis and residual disability; for these purposes as well as for retrospective evaluation of the whole acute period there are often other aspects on the observation time for representative information.—It was in this context the recommendation of a repeated AIS-EIS-scaling at discharge or after 2–4 weeks after trauma was discussed above in this supplement.

The AIS-85 has now moved in the direction of more complicated coding with more precision of body regions etc, but still inefficiently describes injury differentiation to be a diagnostic coding; as an example it is more difficult there to substitute for the addition of 1.1 for "neurological deficit" with a defined diagnostic term than in the ICD.—The merit of the AIS is its severity coding.

Several severity indexes, among them also the AIS and ISS, have been discussed[16] as "subsets of health status indexes" and analysed mathematically regarding "additive value functions". Common deficiencies were discussed, such as patients age (see EIS here) and medical history.—The total body physiological "Trauma score"[7] considers the age up to 60 years, but partly relies on the GCS-sum score method in only five subgroups.

Considering the numbers of influencing factors Krischer[16] recommends a less restrictive approach to the formulation of severity indexes.—This may also be of value for the construction of DRG-groups mentioned above.

Conclusions

Tt seems that the most simple and practical procedure is to combine the severity coding advantages of the original AIS at bedside with the advantage of precise diagnoses of an improved ICD 10 (see Fig. 2).—

ICD—AIS—Neurotraumatology Contents suggested for ICD 10			ICD-9 rev (chapter XVII) (partly present Swedish codes)		

AIS			ICD-10			
1–4	Trauma capitis (head-trauma) (regio spec.)		*new*			
	Vulnus capitis (scalp-wound) (regio spec.)		873.00			
	Vulnus colli (neck-wound) (regio spec.)		874.00			
	Vulnera facei (face-wounds) (regio spec.)		879.00			
			non-compl.		*compl.*	*sequele*
2	Fractura cranii (skull fracture) (regio spec.)		800.00		800.10	800.90
3	Fractura cranii baseos (skull base fracture)		801.00		801.10	
4	Fractura cranii baseos (?) cum liquorrhea			*new*	801.10	
3	Fractura cranii cum impressione		803.00		803.10	803.90
3	Fractura cranii sive oss. facei mult.		804.00		804.10	
I: 1	Amnesia-confusio, vertigo, dizziness, vomiting, lethargia—posttraumat. (intoxicatio)		*new*	( )		
II: 2–3	Coma breve posttraumaticum (brief posttraumatic coma)					
	(commotio cerebri—concussion) (< 30 min)		850.00			
III: 3–4	Coma intermedium posttraumaticum					
	(intermediate posttr. coma 30 min–6 hrs)		*new*	(850.001)		
IV: 4–5	Coma longum posttraumaticum					
	(long posttraumatic coma 6 hrs–24 hrs)		*new*	(850.005)		
V: 4–5	Coma prolongatum posttraumaticum (24 hrs–2 w)		*new*	(850.007)		
VI: 5–6	Coma persistence posttr. (> 2 w)		*new*	(850.008)		
	Vegetating state etc (> 2 w)		*new*	(850.009)		
2	Syndroma posttraumatica					850.90
2–3	Hydrocephalus posttraumat.					*new* ( )
5	Varia (oedema malign, contus. mult.)		*new*	( )		
3–5	Fat embolism—brain		995.10			
3	Laesio cerebri focalis non expansiva (symptomatic diagnosis) (Focal nonexp. cer. lesion)		*new*	(851.00)		
3–4	Contusio cerebri focalis s. hemat. intracerebr. expansiva (Focal expans. cer. contus. or hematoma)		*new*	( )	*new*	(c. corp. alien) (vuln. sclop)
3–4	Pneumocephalus				*new*	
4–5	Hematoma extradurale		852.00			
4–5	Hematoma subdurale ac. (hydroma-hygroma)		853.00			
3	Hematoma subdurale subacuta		*new*	853.001		
3	Hematoma subdurale chron. traumat.					853.90
	[Hematoma subdurale non traum. (431.91)]					
3	Aneurysma (art. ven) traum. (Fist. carot.-cav.)		995.30			
			non-compl.		*compl.*	*sequele*
	Laesio nerv. intracran. sive cranialis n. II		950.00			
	Laesio nerv. intracran. n. III, IV, VI		951.00			
	Laesio nerv. intracran. others		951.01			
	Laesio nervus perif.		959.22		959.32	959.92
2	Defectus cranii posttraum.				800.10	800.90
3	Osteitis cranii posttraum.				800.10	800.90
3–5	Abscessus cerebri posttraum.				800.10	800.90
3	Fractura et luxatio vert.	cerv	805.00		805.10	
3	(without spinal cord symptoms)	thor	805.21		805.31	
2		lumb	805.21		805.31	
4–5	Fractura et luxatio vert.	cerv	806.00		806.10	
4	(with spinal cord damage incl. hematoma)	thor	806.21		806.31	
4		lumb	806.22		806.32	
4–5	Myelopathia traum. ac. (spinal cord damage—	cerv	958.00			
4	acute—incl hematoma)	thor	958.21			
4		lumb	958.22			
4	Myelopathia traum. chron.	cerv				958.90
3	(spinal cord damage—chronic)	thor				958.91
3		lumb				958.92

1–6 AIS: severity grading—threat to life; I–VI AIS: duration grading; new and ( ): new code numbers for ICD necessary.

Fig. 2 a

	ICD—AIS—Neurotraumatology Contents suggested for ICD 10		*ICD-9 rev (chapter XVII)* (partly present Swedish codes)		
AIS		**ICD-10**			
1–4	Head trauma (trauma capitis) (spec. reg.)	new			
	Wound, scalp (vulnus capitis) (spec. reg.)		873.00		
	Wound, neck (vulnus colli) (spec. reg.)		874.00		
	Wounds, face (vulnera facei) (spec. reg.)		879.00		
			closed	*open*	*sequels*
2	Fracture, skull (fractura cranii) (spec. reg.)		800.00	800.10	800.90
3	Fracture skull base (fractura baseos cranii)		801.00	801.10	
4	Fracture skull base with CSF fistula			new 801.10	
3	Fracture skull depressed, displaced		803.00	803.10	803.90
3	Fracture skull or face, multiple		804.00	804.10	
I: 1	Amnesia-confusion, vertigo, dizziness, vomiting lethargy posttraumat. (intoxication)	new	( )		
II: 2–3	Coma, posttraumat., brief (coma breve ptr.) 0–30 min brain concussion, commotio cerebri		850.00		
III: 3–4	Coma, posttraumat., intermediate 30 min–6 hrs (coma intermed. ptr.)	new			
IV: 4–5	Coma, posttraumat., long (coma longum ptr.) 6 hrs–24 hrs	new			
V: 4–5	Coma, posttraumat.-prolonged coma prolong. ptr.) 24 hrs–2 w	new			
VI: 5–6	Coma—persistent > 2 w	new			
	Coma—persistent vegetating state > 2 w (and other specified syndromes)	new			
2	Posttraumat., syndrome (syndroma posttraumat.)				850.90
2–3	Posttraumatic hydrocephalus			new	( )
5	Varia (malign. oedema; mult. contus.)	new	( )		
3–5	Fat embolism—brain		995.10		
3	Focal nonexp. cer. lesion ptr. (sympt. diagnosis)	new	(851.00)		
3–4	Focal expans. cer. contusion or hematoma, intracer. ptr.	new		new	(c. corp. alien) (vuln. sclop) (bullet wound)
3–4	Pneumocephalus			new	
4–5	Hematoma, extradural		852.00		
4–5	Hematoma subdural ac. (hydrom-hygrom)		853.00		
3	Hematoma subdural subacuta	new	853.001		
3	Hematoma subdural chron. ptr. [Hematoma subdural non-traumat. (431.91)]				853.90
3	Aneurysma (art. ven.) traum. (carotid-cav. fist.)		995.30		
			closed	*open*	*sequels*
	Lesion, nerv. intracran. or cranial n. II		950.00		
	Lesion nerv. intracran n. III, IV, VI		951.00		
	Lesion nerv. intracran. others		951.01		
	Lesion, nerve, peripheral nerves		959.22	959.32	959.92
2	Defect, cranial posttraumat.			800.10	800.90
3	Osteitis, cranial posttraumat.			800.10	800.90
3–5	Abscess, cerebral posttraumat.			800.10	800.90
3	Fracture and luxation, vertebral cerv		805.00	805.10	
3	(without spinal cord symptoms) thor		805.21	805.31	
2	lumb		805.21	805.31	
4–5	Fracture and luxation, vertebral cerv		806.00	806.10	
4	(with spinal cord damage incl. hematoma) thor		806.21	806.31	
4	lumb		806.22	806.32	
4–5	Myelopathy, traumat. acute (spinal cord damage cerv		958.00		
4	—acute—incl hematoma) thor		958.21		
4	lumb		958.22		
4	Myelopathy, traumat. chron. cerv				958.90
3	(spinal cord damage—chronic) thor				958.91
3	lumb				958.92

1–6 AIS: severity grading—threat to life; I–VI AIS: duration grading; new and (   ): new code numbers for ICD necessary.

Fig. 2 b.

It will facilitate comparison of clinical materials to apply severity grades to the ICD diagnostic coding, the understanding of which is also facilitated by its clinical terms.

This will also avoid two parallel and different codes for partly similar and partly different purposes, which may cause confusion.—This study has only dealt with head injuries and it will be seen if similar directions for the future also are applicable to other areas.

References

1. AIS 1976; The Abbreviated Injury Scale AMA, AAAM, Morton Grove, IL.
2. AIS 1980; The Abbreviated Injury Scale AAAM, Morton Grove, IL.
3. AIS 1985; The Abbreviated Injury Scale, Arlington Heights, IL. (60005)
4. Berki SE (1984) Grading DRGs. Med Care 22: 1065–1066
5. Blomert DM, Sisler GC (1974) The measurement of retrograde post-traumatic amnesia. Can Psychiatr Assoc J 19: 185–192
6. Cabezudo JM, Olabe J, Lopez-Anguera A (1986) Recovery from locked-in syndrome after posttraumatic bilateral distal vertebral artery occlusion. Surg Neurol 25: 185–190
7. Champion HR, Sacco WJ, Carnazzo AJ, Copes W, Fouty WJ (1981) Trauma score. Crit Care Med 9: 672–676
8. Courville CB (1953) Commotio cerebri. San Lucas Press, Los Angeles, pp 161
9. Evans CD, Bull CPI, Devenport MJ, Hall PM, Jones J, Middleton FRI, Russel G, Stichbury JC, Whitehead B (1977) Rehabilitation of the brain-damaged survivor. Injury 8: 80–97
10. Garthe EA (1982) Compatibility of ICD-9-CM with AIS-80. AAAM The Quarterly/Journal 4: 42–46
11. Gennarelli TA, et al. (1982) Influence of the type of intracranial lesion on outcome from severe head injury. A multicenter study using a new classification system. J Neurosurg 56: 26–32
11 a. Gentleman D, Jennett B (1981) Harards of inter-hospital transfer of comatose head-injured patients. Lancet 2: 853–855
12. Glossary of Neurotraumatology (1979) Acta Neurochir (Wien) [Suppl] 25
13. International Classification of Diseases (ICD 9). World Health Organization, Geneva, 1977
14. International Classification of Diseases Clinical Modification (ICD CM), 1979
15. Jennett B (1976) Assessment of the severity of head injury. J Neurol Neurosurg Psychiatry 39: 647–655
16. Krischer P (1976) Index of severity: Underlying concepts. Health Services Research 11: 143–157
17. Langley J (1982) The international classification of disease's codes for describing injuries and the circumstances surrounding injuries: A critical comment and suggestions for improvement. Accid Anal Prev 14: 195–197
18. Lindgren SO (1960) Acute severe head injuries. Acta Chir Scand [Suppl] 254
19. Lindgren SO (1983) Coma scales—awareness of reaction levels as part of commonly used severity grading. Scot Med J 28: 203
20. Lishman WA (1978) Organic psychiatry. The psychological consequences of cerebral disorder. Blackwell Scientific Publications, Oxford, pp 999
21. Ommaya AK (1985) Biomechanics of head injury: experimental aspects. In: Nahum A, Melvin J (eds) The Biomechanics of trauma. Apple-Century-Crofts, Connecticut, USA, pp 225–269
22. Plum F, Brennan RW (1982) Differential diagnosis of altered states of consciousness. In: Youmans J (ed) Neurological surgery, vol 1. W. B. Saunders Company, pp 63–73
23. Punch L (1984) DRG's first 6 months: Many hospitals are doing better than they'd expected. Modern Health Care 14: 42–44
24. Stuss TD, Ely P, Hugenholtz H, Richard MT, LaRochelle S, Poirier CA, Bell I (1985) Subtle neuropsychological deficits in patients with good recovery after closed head injury. Neurosurgery 17: 41–47
25. Stålhammar D, Holmgren E, Lindgren SO, Lindström L (1983) Brain injury scaling. Ircobi, Salon de Provence
26. Teasdale G, Brooks DN (1985) Traumatic amnesia. Handbook of clinical neurology, vol 1 (45), 185–191

Author's address: Prof. S. Lindgren, Department of Neurosurgery, Sahlgren's Hospital, University of Göteborg, S-413 45 Göteborg, Sweden.

Acta Neurochirurgica, Suppl. 36, 81–85 (1986)

Experimental Animal Physiology Related to Brain Stem Control of Wakefulness

S. Lindström

Department of Physiology, University of Göteborg, Sweden

Summary

Animal experiments indicate that the awake state is supported by activating structures in the caudal reticular core of the mesencephalon and in the caudolateral hypothalamus. Different aspects of the normal wakefulness may be mediated by separate neuronal subsystems. This segregation may explain why atypical combinations of symptoms may occur in head injured patients.

Keywords: Brain stem; lesions; wakefulness; arousal.

From animal experiments it is well known that brain stem structures are deeply involved in the control of sleep and wakefulness (see Ulf Norrsell, this supplement). This brief review will concentrate on a few critical experiments, mainly involving lesions, that in my view set the stage for our present understanding of the problem. It is hoped that insight from these studies may help to cast some light over diagnostic problems that may occur with head injured patients. More detailed accounts can be found in reviews by Moruzzi[16], Żernicki[25] or for modern electrophysiological studies by Hobson[7] and Steriade[23].

The Classical Experiments

The first indication that brain stem structures might be important for the control of wakefulness came through experimental work of Bremer in the mid-1930's[4]. He transected the neuroaxis of cats at two levels, between the medulla oblongata and the spinal cord and between the superior and inferior colliculi. The low transection, giving a so-called "encéphale isolé" preparation, resulted in animals with essentially normal EEG that changed cyclically between episodes of low amplitude, high frequency activity similar to the desynchronized EEG of awake humans and episodes with high amplitude, low frequency activity similar to the synchronized EEG of sleep. After the high, "cerveau isolé", transection the animals displayed a continuous pattern of slow-wave EEG activity and had constricted pupils, as if the forebrain remained in lasting sleep.

Like most of his contemporaries, Bremer believed that the normal transition from the awake to the sleeping state was a passive event following a reduced afferent inflow to the brain. Thus, he proposed that the lack of wakefulness in the cerveau isolé preparation could be explained by the elimination of the trigeminal and vestibulocochlear inflow to the forebrain by the high transection.

The next step forward came with the famous experiments of Moruzzi and Magoun, published in 1949[17]. They demonstrated that high frequency, low intensity electrical stimulation of the central reticular core of the brain stem was more effective than direct stimulation of specific afferent pathways in inducing EEG desynchronization. The effective region extended all the way from the caudal medulla up through the mesencephalon on both sides of the midline. The stimulation effect remained after large bilateral lesions of the lateral parts of the mesencephalic tegmentum, which transected all the specific ascending sensory pathways to the forebrain. Lesions of the medial tegmentum at the same level abolished, however, the effect of stimulation at more caudal levels.

These original experiments were performed on encephale isolé or lightly anesthetized cats but they were soon repeated on intact unanaesthetized animals. It was then found that similar weak brain stem stimuli also induced behavioural arousal in spontaneously sleeping animals[12]. Likewise, both cats and monkeys became comatose after large central mesencephalic lesions[6, 11]. These lesions presumably interrupted an ascending reticular projection but spared the classical sensory pathways to the forebrain. Lesions of the latter pathways or of the central grey resulted in awake animals that were even able to stand and walk. Together these experiments indicated that central reticular structures of the brain stem, rather than specific sensory pathways, were important for the maintenance of wakefulness and for the induction of both behavioural and EEG arousal. As a result the well known concept of an "ascending reticular activation system" was born.

The Mesencephalic Activating Structure

The experiments described so far did not exclude that afferent inflow from the cranial nerves was required to maintain the awake state, as believed by Bremer; they only demonstrated that any such effect was relayed through the brain stem reticular formation rather than through specific ascending pathways. That a sensory isolated brain stem could support an awake state was demonstrated much later by Batini and collaborators[3]. They devised a cat preparation with the brain stem transected in the middle of the pons, rostral to the entry of the trigeminal nerve. This "pretrigeminal" preparation displays continuous EEG desynchronization for the first day, even if also the olfactory and optic nerves are transected. After 12–24 hours short episodes of EEG synchronization reappear and alternate with periods of desynchronization.

The important question whether the different EEG patterns of the pretrigeminal preparation are in any way related to normal behavioural states was addressed in a series of studies by Żernicki and his collaborators[26]. They obtained strong support for the view that the forebrain of such animals is in fact awake during periods of EEG desynchronization. The occulomotor nerves leave the brain stem rostral to the mid-pontine transection which means that the animals can move their eyes in the vertical plane. They also have pupillary and accommodation reflexes. Utilizing these facts the experimenters could demonstrate that pretrigeminal animals follow objects moved in the vertical plane with their eyes during periods of EEG desynchronization. Conditioned reflexes based on pupillary reactions can also be elicited during such periods. Both reactions are lacking during episodes of slow-wave synchronized EEG. This behavioural inactivity suggests that the forebrain is at a state of sleep during these episodes. Such sleep periods can be interrupted by strong olfactory stimuli implying that this restricted preparation also has an essentially normal mechanism for sensory arousal. The pretrigeminal preparation differs from the

encephale isolé preparation in only one important aspect—after this pontine transection the animals seem to be entirely devoid of REM sleep.

When the reactions of the pretrigeminal and cerveau isolé preparations are compared, it is clear that some brain stem structures between the middle of pons and the middle of mesencephalon are able to support the awake state. It may be asked how much of the remaining structures is required for this function. Ślósarska and Żernicki[22] found that, when carefully done, the brain stem could be transected up to the border between the pons and the mesencephalon before the pretrigeminal preparation changed into a typical cerveau isolé preparation. The transition zone is quite narrow suggesting that the critical activation structure is located in the mesencephalic tegmentum within a few millimetres from the ponto-mesencephalic junction (Fig. 1). In most mammals, including man, this will be

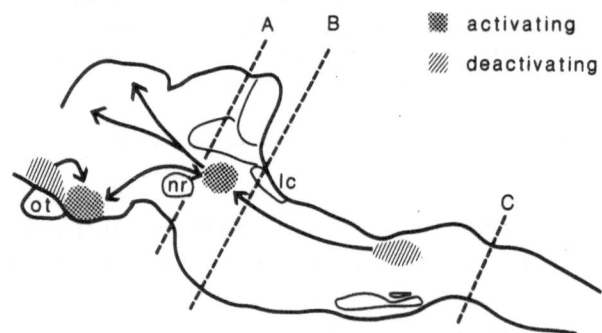

activating

deactivating

Fig. 1. Schematic figure of structures in the brain stem and hypothalamus that control wakefulness. A–C indicate brain stem transections that give rise to the cerveau isolé, pretrigeminal and encéphale isolé preparations. ot optic tract, nr nucleus ruber, lc locus coeruleus

just below the tentorium at a likely stress point during blow towards the head. Neurones in this activating structure are believed to keep the forebrain awake through tonic ascending activity. Combined caudal and rostral lesions indicate that this tonic activity is in turn supported by descending activity from rostral brain structures.

The mesencephalic activating system remains to be identified at the neuronal level. The monoaminergic nuclei near the critical region, the noradrenergic locus coeruleus and the serotonergic midline raphe nuclei have often been implicated since they have a widespread projection to the forebrain. However, none of these structures seem to be directly involved. The neuronal activity of these nuclei in free moving animals is not easily related to the state of wakefulness[5, 14, 23] and there is no dramatic loss of wakefulness after chemical or electrolytic destruction of them[9, 16, 23]. The involved neurones may be located in the peribrachial region surrounding the mesencephalic path of the fibres of the superior cerebellar peduncle. This region contains a mixture of cells projecting either to the specific sensory[1] or to the intralamina nuclei of thalamus, the latter with further projections to wide regions of the cerebral cortex[23]. At least some of these cells are activated in relation to spontaneous or induced arousal[20, 23]. Those neurones which project to the specific thalamic nuclei seem to have a disinhibitory effect[2] and may be responsible for the EEG desynchronization while those with intralaminar projection may be responsible for the behavioural aspect of the arousal[23]. It is not unlikely that separate neuronal mechanisms underly these components of the normal arousal reaction (*cf.* below), although our understanding of the exact mechanisms will have to await a positive identification of the responsible cells.

The idea of a spatially restricted activating structure in the lower mesencephalon is compatible with the widespread activation region found in the stimulation experiments of Moruzzi and Magoun[17]. The brain stem reticular formation is an extremely complicated part of the central nervous system with an entangled network of passing fibres, collateral branches and neurones of different forms and functions, some with very extensive branching patterns[21]. Thus, it is likely that electrical stimuli applied to caudal regions may activate fiber systems with excitatory effects on the more rostrally located activation structure[1]. Such fibers may be interposed between the specific sensory pathways and the mesencephalic activating neurones and mediate the effects of sensory arousing stimuli.

Other Structures Affecting Wakefulness

In the early lesion experiments it was frequently found that the coma induced by central tegmental lesions, even very large ones, was not permanent[12]. After about a week short episodes of EEG desynchronization could be induced by auditory or painful stimuli. The effect did not outlast the stimulation and was only occasionally associated with motor effects such as lifting or shaking the head. The same kind of recovery with episodes of EEG desynchronization may be seen after complete precollicular brain stem transections if the animals are followed for a long enough time (several weeks)[25]. Transitions from synchronized to desynchronized EEG may occur spontaneously or as a result of strong olfactory stimulation. This recovery

points to the existence of other activating structure(s) rostral to the mesencephalon.

Several observations indicate that the responsible system is located in the caudolateral hypothalamus, between the optic chiasm and the mammilary body (Fig. 1). Already in the 1930's Ranson[19] found that bilateral lesions in this region resulted in somnolent or lethargic animals. Modern experiments with EEG recordings have confirmed that animals with such lesions are constantly asleep with slow-wave synchronous EEG activity[18]. Upon sensory stimulation they only respond with transient EEG desynchronization. In contrast to animals with mesencephalic lesions these hypothalamic cats display normal episodes with REM sleep.

Conversely, bilateral lesions of the more rostrally located preoptic region of the hypothalamus induced severe insomnia[15]. Some neurones in this region may thus have a sleep promoting effect, possibly via an antagonistic effect on the more caudal activating region (Fig. 1). If the preoptic area is stimulated electrically in an awake cat the animal goes to sleep within a few seconds[24]. Another sleep promoting region has been identified in the caudal medulla oblongata near the nucleus of the solitary tract[16]. This region was identified when it was realized that pretrigeminal animals spend far more time in the awake state than encephale isolé animals. Accordingly, it was proposed that some caudal brain stem structure had a tonic inhibitory action on the mesencephalic activation structure. In agreement with this proposition sleeping animals are aroused when this region is selectively anaesthetized or inactivated by cooling[13, 16]. Stimulation in the same region rapidly induces sleep in awake animals, just as is the case for the analogous hypothalamic region[18].

So it seems that the awake state is maintained by two activating structures, one in the mesencephalic reticular formation near the junction with pons, the other in the caudolateral hypothalamus, both structures equipped with antagonistic systems. In normal animals the two activating structures probably operate in conjunction. There is at least anatomical evidence for reciprocal connexions between these regions that may subserve such a function. The reappearance of periods of wakefulness after lesions of either structure may be due to a gradual take over of the control from the remaining part just like segmental reflexes recover after spinal shock.

The actual mechanism behind the partial recovery is as little known as is the normal operation of the activation systems. As pointed out above, our knowledge of these structures is still very rudimentary and the diagram in Fig. 1 is almost certainly a gross oversimplification. The responsible cells have not been identified with certainty and as a consequence we have no hard facts about the operating circuitry or its mode of activation and inhibition. This ignorance calls for care in interpreting the findings of stimulation and lesion experiments.

Dissociation of EEG Desynchronization and Wakefulness

In the described experiments there has been a close correlation between different physiological signs of wakefulness, such as EEG desynchronization, and awake behaviour. This is not necessarily the case, especially not after brain lesions. REM sleep may serve as a good example to illustrate this point. This sleep stage seems to be generated by neuronal systems in the pons[10] (which explains why there is no REM sleep in pretrigeminal animals) and it is characterized by many electrophysiological changes typical of the awake state[7]. There are rapid saccades of the eyes (REM = rapid eye movements), theta activity in the hippocampus, facilitation of impulse transmission through specific sensory nuclei and EEG desynchronization. Not surprisingly, the cerebral cortex seems to be active as suggested by the frequent dreams. Yet, the individuals are behaviourally asleep and in fact more difficult to arouse by sensory stimuli than during deep slow-wave sleep. We do not know why the brain in this state, despite a facilitated sensory transmission and a seemingly aroused cortex, is so unaccessible to peripheral inputs.

With lesions the situation may be even more complicated. During REM sleep there is a pronounced inhibition of spinal motoneurones resulting in a characteristic muscular atonia. This inhibition is relayed from the pons to the spinal cord via inhibitory neurones in the caudal medulla[20]. By certain pontine lesions in the cat, it is possible to eliminate this inhibitory effect without affecting other components of the REM activity. Animals with such lesions have REM episodes without atonia. This means that their REM episodes are practically indistinguishable from the awake state with electrophysiological techniques. What is worse, these animals may have normal reflexes and display well coordinated motor behaviour during the REM episodes. They have been observed to rise, to walk around and to jump after imaginary objects as if they were acting out some dreams. Yet, it is easy to demonstrate that they are not awake in the common

sense of the word. They pay no attention to real objects in the world around them such as a living mouse or food. Like normal animals during REM they are also difficult to wake up.

A behaviourally similar phenomenon in humans is somnambulism. The individuals move around with open eyes and usually avoid obstacles, like a wellprogrammed robot. Even so, they are clearly unaware of the surroundings and very difficult to wake up. Interestingly, these coordinated motor activities occur in man during episodes of deep slow-wave sleep, not during REM[8].

These drastic examples may illustrate that neither EEG desynchronization nor seemingly purposeful motor acts are necessarily associated with wakefulness and awareness of ourselves or events in the surrounding world. The explanation may be that different neuronal subsystems are responsible for various aspects of the normal awake state and that these subsystems may be selectively activated in certain behavioural situations. Needless to say these different subsystems may also be more or less selectively affected by traumatic head injuries. Thus, it is not surprising that many patients with head injuries have symptoms that do not fit into simple general schemes intended to describe the severity of the damage.

Acknowledgements

Work in the author's laboratory was supported by the Swedish Medical Research Council (Project No. 4767).

References

1. Ahlsén G (1984) Brain stem neurones with differential projection to functional subregions of the dorsal lateral geniculate complex of the cat. Neurosci 12: 817–838
2. Ahlsén G, Lindström S, Lo F-S (1984) Inhibition from the brain stem of inhibitory interneurones of the cat's lateral geniculate nucleus. J Physiol (Lond) 347: 593–605
3. Batini C, Moruzzi G, Palestini M, Rossi GF, Zanchetti A (1959) Effects of complete pontine transections on the sleep-wakefulness rhythm: the midpontine pretrigeminal preparation. Arch Ital Biol 97: 1–12
4. Bremer F (1937) L'activité cérébrale au cours du sommeil et de la narcose. Contribution à l'étude du mécanisme du sommeil. Bull Acad Roy Méd Belg 4: 68–86
5. Foote SL, Bloom FE, Aston-Jones G (1983) Nucleus locus coeruleus: New evidence of anatomical and physiological specificity. Physsiol Rev 63: 844–914
6. French JD, Magoun HW (1952) Effects of chronic lesions in central cephalic brain stem of monkeys. Arch Neurol Psychiatry (Chic) 68: 591–604

7. Hobson JA (1984) How does the cortex know when to do what? A neurobiological theory of state control. In: Edelman GM, Gall WE, Cowan WM (eds) Dynamic aspects of neocortical function. J. Wiley & Sons, New York, pp 219–257

8. Jacobson A, Kales A, Lehmann D, Zweizig JR (1965) Somnambulism: All-night electroencephalographic studies. Science 148: 975–977

9. Jones BE, Harper ST, Halaris AE (1977) Effects of locus coeruleus lesions upon cerebral monoamine content, sleep-wakefulness states and the response to amphetamine in that cat. Brain Res 124: 473–496

10. Jouvet M (1962) Recherches sur les structures nerveuses et les mécanismes responsables des différentes phases du sommeil physiologique. Arch Ital Biol 100: 125–206

11. Lindsley DB, Bowden JW, Magoun HW (1949) Effect upon the EEG of acute injury to the brain stem activating system. Electroenceph Clin Neurophysiol 1: 475–486

12. Lindsley DB, Schreiner LH, Knowles WB, Magoun HW (1950) Behavioural and EEG changes following chronic brain stem lesions in the cat. Electroenceph Clin Neurophysiol 2: 483–498

13. Magni F, Moruzzi G, Rossi GF, Zanchetti A (1959) EEG arousal following inactivation of the lower brain stem by selective injection of barbiturate into the vertebral circulation. Arch Ital Biol 97: 33–46

14. McGinty DJ, Harper RM, Fairbanks MK (1973) 5-HT-containing neurons: Unit activity in behaving cats. In: Barchas J, Usdin E (eds) Serotonin and behaviour. Academic Press, New York, pp 267–269

15. McGinty DJ, Sterman MB (1968) Sleep suppression after basal forebrain lesions in the cat. Science 160: 1253–1255

16. Moruzzi G (1972) The sleep-waking cycle. Rev Physiol 64: 1–165

17. Moruzzi G, Magoun HW (1949) Brain stem reticular formation and activation of the EEG. Electroenceph Clin Neurophysiol 1: 455–473

18. Naquet R, Denavit M, Albe-Fessard D (1966) Comparison entre le rôle du subthalamus et celui des différentes structures bulbo-mésencéphaliques dans le maintien de la vigilance. Electroenceph Clin Neurophysiol 20: 149–164

19. Ranson SW (1939) Somnolence caused by hypothalamic lesions in the monkey. Arch Neurol Psychiatry (Chic) 1–23

20. Sakai K (1980) Some anatomical and physiological properties of ponto-mesencephalic tegmental neurones with special reference to the PGO waves and postural atonia during paradoxical sleep in the cat. In: Hobson JA, Brazier MAB (eds) The reticular formation revisited. Raven Press, New York, pp 427–447

21. Scheibel ME, Scheibel AB (1958) Structural substrates for integrative patterns in the brain stem reticular core. In: Jasper HH, Proctor LD, Knighton RS, Noshay WC, Costello RT (eds) Reticular formation of the brain. Little, Brown and Co, Boston, pp 31–55

22. Ślósarska M, Żernicki B (1973) Sleep-waking cycle in the cerveau isolé cat. Arch Ital Biol 111: 138–155

23. Steriade M (1984) The excitatory-inhibitory response sequence in thalamic and neocortical cells: State-related changes and regulatory systems. In: Edelman GM, Gall WE, Cowan WM (eds) Dynamic aspects of neocortical function. J Wiley & Sons, New York, pp 107–157

24. Sterman MB, Clemente CD (1962) Forebrain inhibitory mechanisms: Sleep patterns induced by basal forebrain stimulation in the behaving cat. Exp Neurol 6: 103–117

25. Villablanca J (1965) The electrocorticogram in the chronic cerveau isolé cat. Electroenceph Clin Neurophysiol 19: 576–586

26. Żernicki B (1968) Pretrigeminal cat. Brain Res 9: 1–14

Author's address: S. Lindström, M.D., Department of Physiology, University of Göteborg, Box 33031, S-400 33 Göteborg, Sweden.

Acta Neurochirurgica, Suppl. 36, 86–88 (1986)

Awareness, Wakefulness and Arousal

U. Norrsell

Department of Neurology, Sahlgren's Hospital, University of Göteborg, Sweden

Summary

The concepts awareness, wakefulness, and arousal are compared, and some neurophysiological and neuropsychological studies of awareness are described. The different studies are suggested to show that awareness depends on neural activity of the cerebral cortex, but the relationship between cortical activity and awareness is found to be conditional. Consequently, the presence of awareness can only be established with behavioural methods.

Keywords: Awareness; evoked potentials; brain stimulation; cerebral commissurotomy.

People who work with head injured patients have to use words like awareness (or consciousness), wakefulness and arousal quite frequently. An obvious reason is the need to tell colleagues or the patient's relatives about his state, and its implications for the prognosis. Consequently, it is perhaps appropriate to include some comments on the conceptual basis of those words among the papers of the symposium. The approach will be concrete and restricted to clinical aspects, however, and the reader who is interested in the general aspects of the concepts is directed elsewhere. Different views may be obtained from essays by, *e.g.* Hebb[6], Kubie[7], and Weiskrantz[22]. Enlightening discussions of the inconvenient, albeit recurrent idea of the consciousness as an epiphenomenon have been published by Smith[15], and Sperry[18]. The two words consciousness and awareness will be treated here as synonyms, although some authors think otherwise (*cf.* Griffin[5]). The particular word consciousness will be avoided, since it is open to several interpretations when used in connexion with the variable condition of a head injured patient with the comatous state (or unconsciousness) at one end.

The three words of the above title are used normally in such a way that they may be regarded to indicate three partially independent, but at the same time hierarchically arranged concepts with awareness above the two others. This means that signs of wakefulness and/or arousal do not necessarily indicate the presence of the individual's awareness of a situation or condition. The term wakefulness is probably best used to indicate the level of reactivity, whereas the term arousal is probably best saved for the changes of reactivity. The suggestion may be illustrated by the example of a man lying in bed at night whose wakefulness is being maintained by a series of noises, but who becomes aroused first at the actual appearance of a burglar. The term arousal is used, however, for both neurophysiological and psychological concepts: In neurophysiology to indicate the desynchronization of the cerebral EEG. In psychology to indicate the degree of mental and emotional activation in connexion with the performance of a behavioural transaction.

The desynchronization of the cortical EEG is caused by a change of cortical neuronal activity, and this change of activity may be either the cause or the effect of a correlated behavioural transaction. The true relationship, however, between an EEG desynchronization and an allied behavioural transaction remains obscure[13]. The mechanisms of EEG arousal have been studied to a great extent in subhuman mammals like the cat. Whatever its relation to behaviour it therefore is unlikely to be a specific indicator of an individual's awareness of a situation, at least in the common usage of the word[1].

At present, awareness is probably best discussed relative to man and there are some interesting observations. It is quite well known that depending on its character, a behavioural transaction may be more or less dependent on the neuronal activity of the cerebral cortex. There are also reasons to believe that the awareness of an event always depends on certain kinds of cortical neuronal activity. We all know, however, that a person is not always aware of everything which happens to him, and one may then ask if one is always aware of events which cause cortical activity. One can also ask, when performing a transaction of which one is aware, if the awareness precedes the transaction. The answer appears to be no in both instances, at least sometimes.

Libet and colleagues[8–10] have recorded from the postcentral gyrus of the cerebral cortex, or stimulated the postcentral gyrus or the thalamic somatosensory relay of human patients undergoing neurosurgical therapy in local anesthesia. They recorded potentials which were evoked by single epidermal electrical stimuli of varying intensities, and found a dissociation between the thresholds for the appearance of a primary cortical evoked potential, and the patients' subjective awareness of the stimulus. The threshold for subjective awareness was found to be 110–130% of the threshold for the evoked potential[8]. The patients' awareness of the skin stimuli was correlated to the appearance of suprathreshold, longer latency components of the cerebral somatosensory evoked potential. Libet[8] concluded: "It follows . . . that the presence or amplitude of an evoked potential, particularly of the primary component, cannot be assumed to be an indicator of the occurrence or intensity of subjective sensory experience . . ."

There are earlier observations[3, 4] which support Libet's conclusion, but the essential dissociation between the evoked potential and awareness thresholds has also been denied[11]. The failure of Leuders et al.[11], however, to replicate the findings of Libet et al.[9] in a single patient, when using a different type of peripheral, electrical stimulation technique, appears to be of subordinate interest at present. Nevertheless, the choice of peripheral stimulus may be critical[16], but need not concern us here.

Libet and his colleagues[8, 10] also found that they could interfere with the awareness of a peripheral skin stimulus by direct, electrical stimulation of the cerebral, postcentral gyrus. They used a peripheral stimulus which was above the awareness threshold when used alone. The peripheral stimulus was not percieved, however, when it was administered in connexion with electrical stimulation of the postcentral projection area. The masking presumably was caused by interference with the cerebral processing of the neural activity which had been elicited by the peripheral stimulus. The cerebral stimulation caused retroactive masking of the peripheral stimulus for several hundred ms and in one patient even when it was applied half a second after the former. This is a very long time when compared to, e.g.

the reaction time to a simple somatosensory stimulus, which is of the order of magnitude of 100–150 ms, and the findings seem to indicate, that under some circumstances we may perform a behavioural transaction before having percieved the causal event. Anyway, the findings of Libet and his colleagues[8–10], as well as others[14], have indicated that awareness is not an unconditional correlate of behavioural functions which include cerebral, cortical activity. It is thus possible, that our awareness of behavioural transactions may be a special cerebral function which is only necessary under certain conditions.

The suggestion that our awareness depends on cerebral activity is supported by various evidence. The observations of Weiskrantz and other investigators[21] of so-called "blind sight", i.e. the loss of visual awareness despite retained visual function after lesions of the cerebral visual projection areas, have provided one type of evidence. Other, even more compelling evidence comes from observations of epileptics, who have undergone cerebral commissurotomies for therapeutical reasons. The larger commissurotomies involve transections of the entire corpus callosum, and the anterior and hippocampal commissures[2], and produce the so-called "split brain" condition. This means, among other things, that the somatosensory and visual half fields fail to unite at the longitudinal midline, and are independent with regard to perceptual processes which are executed at the cerebral level. Thus, the appearance of a "split" or disconnexion symptom for a task involving such a sensory function after commissurotomy provides evidence for the participation of the cerebral cortex in that particular task[17].

The "split brain" patients are usually lateralized for the speech functions, which are unevenly distributed between the two cerebral hemispheres. They are able to read and understand spoken language to a certain extent with both hemispheres, but are restricted to an almost negligible level with regard to expressive language for their right hemispheres[12]. The patients' verbal reports of their intentions and memories therefore reflect the opinions of their left hemispheres. It is possible, however, to glean what appears to be independent opinions which belong to their right hemispheres by means of nonverbal communication or through the patients' emotional reactions[19]. The latter findings have indicated the presence of independent awareness for the two hemispheres.

The evidence for the presence of "the higher reflective self-conscious type of mental awareness that characterizes the human brain" in the linguistically subordinate hemisphere has not always been accepted, and was examined by Sperry *et al.*[20] in a special investigation. They were able to present complicated pictures for detailed examination by the commissurotomized patients' right hemispheres alone by means of a contact lens technique, which was developed by Zaidel[23]. The pictures contained abstract symbols, or photographs of public and historical figures etc. The patients' verbal comments of the proceedings showed that their left hemispheres were unaware of the presented material. In such a way it became clear that their nonverbal responses, and emotional reactions reflected the sentiments of their right hemisphers. The descriptions of the patients behaviour[20] makes interesting reading, which argues convincingly for a cognitive and conative capacity of their right hemispheres, which is comparable to that of their left, speaking hemispheres.

A final statement based on the presented evidence ought to be, that awareness is a function which depends on neural activity of the cerebral cortex, and that consequently any behavioural transaction which includes awareness by necessity indicates activation of the cerebral cortex. There are other behavioural transactions which depend on neural activity of the cerebral cortex, however, which may not include awareness. Consequently nonbehavioural (*e.g.* electrophysiological) tests of cortical activation are insufficient to provide conclusive evidence of awareness. The behavioural tests of the awareness of a brain damaged patient may obviously sometimes be confounded by simultaneous disabilities like aphasia. The work with commissurotomized patients has shown, however, that it may be possible even in such cases, to judge the patients' awareness by studying the consistency of his reactions to objects or people about which he must be expected to have an opinion on the basis of his premorbid background, and developmental level.

References

1. Bullock TH (1982) Afterthoughts on animal minds. In: Griffin DR (ed) Animal mind—Human mind. Springer, Berlin Heidelberg New York, pp 407–414
2. Bogen JE, Sperry RW, Vogel PJ (1969) Commissural sections and the propagation of seizures. In: Jasper HH *et al.* (eds) Basic mechanisms of the epilepsies. Little, Brown, Boston, pp 439–440
3. DeBecker J, Desmedt JE, Manil J (1965) Sur la relation entre le seuil de perception tactile et les potentiels évoqués de l'écorce cérébrale somato-sensible chez l'homme. CR Acad Sci (Paris) 260: 687–689
4. DeBecker J, Desmedt JE, Manil J (1965) Corrélations psychologiques des potentiels évoqués cérébraux. J Physiol (Paris) 57: 595
5. Griffin, DR (1982) Introduction. In: Griffin DR (ed) Animal mind—human mind. Springer, Berlin Heidelberg New York, pp 1–12
6. Hebb DO (1954) The problem of consciousness and introspection. In: Delafresnaye J *et al.* (eds) Brain mechanisms and consciousness. Blackwell, Oxford, pp 402–417
7. Kubie LS (1954) Psychiatric and psychoanalytic considerations of the problem of consciousness. In: Delafresnaye JF *et al.* (eds) Brain mechanisms and consciousness. Blackwell, Oxford, pp 444–467
8. Libet B (1973) Electrical stimulation of cortex in human subjects, and conscious sensory aspects. In: Iggo A (ed) Handbook of sensory physiology, vol 2. Springer, Berlin Heidelberg New York, pp 743–790
9. Libet B, Alberts WW, Wright EW, jr, Feinstein B (1967) Responses of human somatosensory cortex to stimuli below threshold for conscious sensation. Science 158: 1597–1600
10. Libet B, Alberts WW, Wright EW, jr, Feinstein B (1972) Cortical and thalamic activation in conscious sensory experience. In: Somjen GG (ed) Neurophysiology studied in man. Excerpta Medica, Amsterdam, pp 157–168
11. Lueders H, Lesser RP, Hahn J, Dinner DS, Klem G (1983) Cortical somatosensory evoked potentials in response to hand stimulation. J Neurosurg 58: 885–894
12. Norrsell U (1982) Comment on the partial roles of the cerebral hemispheres for speech. In: Grillner S *et al.* (eds) Wenner-Gren center international symposium series, vol 36. Pergamon Press, Oxford New York Toronto Sydney Paris Frankfurt, pp 67–73
13. Schlag J (1974) Reticular influences on thalamo-cortical activity. In: Remond A *et al.* (eds) Handbook of electroencephalography and clinical neurophysiology, vol 2 C. Elsevier, Amsterdam, pp 119–134
14. Shevrin H, Fritzler DE (1968) Visual evoked response correlates of unconscious mental processes. Science 161: 295–298
15. Smith HW (1959) The biology of consciousness. In: Brooks C McC *et al.* (eds) The historical development of physiological thought. Hafner, New York, pp 109–136
16. Soininen K, Järvilehto T (1983) Somatosensory evoked potentials associated with tactile stimulation at detection threshold in man. EEG Clin Neurophysiol 56: 494–500
17. Sperry RW (1961) Some developments in brain lesion studies of learning. Federation Proc 20: 609–616
18. Sperry RW (1965) Mind, brain, and humanist values. In: Platt JR (ed) New views of the nature of man. University of Chicago Press, Chicago, pp 71–92
19. Sperry RW, Gazzaniga MS, Bogen JE (1969) Interhemispheric relationships: the neocortical commissures; syndromes of hemisphere disconnection. In: Vinken PJ, *et al.* (eds) Handbook of clinical neurology, vol 4. North-Holland, Amsterdam, pp 273–290
20. Sperry RW, Zaidel E, Zaidel D (1979) Self recognition and social awareness in the deconnected minor hemisphere. Neuropsychologia 17: 153–166
21. Weiskrantz L (1980) Varieties of residual experience. Quart J Exp Psychol 32: 365–386
22. Weiskrantz L (1985) Introduction: categorization, cleverness and consciousness. Phil Trans R Soc (Lond) B 308: 3–19
23. Zaidel E (1975) A technique for presenting lateralized visual input with prolonged exposure. Vision Res 15: 283–289

Author's address: U. Norrsell, M.D., Department of Neurology, Sahlgren's Hospital, University of Göteborg, S-413 45 Göteborg, Sweden.

Acta Neurochirurgica, Suppl. 36, 89 (1986)

Electrophysiological Assessment of Conscious Level

A. Bricolo

Department of Neurosurgery, University Hospital, Verona, Italy

Consciousness and vigilance shift continuously and their behavioral and clinical manifestations are implemented somewhat gradually, each shift corresponding to a different level of activity: waking, various degrees of attentiveness, light, deep and paradoxical sleep, various levels of coma and of altered states of responsiveness, etc. Each of these states is associated with a certain working mode in the brain—though on account of our limited semiologic methods we are not always able to detect each of them or assess it accurately. In comatose states, apart from the clinical data emerging from neurological examination, electrophysiologic techniques such as electroencephalogram (EEG) and evoked potentials (EPs) remain the best possible sources of objective information concerning the functional level of cerebral activity. Essentially the EEG represents the only biological activity suitable for continuous noninvasive monitoring of brain function. This property is especially instrumental in the acute phase of posttraumatic coma where the most important task is to keep the patient's course under strict control in order to obtain earlier detection of CNS functioning deterioration. EPs provide reliable and objective data about the integrity of the involved pathways and level of functioning of CNS structures. Short latency somato-sensory (SEP) and brain-stem uditory EP (BAEP) have very close anatomic correlations and are resistant to alteration by anything except structural abnormality. They are unchanged in barbiturate iatrogenic coma even when EEG becomes iso-electric and the clinical examination absent. Because of their anatomic specificity and physiologic and metabolic immutability, EPs provide a reliable look at "physiologic anatomy". To complement the clinical neurologic data with EEG monitoring and serial multimodality EP examinations allows a better assessment of brain function in patients with altered level of consciousness and affords finer diagnosis of the location and extent of CNS damage not otherwise obtainable. Furthermore, electrophysiologic techniques can replace the neurologic examination in iatrogenically comatose and/or paralysed patients.

Reference

1. Bricolo A, Faccioli F, Turazzi S, Pasut ML (1983) EEG and evoked potentials in brainstem traumatic lesions. In: Villani R, Papo I, Giovanelli M, Gaini SM, Tomei G (ed) Advances in neurotraumatology, pp 79–84. Excerpta Med, Int congr ser no 612. Elsevier Science Publishers B.V.

Author's address: A. Bricolo, M.D., Department of Neurosurgery, University Hospital, Verona, Italy.

Acta Neurochirurgica, Suppl. 36, 90 (1986)

Clinical Assessment of Consciousness

Introduction

B. Jennett

Department of Neurosurgery, The Southern General Hospital, University of Glasgow, Scotland

The last decade has seen clarification in the definition of coma and other altered states of responsiveness (vegetative state, confusion, posttraumatic amnesia). A distinction should be made between hour to hour assessments in the acute stage, as a basis for detecting complications, and assessment on a longer timescale in order to assess the duration of coma and predicting ultimate outcome. Where standardized methods of assessment in the acute stage are used it is now possible to assess the outcome of many patients and that makes it possible to compare the results of alternative methods of management by comparing the outcome of patients whose outlook was predicted to be similar. This also requires simple and standardized classification of outcome. Such classification makes it possible to assess the economic and social impact of injury and so in turn the influence of various management methods on this. The aggregate of disability from the many mildly or moderately injured patients is probably much greater than that of the few severely injured patients who attract most attention both in the acute and in the rehabilitation phase[1].

Reference

1. Jennett B, Teasdale G (1981) Management of head injuries. F. A. Davis Company, Philadelphia, pp 361

Author's address: B. Jennett, Department of Neurosurgery, The Institute of Neurological Sciences, Glasgow G12 4TF, Scotland.

Acta Neurochirurgica, Suppl. 36, 91–94 (1986)

Assessment of Responsiveness in Head Injury Patients

The Glasgow Coma Scale and Some Comments on Alternative Methods

D. Stålhammar[1] and **J. E. Starmark**[1, 2]

[1] Department of Neurosurgery, Sahlgren's Hospital, University of Göteborg, Sweden
[2] Department of Psychiatry III, Lillhagen's Hospital, University of Göteborg, Sweden

Summary

The last twelve years history of coma scaling, *i.e.* reaction level scaling is reviewed. Examples are given of different Glasgow Coma Scale sum scores. The common use of these "sum scores", aggregations of various features, may give an impression of corresponding conscious levels with different functions tested. A more direct approach with mention of varied responses in a reaction level scale may be more reliable and this is also possible to use in a neurological observation chart at bedside.

Keywords: Head injury assessment; mental responsiveness; modernized coma scales; reaction level scales.

Among all systems for assessment of responsiveness in head injury patients the Glasgow Coma Scale (GCS) is the most widely spread[7]. By this scale three features

Table 1. *The Glasgow Coma Scale*

Eye Opening		
spontaneous	E	4
to speech		3
to pain		2
nil		1
Best motor response		
obeys	M	6
localizes		5
withdraws		4
abnormal flexion		3
extensor response		2
nil		1
Verbal response		
orientated	V	5
confused conersation		4
inappropriate words		3
incomprehensible sounds		2
nil		1

Coma score (E + M + V) = 3 to 15

are independently observed: eye opening, motor response, and verbal performance. See Table 1. On the observation chart these three coma scale scores are displayed separately on one chart as seen in Fig. 1.

The Glasgow Coma Scale indeed introduced a new application of the findings during observation for the assessment of impaired responsiveness of head injuries. Its operational definitions are precise, and careful studies of interobserver agreement and of predictive validity have been performed and proved its usefulness[1, 4, 9].

However, the GCS has not been adopted in all countries. In Scandinavia this has been done only in a few clinics, and in Sweden there was a decision 1984 among neurosurgeons and anesthesists to introduce a traditional single line scale[3].

One aspect of the recent twelve years' history of coma scaling is presented in Fig. 2. The GCS was published in 1974 with its three aspects. 1976[8] the GCS sum score appeared, constructed by adding the scores from these aspects, even when one or two features were untestable. Still later these 13 GCS Sum Score levels have been aggregated in various ways as illustrated in Fig. 3.

In scientific studies there is a need to make an overall assessment of responsiveness in order to group the patients in terms of severity. With a scale constructed like the GCS there are however problems when combining the scores from the three components. Although it is not correct simply to add these three nonparametric scores, most investigators still do so. Therefore, although the GCS evidently is a most practical and reliable method for individual patient monitoring and provides very valid information for prediction of outcome when it is used correctly[2], there are some

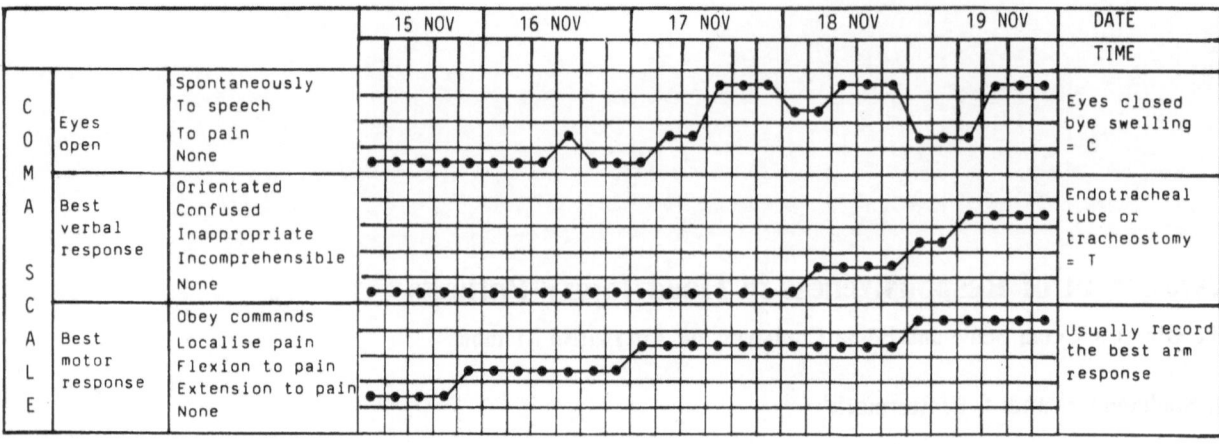

Fig. 1. Observation chart for Glasgow Coma Scale

---

12 years history of assessment of impaired responsiveness

1974[7]	1976[8]	1976–1986	1986
GCS Independently evaluated aspects in *three separate scales:* eye (4), motor (5), verbal (5) "EMV-profile"	The 3 GCS scales *secondarily combined in a sum* [eye (4), motor (6), verbal (5)]	The GCS *sum scores aggregated* in various ways see Fig. 3	*RLS 85* Independently evaluated aspects (eye, motor, verbal and other) *primarily combined in one scale* see Fig. 5
	(4 + 6 + 5) 3–15:		
4 + 5 + 5 levels	*13 levels*	*3 or 4 levels*	*8 levels*

Fig. 2. Twelve years history of coma scaling

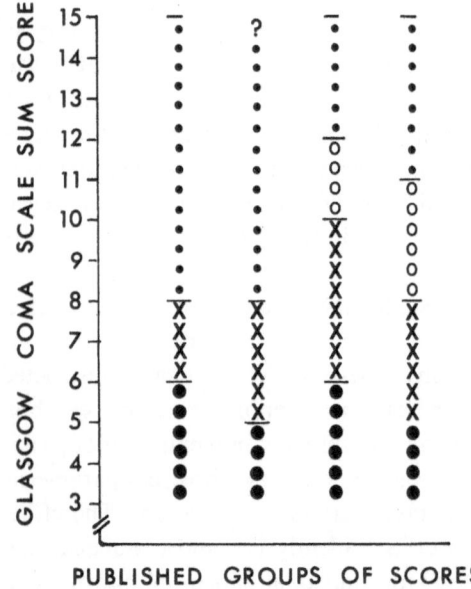

PUBLISHED GROUPS OF SCORES

Fig. 3. Varying aggregation of GCS sum scores

problems regarding its use for assessing overall responsiveness.

The occurrence of untestable features is another source of error when a sum score of several aspects is used. In spite of these problems the GCS sum score is

Reaction level scales (RLS 85)

1 Alert. No delayed response.
2 Drowsy or confused. Response to light stimulation.
3 Very drowsy or confused. Response to strong stimulation.
4 Unconscious. Localizing but does not ward off pain.
5 Unconscious. Withdrawing movements at pain stimulation.
6 Unconscious. Stereotype flexion movements at pain stimulation.
7 Unconscious. Stereotype extension movements at pain stimulation.
8 Unconscious. No response to pain stimulation.

Fig. 4. The Reaction Level Scale presently under investigation in Göteborg regarding its reliability and validity. Operational definitions in Fig. 5

REACTION LEVEL SCALE, RLS 85

1 **Alert.**
No delay in response.

Alert: Not drowsy, orientated.
(Intubated patient: No signs of delay in reaction)

2 **Drowsy or confused.**
Responsive to weak stimulation.
Weak stimulation: Approaching the patient verbally or by touch.

Drowsy: The patient is drowsy if he feels or seems drowsy and shows delay in reaction.

Confused: If the patient gives the wrong answer to at least one of the three questions below, he will be recorded as being confused: a) "What is your name?" (first and second name), b) "Where are you?" (place, e.g. name of town, or "in hospital"), c) "What year and month is it?".

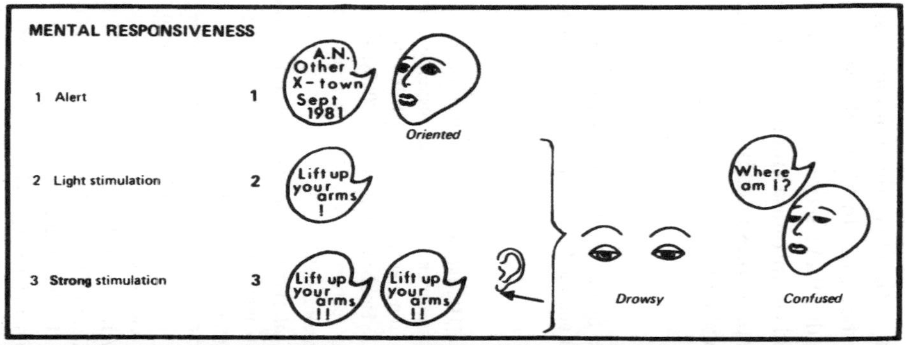

3 **Very drowsy or confused.**
Responsive to strong stimulation.
Strong stimulation: Repeated loud verbal approach, shaking, or pain stimulation.

MENTALLY RESPONSIVE
NOT MENTALLY RESPONSIVE

Mental responsiveness: Arousable. Performs at least one of the following functions: oral response with words – oriented eye movements – obeying commands – warding off pain.

Oriented eye movements: Eye opening with eye contact and some attempt at oriented eye movements.

Obeying commands: At request the patient performs a specific movement, e.g. "Lift up your arms", "put out your tongue", "open/close your eyes"

Warding off pain: The patient localizes pain and makes an active attempt to remove the painful stimulus.

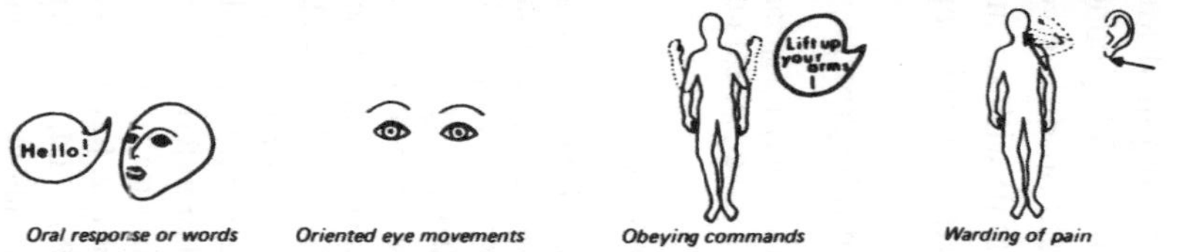

4 **Unconscious.**
Localizes but does not ward off pain.

Unconscious: No response. Cannot perform any activity defined under mental responsiveness.

Localizes pain: The patient is examined lying on his back with arms resting along the sides of his body. a) on retromandibular pain stimulation, the patient moves one hand above chin level, b) on pain stimulation of the fingertips (nailbed) of one hand, the patient moves the other hand across the midline.

5 **Unconscious.**
Withdrawing movements on pain stimulation

Withdrawing movements: a) on retromandibular pain stimulation, the patient turns away his face, or b) on pain stimulation of the fingertips (nailbed), the patient does not localize the pain stimulus but makes clear withdrawing movements.

6 **Unconscious.**
Stereotyped flexion movements on pain stimulation.

Stereotyped flexion movements: a) on retromandibular pain stimulation, or b) on pain stimulation of the fingertips (nailbed), the patient makes slow and mechanical flexion movements of elbows and wrists, but no localizing or withdrawing movements.

7 **Unconscious.**
Stereotyped extension movements on pain stimulation.

Stereotyped extension movements: a) on retromandibular pain stimulation, or b) on pain stimulation of the fingertips (nailbed), the patient makes extension movements, straightening his arms or legs. NB: No flexion movement must be observed. If both flexion and extension movements occur the flexion movement, i.e. the best response will be recorded.

8. **Unconscious.**
No response to pain stimulation.

No response to pain stimulation: On repeated strong pain stimulation, retromandibular or fingertip, the patient does not respond with any movement of either arms, legs or face.

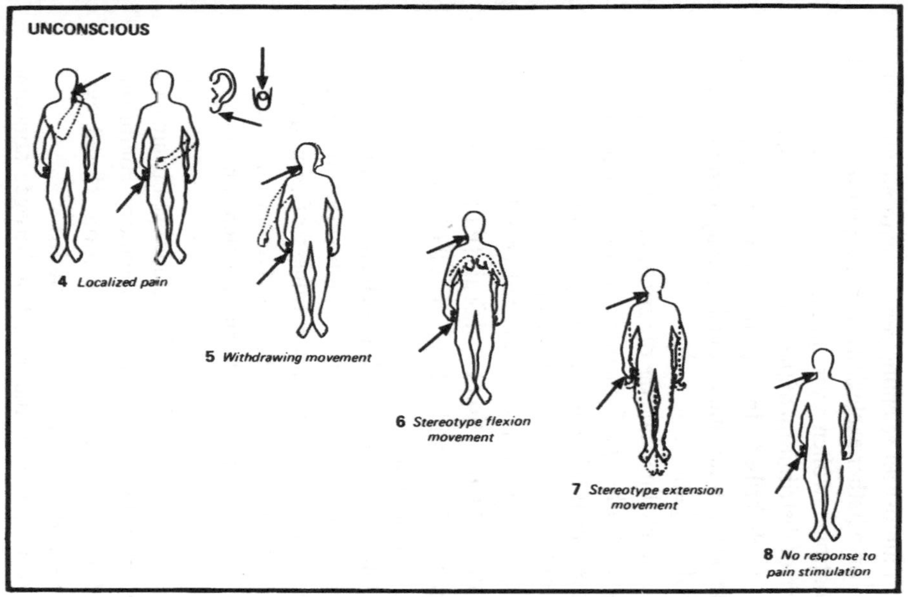

EH, JES, DS, MS, IBS

Fig. 5. The Reaction Level Scale presently under investigation in Göteborg regarding its reliability and validity used in almost all scientific reports without any comments on whether exclusions or pseudoscores are used (intubation, swollen eyes, aphasia etc). Neither the pattern of distribution of the three aspects at each "sum level" is described. In a population of severe head injuries for instance such exclusions may amount to 10–20% of the patients.

In a single line scale the observations of eye, verbal, motor and other performances are directly combined for assessment of the level of responsiveness. Thereby the problems with untestable features may be reduced.

In Göteborg we have elaborated a single line scale in eight steps, the Reaction Level Scale (RLS 85) which is presented in Fig. 4 and in Fig. 5. The RLS 85 is based on the following logics:

1. One single scale with two hierarchially ordered sections. A neuropsychiatric section with three levels, based on latency and purposefulness of response. A motor section with five levels based on motor response (localizing, withdrawal, flexion, extension and no movements to pain).

The definitions of the levels include eye opening and verbal responses but not as obligatory conditions. Therefore "difficult cases" (intubation, closed eyes, dysphasia) do not have to be excluded.

2. A definition of the transition between noncoma and coma to allow for estimation of coma duration.

Although no exclusions will occur with this scale the investigator encounters other difficulties, *i.e.* considering the comparative importance of the different features and assessing which is the actual level of responsiveness. It will depend on the operational definitions used, the kind of personnel and the quality of the instructions, whether acceptable reliability will be achieved with such a single scale. According to our investigations[6] the interobserver agreement is better for RLS 85 than that for the GCS.

Other criticism of the GCS regards its sensitivity for early detection of deterioration[10]. In an analysis of this problem Price and Marsden considered the three factors; interobserver variability, the minimum sensitivity required and the effort to assess the separate features[5]. They concluded that a score span of about 30 should produce a good compromise and they designed the scale with seven aspects presented in "management charts"—in this supplement.

Acknowledgement

This study is supported by Swedish Medical Research Council proj no B86-27X-6613-03B and the Folksam Insurance Company.

References

1. Braakman R, Avezaat CJJ, Maas AIR, *et al.* (1980) Interobserver agreement in the assessment of the motor response of the Glasgow Coma Scale. Clin Neurol Neurosurg 80: 100–106
2. Braakman R, Gelpke GJ, Habbema JDF, *et al.* (1980) Systematic selection of prognostic features in patients with severe head injury. Neurosurgery 6: 362–370
3. Gordon E, Pontén U *et al.* (1984) Behandlingsprinciper för akut skall-hjärnskadade patienter vid sjukhus utan neurokirurgisk expertis. Läkartidningen 81: 1521–1523
4. Jennett B (1979) Predictors of recovery in evaluation of patients in coma. In: Thompson R, Green J (eds) Advances in neurology, vol 22. Raven Press, New York
5. Price, DJ, Marsden AK (1982) A practical coma scale for monitoring head injuries. In: Wilson, Marsden (eds) Care of the acutely ill and injured. J. Wiley and Sons Ltd
6. Starmark J-E, Stålhammar D, Holmgren E, Rosander B Assessment of responsiveness at acute impairment of brain function. A comparison between the Glasgow Coma Scale and the Reaction Level Scale. 1986 in preparation.
7. Teasdale G, Jennett B (1974) Assessment of coma and impaired consciousness. A practical scale. Lancet 2: 81–84
8. Teasdale G, Jennett B (1976) Assessment and prognosis of coma after head injury. Acta Neurochir (Wien) 34: 45–55.
9. Teasdale G, Knill-Jones R, van der Sande J (1978) Observer variability in assessing impaired consciousness and coma. J Neurol Neurosurg Psychiatry 41: 603–610
10. Cranswick T, Smith BJ, *et al.* (1979) Recherche d'une échelle de coma de sensibilité optimale. Le Journal de l'Infirmière de Neurochirurgie 23: 16–20

Author's address: Ass. Prof. D. Stålhammar, Department of Neurosurgery, Sahlgren's Hospital, University of Göteborg, S-413 45 Göteborg, Sweden.

Acta Neurochirurgica, Suppl. 36, 95–102 (1986)

Acute Head Injury

Management Charts

S. Lindgren

Department of Neurosurgery, Sahlgren's Hospital, University of Göteborg, Sweden

Summary

Some guidelines for standardization of management charts for head injured patients are exemplified.

The acute head injury record—"admission chart"—needs special attention to facilitate continuous management of each patient.

The "observation chart" shows traditiōnally more similarity in the different clinics.

The diagnostic terminology and diagnostic classification during management and at discharge of the patients need modernization in relation to ICD and to severity—which is discussed elsewhere in this supplement.

Keywords: Acute head injury; admission charts; observation charts; diagnostic charts.

The need for standardization of judgement of deficits of patients with acute head injuries has been discussed elsewhere in this supplement.

It may be used in the ordinary daily routine according to a similar terminology and type of description at each management level and station a patient may pass in a geographic region.

Here only some examples of practical charts are given as a basis for management decisions, for prediction of outcome and for prediction and detection of complications. They are not primarily considered to be research tools.

Admission Charts

There seems to be a tendency to increase information from the place of accident and during transportation before rhe arrival to the first medical care. This information is usually recorded in the first part of the admission chart and is of extreme importance for later epidemiological studies and prevention of further accidents and injuries.

I. The first admission chart (I) from Gothenburg, used during the last ten years, was made very simple and comprises only one page (Fig. 1).

A. Place of accident, accident type, type of road-user, safety measures used, and object impacting the head are mentioned.

B. The patients condition is then mentioned and related to transportation.

C. Examination of the impact site injury as well as neurological signs and respiratory and cardiovascular findings are reported in the next section and the most important record is on the conscious or reaction level. It should be described rather than codified which here is an application of Glasgow Coma Scales on AIS basis!

D. The last section describes focal symptoms with bilateral differences of extremity power and movement. Eye movements and fixation and abnormalities of pupils are also notified.

This type of admission chart sections will be found better developed in the following more extensive admission charts. An improvement is drawings of the human body and of the head where the location of injuries can be pointed out.

II. The next admission chart (II) is comprising two pages, also from Gothenburg (Fig. 2 a, b).

III. The third admission chart (III) is from Pinderfield Hospital (David Price). The assessment of conscious level is partly an extension of the Glasgow Coma Scale, but considers several other functions, vital functions etc (seven aspects) together 34 scores (Fig. 3 a, b).

IV. The last admission chart (IV) shown here is from Uppsala, Sweden, and is similar to admission chart II (Fig. 4 a, b). In both the conscious or reaction level grading is based on the RLS (Reaction Level Scale) 1–8—(see Stålhammar, this supplement).

RECORD: HEAD INJURIES, ACUTE   ADMISSION CHART I (Gothenburg)

A

Inst., Clinic, Ward, OPD	Pt ID

ACCIDENT | date | time

Place of acc. | age

☐ Home ☐ Work ☐ Other...............   ☐ Male ☐ Female

ACCIDENT TYPE   Information from:

Fall
☐ on the level
☐ from height
☐ steps
☐ after fainting

☐ no information

☐ other..................

Collision
☐ pedestrian
☐ cycle
☐ moped or mc
☐ car driver
☐ passenger front
☐   "   back
☐ safety belt used
☐ helmet

Head impact by
☐ floor, wood, concrete
☐ ground, road surface
☐ windshield
☐ dashboard
☐ steering-wheel
☐ blow?

B

Unconscious   TRANSPORT:...........
☐ at accident   ☐ later   ☐ answers   ☐ moved   ☐ vomited

☐ intoxication?........... ☐ Airway; free   Resp. support:...........

C

EXAMINATION | date | time | ☐ 1st hospital ☐ 2nd hospital | General condition

Head injuries   ☐   ☐   ☐   ☐

Site of impact face frontal occip. right left vertex
                                       side   side

Airway   Intub. ☐

REACTION LEVEL

on request	on pain-movem.	Opens eyes
0 ☐ alert	0 ☐ normal	0 ☐ spontaneous
1 ☐ simple answers drowsy occasionally	1 ☐ agitated movements	1 ☐ to speech; fixation
☐ amnesia PTA RA duration:		
☐ disorientated		
☐ restless, confused		
2 ☐ drowsy, delayed react.	2 ☐ irritated localizing	2 ☐ on command; fixation
3 ☐ irrelevant sounds	3 ☐ withdrawal	3 ☐ to pain
4 ☐ nil	4 ☐ stereotype: -flexion	4 ☐ nil
5 ☐ nil	5 ☐ -extension	5 ☐ nil
6 ☐ nil	6 ☐ nil	6 ☐ nil

Respir. ☐ normal....rate/min
☐ shallow ☐ deep ☐ irreg.

BP   pulse rate

Shock   temp.

Other injuries   Wounds

Previous neurol.dis.

D

FOCAL SYMPTOMS   ☐ Dysphasia   ☐ Pain

Note side differences:
ability to move impaired in
power " "   "   " right left
        arm   ☐   ☐
        leg   ☐   ☐
        face   ☐   ☐

Tonus reduced in
        arm   ☐ . ☐
        leg   ☐   ☐

Plantar resp. - ext.   ☐   ☐

Neck stiffness (caution!) ☐

Eye movements   ☐ follows

☐ fixed forward ☐ deviat. ☐ undul.

Pupils   right   left
    large   ☐   ☐
    small
    equal   ☐

Reaction to light
    direct   ☐   ☐
    indirect   ☐   ☐

Reaction level: _____ Changes?   Measures: Examiner:
Focal symptoms: _____

Fig. 1

Acute Head Injury record   **ADMISSION CHART II** (Gothenburg)

Hospital	Clinic	
Accident day	Hour	
Arrival day	Hour	Age

☐ male ☐ female

Accident - Injury   According to ☐ Patient ☐ Ambulance ☐ Accompanying

		Patient involved		Protective device
1 Work	1 ☐ Pedestrian	0 ☐ No	1 ☐ Pedestrian	0 ☐ None
2 Leisure	2 ☐ Cycle		2 ☐ Cycle	
Fall	3 ☐ Moped		3 ☐ Moped	1 ☐ Seatbelt
1 At same level	4 ☐ MC-driver		4 ☐ MC	
2 From height	5 ☐ MC-pass		5 ☐ Car	2 ☐ Helmet
3 Steps	6 ☐ Car-driver		6 ☐ Lorry	
Fainting	7 ☐ Car-pass frontseat		7 ☐ Bus	3 ☐ Both
1 Assault	8 ☐ " " backseat		8 ☐ Tram	
2 Sports	9 ☐ Others		9 ☐ Others	
3 Other				

Patients condition	awake	"unconscious"	respiratory distress	large hemorrhage	convulsions
Site of accident	1 ☐	2 ☐	3 ☐	4 ☐	5 ☐
During transport	☐	☐	☐	☐	☐
At arrival	☐	☐	☐	☐	☐

pulse ☐   bloodpressure | syst | diast |

Breathing
☐ Normal
☐ Intubation

At arrival (hour   )

Pupils light reaction
1 ☐ Normal
2 ☐ No reaction
3 ☐ Not evaluated

Movement reaction bilat. difference?
☐ No
1 ☐ Right worse
2 ☐ Left worse

Intox/medicine
0 ☐ No
1 ☐ Alcohol
2 ☐ Sedation
3 ☐ Muscle relaxant
4 ☐ Other

REACTION LEVEL SCALE (RLS 82) Reaction level
1 Alert. No delayed response.
2 Drowsy or confused. Arousable at slight stimulation.
3 Very drowsy or confused. Arousable at strong stimulation
4 Unconscious. Localizing but not warding off.
5 Unconscious. Withdrawing at pain stimulation.
6 Unconscious. Stereotype flexion at pain stimulation
7 Unconscious. Stereotype extension at pain stimulation
8 Unconscious. No response to pain.

6 hrs after first evaluation

pupils light
1 ☐ Normal
2 ☐ No reaction
3 ☐ Not evaluated

Movement reaction bilat. difference?
☐ No
1 ☐ Right worse
2 ☐ Left worse

Intox/medicine
0 ☐ No
1 ☐ Alcohol
2 ☐ Sedation
3 ☐ Muscle relaxant
4 ☐ Other

or reaction level	0-6 hrs	6-24 hrs	2-3 day	4-7 day after arrival
best				
worst				

Form checked, sign   Nr ☐   Fil nr ☐☐☐☐   Computerized, sign:

Fig. 2a

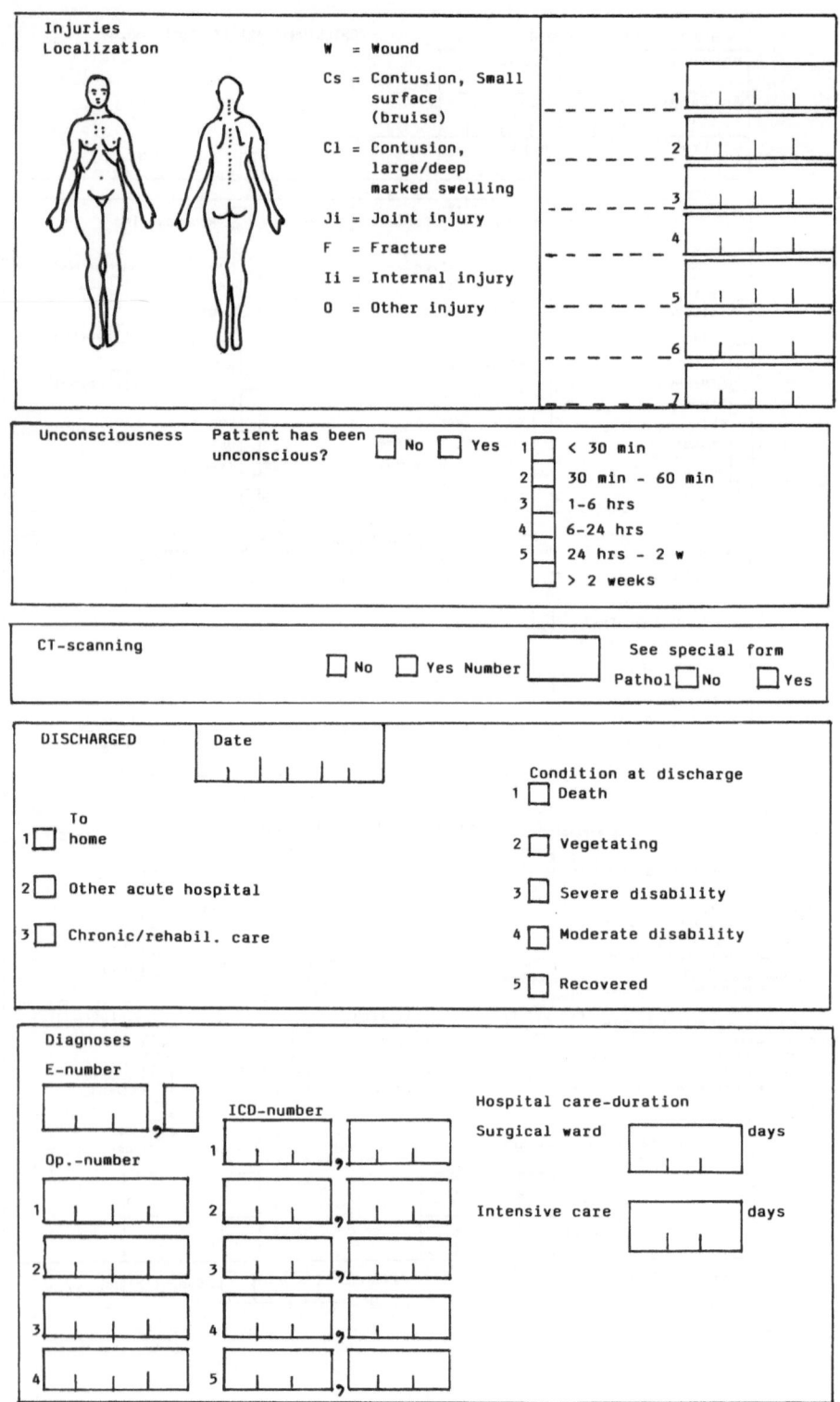

Fig. 2 b (continued from 2 a)

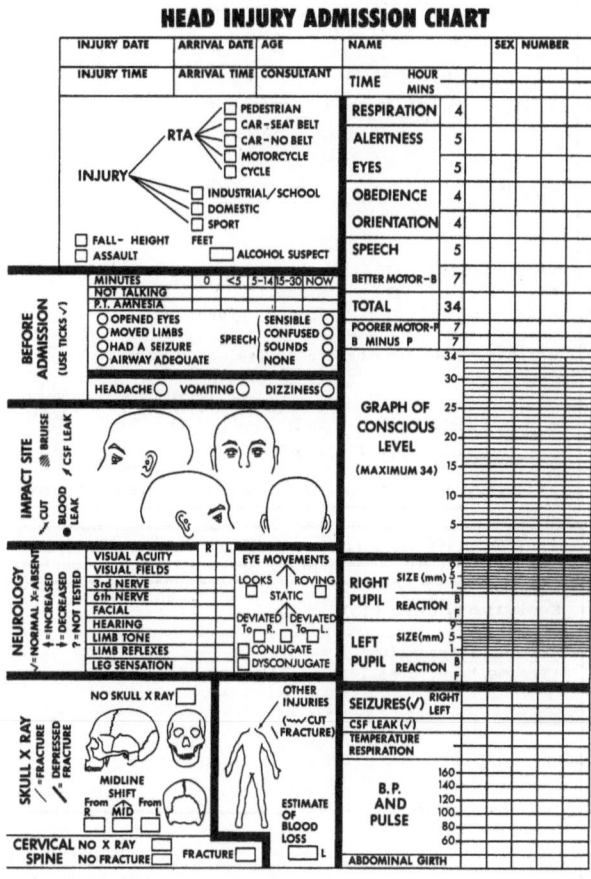

HEAD INJURY ADMISSION CHART

Fig. 3 a (Pinderfields Gen. Hospital—D. Price)

ASSESSMENT OF CONSCIOUS LEVEL

RESPIRATION
4. Normal spontaneous and regular
3. Hyperventilation or shallow but regular
2. Cheyne Stokes (periodic) or variably irregular (ataxic)
1. Inadequate spontaneous ventilation requiring support

ALERTNESS (A measure of rousability shown by flinching facial, respiratory or limb movements)
5. Fully alert — immediately responds to name
4. Drowsy but easily roused by speech or gentle shaking
3. Rousable by shout or firm shaking
2. Unrousable by shout but rousable by superficial pain
1. Rousable by deep pain only
0. Unrousable

EYES
5. Spontaneous eye-opening and looks at people
4. Spontaneous eye-opening but not looking at people
3. Opens eyes in response to normal speech
2. Opens eyes to shout
1. Not looking at people and only opens eyes to pain
0. No eye-opening even to pain

OBEDIENCE
4. Obeys complex commands
3. Immediate appropriate response to simple commands
2. Delayed response to repeated simple commands
1. Doubtful or inappropriate response to simplest commands
0. No obedience to simplest commands

ORIENTATION
4. Fully orientated in all respects with good memory of today's events
3. Aware of who he is and where he is but has poor memory of today's events
2. Moderately confused and uncertain as to where he is
1. Very confused and even unsure of who he is
0. Too drowsy to assess

SPEECH
5. Spontaneous conversation — answering all questions with quite elaborate answers such as 'I am all right apart from my headache'
4. As above but with no spontaneous conversation
3. Answers only simple questions with several appropriate words
2. Answers simple questions with monosyllabic and often inappropriate words
1. Incomprehensible sounds (in response to speech or pain)
0. No sounds in response to speech or pain

BETTER MOTOR RESPONSE (B.M.R)
(Stronger side)
7. Brisk movement with full power or if less conscious, localising immediate purposeful and useful responses (against resistance to pain)
6. Impaired postural maintenance, or some weakness, or if less conscious, sluggish localising purposeful response to pain with effective withdrawal
5. Non-localising effective withdrawal from pain
4. Abnormal flexion with non-purposeful response to pain
3. Brisk extensor posturing without either purpose or effective withdrawal
2. Sluggish extensor posturing without effective withdrawal
1. Only a flicker to pain
0. None

POORER MOTOR RESPONSE (P.M.R.)
(Weaker side)

B.M.R. minus P.M.R.
This gives a measure of the severity of hemiparesis

TOTAL SCORE 34

Fig. 3 b (continued from 3 a)

Acute Head Injury record

ADMISSION CHART IV
AKADEMISKA HOSPITAL, UPSALA

Pat. ID

Accident injury information from

Patient ☐ Ambulance ☐ Accompanying ☐
           personnel

Accident   19   -   -   hr
Found   19   -   -   hr

Accident description:

Traffic accident ☐   Not specified ☐
Other accident ☐   Assault ☐
Fall ☐   Police inform. ☐

Patients condition before arrival to hospital:

	Awake	Unscious	Respiratory distress	Large hemorrh.	Convulsion	Vomiting
At site of accident	☐	☐	☐	☐	☐	☐
During transport	☐	☐	☐	☐	☐	☐

Measures: Resuscitation ☐   Intub. ☐ Ass. ventil.☐   Spont. respir. ☐   Oxygen ☐

REACTION LEVEL (RLS 1-8) at arrival   Acad. hospi. RLS= /   Sign. receiv. nurse

---

Examination by doctor (RLS):   19   -   -   hr

Further information:
(Trauma type, complicating illness)

Right-handed ☐

Susp. intoxication   ☐ What?_____   Left-handed ☐

Ventilation   **Circulation** Blooddpressure ———Pulse———
Normal ☐   Aspiration ☐   Chock ☐ Abdominal _____
Insuff. ☐   Obstruction ☐   circumf.
Forced ☐   Thorac. inj.☐

Skull

Impact site   Blood intraorbit R ☐   L ☐
(Localisation)
                         Blood - ear   R ☐   L ☐

                         Blood from   nose ☐   mouth ☐

                         CSF from   _____

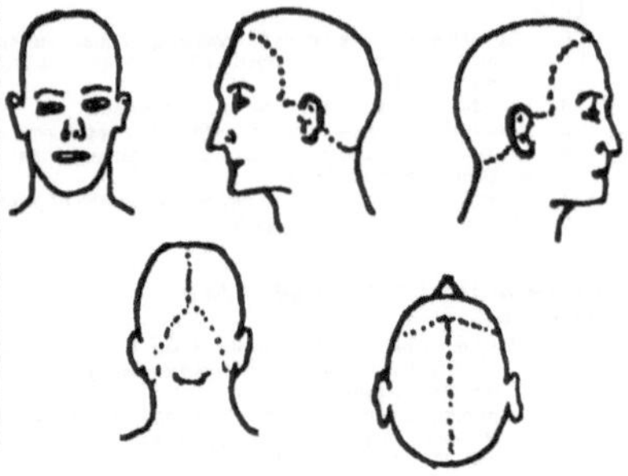

Neck	No	Yes
Neck stiffness	☐	☐
Abnorm.posture	☐	☐
Movem.pain	☐	☐
Tenderness	☐	☐

Fig. 4a

NEUROLOGICAL EXAMINATION:

See encl. Neurological observation chart.

Sensibility impairment marked on Fig. below

Other injuries: Localization in Fig. - Description.

W = Wounds; Cs = Contusion, small surface (bruise)

Cl= Contusion, large/deep, marked swelling

F = Fracture; L = joint injury; Ii = Internal injury; O = Other injury. Which?

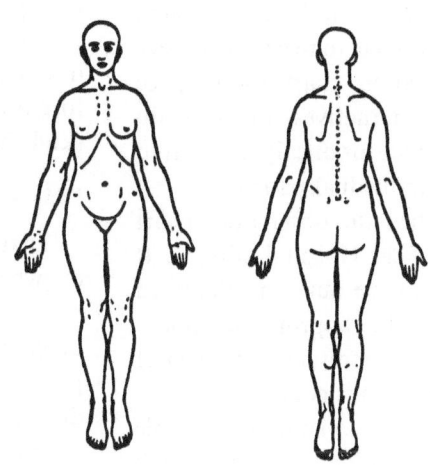

Fig. 4 b (continued from 4 a). Prelim. diagnosis and measures:

NEUROLOGICAL OBSERVATION CHART

SHEET No.
NAME

DATE	MONTH / DAY	
TIME	HOUR / MINS	
RESPIRATION	4	
ALERTNESS	5	
EYES	5	
OBEDIENCE	4	
ORIENTATION	4	
SPEECH	5	
BETTER MOTOR—B	7	
TOTAL	34	
POORER MOTOR—P	7	
B MINUS P	7	

GRAPH OF CONSCIOUS LEVEL (MAXIMUM 34)

34 30 25 20 15 10 5

RIGHT PUPIL — SIZE (mm) 9 5 1 — REACTION B F

LEFT PUPIL — SIZE (mm) 9 5 1 — REACTION B F

SEIZURES(✓) RIGHT LEFT

ICP

TEMPERATURE

RESPIRATION

B.P. AND PULSE

160 140 120 100 80 60

ABDOMINAL GIRTH

Fig. 5 (from Pinderfields Gen. Hospital)

Observation Charts

There is a neurosurgical tradition and care in the wards not only for head injured patients but for all patients, particularly in the postoperative course after intracranial operations. Similar systemic and neurological functions, particularly the so-called vital functions, are examined in a similar way in all clinics. Only the layout will be somewhat different. In some observation charts all functions are graded, from blood pressure, reaction levels, degree of paresis etc to reaction and size of pupils. In other observation charts, less space occupying, the number of alternatives for each observation is given and only space for one figure is left to be filled in in the chart for individual patients.

An example of a part of the latter observation chart is shown here from Pinderfield Hospital (Fig. 5). It requires a good knowledge of the nurses in the ward about the scoring charts and the appropriate choice. Braakman *et al.* in this supplement discuss a number of powerful predictive features and combined scores which must be considered; they also show an example of prediction table for use at bedside at "appropriate" times after trauma.

CT Scanning Evaluation

Due to the increasing importance and frequency of CT scanning in examinations in various hospitals without neurosurgical services as well as for research purposes it has become necessary with standardization charts also regarding findings in CT scanning procedures. The ventricular system, the basal cisterns, shifts of brain tissue, various types of attenuation focal and diffuse as well as revealing different types of hemorrhages etc are mentioned in these charts. Also some types of fractures particularly in the skullbase and anterior and lower part of the head will be elucidated by the investigations.

However, this is partly beyond the scope of this neurosurgical review. The indications for plain X-ray of the skull in the acute stage and later are somewhat different in different hospitals. However, it must not be forgotten that after anterior and vertex impacts to the skull the cervical spine may be involved.

Diagnostic Chart

Diagnostic terminology has already been discussed elsewhere in this supplement. After admission the diagnostic findings may be included in the dynamic diagnostic evaluation of the course of the head injured patient. Particularly at the discharge of the patient the diagnostic standardization is extremely important for international cooperation and comparison in improving the management of the head injury patients.

The international codifying must regard the contents of the diagnostic terms to be reliable and valuable. It must have prognostic as well as management implications.

Author's address: Prof. S. Lindgren, Department of Neurosurgery, Sahlgren's Hospital, University of Göteborg, S-413 45 Göteborg, Sweden.

Acta Neurochirurgica, Suppl. 36, 103–105 (1986)

Is it Possible to Define a General "Conscious Level"?

J. E. Starmark and **S. Lindgren**

Department of Psychiatry III, Lillhagens Hospital, and the Department of Neurosurgery, Sahlgren's Hospital, University of Göteborg, Sweden

Summary

The difficulties in defining a general conscious level are discussed as exemplified by Glasgow Coma Scale and Reaction Level Scale, a new scale recommended by Swedish neurosurgeons. Precise definitions of stimuli and of responses are needed since several studies have shown ambiguity of assessment within the same patient. Some of the difficulties arising from summing up and grouping levels of the Glasgow Coma Scores are discussed and as a consequence a new level for defining coma with a better reliability is proposed. We also briefly discuss the difficulty when to stop assessing conscious level.

Keywords: Consciousness; coma; Glasgow Coma Scale; Reaction Level Scale; inter-rater reliability; coma limit; persistent vegetative state.

There is no good definition of "consciousness" so it is not surprising that much attention has been paid to the question of defining "unconsciousness" or "coma". A good definition would solve many practical, legal and scientific problems.

Some neurosurgeons claim that "one can't be more or less unconscious; it is a question of being in coma or not being in coma".

Judging from that point of view the term "coma scale" would be a misnomer.

At least 40 different scales have been published since Muller's review[2] 1969. In recent years there has been a tendency in the literature to assess several important aspects of responsiveness including an assessment of a conscious level and other important prognostic factors such as different neurological signs and CT-findings etc—all summing up to prognostic scores. The predictive power increases after the inclusion of more factors and as the time epochs after the trauma pass. This paper does not consider the problems of multidimensional scaling and scoring systems—for a recent discussion on the subject see ref 1 and 3.

This discussion will concentrate on some important aspects of assessing conscious level. As examples we have chosen the "Glasgow coma scale (GCS)" published 1974 by Teasdale and Jennet[4] and the "Reaction level scale (RLS)" recommended by Swedish neurosurgeons[5].

The Concept of a Conscious Level

It is widely accepted that there exists a comatose state and that within that state the patients may exhibit different motor reactions after nociceptive stimulation. These reactions have been shown to have high predictive power of prognosis after traumatic and non-traumatic coma states[6, 7]. From direct observation it is obvious that a patient not in coma may display different degrees of somnolence and confusion. The importance of these neuropsychiatric states is that they contribute to the duration of post-traumatic amnesia (PTA).

From these results it seems important to record motor reactions as well as different aspects of somnolence and confusion at each range of reactions recorded to assess overall brain functioning in order to correlate it with overall brain damage.

The GCS and RLS scales are in fact very similar—with few exceptions they evaluate the same aspects of overall brain functioning. Why then are Swedish neurosurgeons unwilling to accept GCS?

Apart from local tradition one main reason might be that it is difficult first to accept the principle of a conscious level and then to abandon the SUM SCORE as an overall measure of brain damage (vide infra).

Teasdale and coworkers showed that the combined contributions of the three subcales of the GCS (Eye, Motor and Verbal) have a better predictive power than the SUM SCORE[9]. How could this astonishing result be possible if one accepts the concept of a conscious level as a basis for severity of brain damage?

The most probable answer is that the different

subscales in the GCS have different error variances of measurement and that the formation of a SUM SCORE has low reliability (this depends on the mathematical fact that the square of error variances is added to create the square of the SUM SCORE error variance).

$$s^2 \text{ (SUM SCORE)} = s^2 \text{ (EYE)} + s^2 \text{ (MOTOR)} + s^2 \text{ (VERBAL)}$$

A practical consequence of this fact is that the same conscious level is represented by different combinations of the three subscales. Another mathematical quality of SUM SCORE is that the number of possible combinations have a maximum in the region of SUM SCORE 8–10, i.e. a group of comatose and noncomatose patients.

Bearing this in mind we propose that the GCS from a theoretical point of view should be a good scale for most severe head injuries and some mild injuries. But we think that nobody has shown that the GCS is adequate for the groups of moderate and some mild head injuries. In fact the discussion in literature between Jagger[10] and the Glasgow group[11] supports our view.

Our conclusion is that if we could use a scale with better reliability of overall functioning it still would be possible to keep to the principle of a conscious level or a reaction level.

Type of Stimuli

Our two examples use different stimulation techniques. In fact in grade 2 and 3 in the RLS, stimuli are defined by "contact by 'talk/touch' and 'shake/shout'". Even the pain stimulation is slightly different—nailbed pressure and supraorbital pressure in the GCS; retromandibular pressure and nailbed pressure in the RLS. Do these differences have any practical consequences? The answer is—we don't know—yet. However it seems quite clear that the type of stimulus and the location of that stimulus on the body have effects on the type and frequency of elicited stereotyped movements[12]. The supraorbital stimulus gives the highest frequencies of responses and a previously bent arm more flexor responses than a stretched arm.

In one of our studies (Starmark, Heath[13]) of intoxications we were able to show that for this etiology the sternal rubbing and retromandibular pressure were significantly better techniques than supraorbital pressure and nailbed pressure in eliciting responses to nociceptive stimuli in coma.

It is not easy to interpret these findings. Of course the etiology of the conditions may have an important impact of the responses—i.e. the pain receptors may have different thresholds for eliciting response in different parts of the body and these receptor thresholds may be differently influenced by toxic agents. However, these findings are an observandum since several studies have shown that about 50–70% of patients with head injuries have an intoxication at admission. Referring again to mild and moderate head injuries, it seems to be very important to know how the impaired consciousness was assessed.

Our conclusion is that too few studies deal with the problem of stimulation techniques. May one of the explanations to the limited predictive power of the GCS in the study of Jaggers[10] depend on the chosen stimulation technique combined with many alcoholics or acute intoxicated patients?

The Reliability of Scales

A good reliability of measurement is a prerequisite for validity and predictive power[4].

In a pilot study[15] we were able to show that the reliability of the three subscales in GCS (with the exception of verbal subscale where only nonintubated patients were assessed) had high reliability which approximately equalled the reliability of RLS. The SUM SCORE only had a moderate reliability.

Defining Coma

In the GCS coma is defined as: no eye opening to pain, not uttering any words and not obeying command indicating a step-level concept at least on this level. This means that all patients with a SUM SCORE less than 7 and about 50% of the patients with SUM SCORE 8 are in coma[16].

For nontraumatic coma a different level has been used for the GCS: Eye opening to pain was permitted; but the patient must not utter any word nor be able to localize pain[8].

The RLS has two coma levels:

a) grade ¾ approximately the same as the one used in Glasgow (criteria: none of i) purposeful warding off pain stimuli, ii) eye opening with fixation, iii) uttering of any word or iv) obey command) and

b) grade $^4/_5$ meaning not be able to localize pain.

No figures of reliability appear in literature concerning coma levels. Preliminary results from intoxications[14] showed low to nonsignificant reliability for all coma levels. This probably reflects both the high variability of patients behaviour at this level and the necessity of combining several requirements in one level. In this respect the single line scale may not have any advantage over the SUM SCORE. Please observe that the definition of coma in GCS has the same effect regarding reliability as forming a SUM SCORE—all three factors must be present at the same time.

The design of a study of reliability of coma levels is very important. This depends on the definition of the coefficient of reliability used and limitations of that coefficient[17].

Our proposal is that a higher reliability would be obtained if the GCS definition of coma was changed to: No eye opening to pain, not any sound to pain and no ability to localize pain. This would be equal to SUM SCORE 6 or lower. The corresponding RLS level is 5.

When to Stop Assessing?

This question is not trivial when considering severe head injuries. It is trivial when the patient dies or is moderately or mildly disabled. But when should one stop recording conscious level when the patient is merging into a persistent vegetative state (which is an outcome category)? Most patients with PVS die in a few weeks or months—and then again the problem is trivial. But the PVS is not a single welldefined syndrome—it is a syndrome of considerable variability[18]. This difficulty is avoided if one stops talking about "conscious levels" and instead starts talking about reaction levels. Perhaps it would be possible to define different PVS: states and thereby maybe elucidate apparent conflict in literature of the eventual PERSISTENCE of "vegetative states"[19].

So we are back to the first question:

IS IT POSSIBLE TO DEFINE A GENERAL CONSCIOUS LEVEL? Our answer is a qualified "Yes" but there are many unsolved problems in using the existing scales both for different severity grades of head injuries and of different etiologies of coma. Much more work ought to be done in defining stimulation and responses, in investigation of long-run reliability of different SUM SCORES of levels, categories and scoring systems in order to achieve better scale construction. Perhaps one should abandon the whole concept of conscious levels and just talk about reaction levels.

Acknowledgement

This study is supported by Swedish Medical Research Council proj no B86-27X-6613-03B and the Folksam Insurance Company.

References

1. Brihaye J, Frowein RA, Lindgren S, Loew F, Stroobandt G (1978) Report on the Meeting of the W.F.N.S. Neuro-Traumatology Committee, Brussels, 19–23 September 1976. Acta Neurochir (Wien) 40: 181–186
2. Müller GE (1974) Classification of head injuries. In: Vinken PJ, Bruyn GW (eds) Handbook of Clinical Neurology, vol 23. North Holland Publ Comp, pp 1–22
3. Anonymous (1983) Panel: Current status of trauma indices. J Trauma 23: 185–201
4. Teasdale G, Jennett B (1974) Assessment of coma and impaired consciousness. A practical scale. Lancet ii: 81–84
5. Starmark JE, Carlsson C, Holmgren E, et al. (1984) Bedömning av medvetande och reaktionsgrad vid traumatiska hjärnskador. Läkartidningen 81: 1528–1529
6. Jennett B, Teasdale G, Braakman R, et al. (1979) Prognosis of patients with severe head injury. Neurosurg 4: 283–289
7. Braakman R, Gelpke GJ, Habbema JDF, et al. (1980) Systematic selection of prognostic factors with severe head injury. Neurosurgery 6: 362–370
8. Levy DE, Caronna JJ, Bates D, et al. (1981) Prognosis in nontraumatic coma. Ann of Int Med 94: 293–301
9. Teasdale G, Murray G, Parker L. (1979) Adding up the Glasgow Coma Score. Acta Neurochir (Wien) [Suppl] 28: 13–16
10. Jagger J, Jane JA, Rimel R (1983) The Glasgow Coma Scale: To sum or not to sum? Lancet ii: 97
11. Teasdale G, Jennett B, Murray L, et al. (1983) Glasgow Coma Scale. To sum or not to sum. Lancet ii: 678
12. Barolat-Romana G, Larson SJ (1984) Influence of stimulus location and limb position on motor responses in the comatose patient. J Neurosurg 61: 725–728
13. Starmark JE, Heath A (1985) Severity grading of intoxications. A comparison between three different coma scales. Manuscript to be published
14. Nunnally JC (1978) Psychometric theory. 2nd ed Mc Graw-Hill Publ Co, New York
15. Starmark JE, Holmgren E, Stålhammar D (1982) Estimation of reaction levels in coma patients. ICRAN
16. Jennett B, Teasdale G (1977) Aspects of coma after severe head injury. Lancet i: 878–881
17. Cohen J (1960) A coefficient of agreement for nominal scales. Educ Psychol Measurement 20: 37–46
18. Jennett B, Plum F (1972) Persistent vegetative state after brain damage. Lancet i: 734–737
19. Shuttleworth E (1983) Recovery to social and economic independence from prolonged postanoxic vegetative state. Neurology 33: 372–374

Author's address: J. E. Starmark, M.D., Department of Psychiatry III, Lillhagens Hospital, University of Göteborg, S-42203 Hisings-Backa 3, Sweden.

Acta Neurochirurgica, Suppl. 36, 106–111 (1986)
© by Springer-Verlag 1986

Factors Restricting the Use of Coma Scales

D. J. Price

Department of Neurosurgery, The General Infirmary, Leeds, Great Britain

Summary

The Glasgow Coma Scale has been well established as the ideal scale for identifying specific levels of consciousness. It is widely used to provide a consistent entry criterion for series of head injuries under study, to create arbitrary thresholds for management decisions and as an important component of the data-set for comparative studies of patients in different centres with specified treatment regimes. Its international reputation for application to these 3 functions is well deserved but the dangers of summing the subscores have been rightly emphasized by the designers. Any further improvements may only cause confusion and it will undoubtedly continue as the recognized standard for many years.

Unfortunately, this scale is very inadequate for monitoring head injured patients at risk of deterioration as it is insufficiently sensitive. The prompt recognition of the first signs of deteriorating consciousness is of paramount importance. A more sensitive scale encompassing more aspects of the response of the patient to the environment is required. For this purpose of trend detection, subscore summation is acceptable and nurses find a single graph easier to interpret.

Keywords: Head injury; coma scale; trends.

Introduction

An alteration in the state of consciousness is the most consistent and characteristic feature of brain damage sustained either as a direct result of acceleration/deceleration trauma or as a consequence of a subsequent complication of such trauma. Half a century ago, Symonds suggested that the duration of unconsciousness might be used as a measure of the degree of cerebral damage after closed head injury[11]. For the last quarter of a century, neurosurgeons have been fascinated by the concept of measuring degrees of consciousness as we continue to support the traditional view that this represents the most important single component of the neurological state. Controversy emanates from the inevitable frustration facing any coma scale designer, as no scale is perfect for every purpose and advantages gained from one aspect of the design are almost invariably counterbalanced by disadvantages from others. The difficulty of expressing the subjective concept of consciousness in objective terms is reflected in the plethora of systems for measuring the so-called "conscious level" that have been proposed over the years[2, 3, 11, 13].

Design Philosophy

The "perfect" scale should be truly linear with a sensitivity related to the requirements and with minimal data redundancy. It should preferably provide a single "number" which accurately represents the proportion of the consciousness remaining and this number should not take into account any associated anatomical or pathological presumptions or any predictive inference (such as "serious"). Words in the coding instructions must be easily understood by the most junior nurse and should relate to what she actually sees and can describe in simple terms. The selection of each subscore should be devoid of any ambiguity by the use of unique and mutually exclusively designations. A change in the score over a course of time should reflect the same equivalent change in consciousness whether it occurs in the lower or the upper part of the scale. A scale must be robust and easily accepted and any trends should be visible at a glance. Inter-observer variability tests should show no more than a 5% inaccuracy. For patients first seen in the emergency department, any scale should facilitate recognition of very mild degrees of disorientation, of variability in alertness or of the suspicion that the patient may not have as yet emerged from his post-traumatic amnesia. A scale should allow for the inevitable missing data due to periorbital hematoma, dysphasia or intubation. Quite clearly, no scale can comply with all these demands and we should perhaps not search for a single "perfect" measurement system for use for all purposes.

Reasons Why Scales Are Required

1. Criteria for inclusion into a series
2. Management decisions
3. Comparative studies
4. Monitoring trends

1. Criteria for Inclusion Into a Series

If one series of head injuries is to be compared with another, the inclusion criteria must be identical. The initial conscious level following any necessary resuscitation is usually considered as the most useful single entry criterion but only a two point (binary) scale is then required. After 3 days of constant and often heated discussion of the Neurotraumatology Committee of the World Federation of Neurosurgical Societies in 1976, we did reach a compromise and this has stood the test of time[4]. Coma may be expressed as a Boolean definition: "No eye-opening in response to pain
and No obedience to any commands
and No recognizable words in response to speech or pain"
A patient is not in coma if:
"Eye-opening in response to speech or pain
or Some obedience to commands
or Recognizable words are spoken when stimulated by speech or pain"
If this definition is not strictly adhered to, comparisons between comatosed head injuries from different centres become virtually impossible. The exclusion of the eye-opening component by workers in one American centre demonstrated the need for identical entry criteria before attempting to compare databases across the Atlantic[1, 6].

The Glasgow Coma Scale (GCS) is more than adequate in providing the information needed for any selected inclusion criteria.

2. Management Decisions

When a patient arrives in a hospital with a head injury, management decisions have to be made within 5 minutes. At this stage, only the conscious level, pupillary signs and crude detection of any lateralizing signs are usually available. In West Yorkshire, this decision is based on a set of Boolean rules. One of these rules is as follows:
"*If* there is respiratory deficiency *or* there are no purposeful motor responses *and* there is no eye opening *and* there is no obedience to commands *then* a blood gas should be taken *and* the patient ventilated on the way to the CT scanner for surgery if necessary *and* he will require intracranial pressure monitoring".

Before the advent of the Glasgow Coma Scale, several workers developed scales with multiple feature definitions. They did have the advantage of simplicity and did provide apparently unambiguous and discrete levels with no necessity for subscore summation. In 1968, this scale was developed for the Birmingham Accident Hospital:

Levels of Response

9. Alert, rational and full orientated
8. Automatism. (Appears fully awake and alert, but gives incorrect information)
7. Drowsy but answers all questions. Mild impairment of orientation
6. Answers simple questions but confused and irritable, obeys most commands
5. Answers only "Yes" or "No". Disorientated, restless and confused. Obeys only simplest commands
4. No obedience to any commands but responds to pain purposefully
3. No obedience to commands and responds to pain without purpose
2. Unrousable by any means
1. Unrousable, no cough reflex and requires artificial respiration.

Such a scale was used for both inclusion and management decisions[10] but when the design was extended beyond those functions, it proved to be inadequate as any subsequent attempts at gaining sensitivity by increasing the number of points on the scale seriously jeopardized the chances of finding patients with particular feature combinations and it was not unusual to be unable to "fit" a particular patient into a single level.

In contrast, the alternative design philosophy of scoring separately for each component aspect of the conscious level with an option of adding the subscores seemed the only way forward.

The Glasgow Coma Scale provides the information relating to the conscious level for management decisions very adequately. The only danger arises when attempts are made to summate the subscores and it is for this reason that our colleagues in Glasgow have rightly resisted the temptation to graph the summation or imply that any specific level of the summed score can be used with impunity[15].

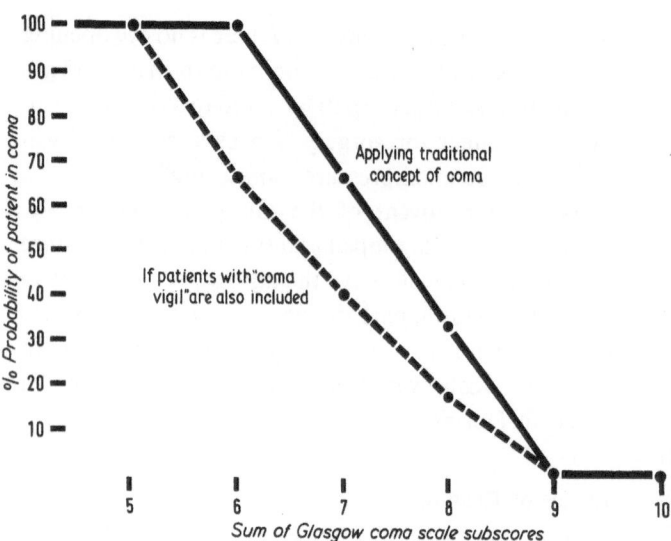

Fig. 1. This graph illustrates the danger of using the sum of Glasgow Coma subscores to identify patients in coma. Those with sums below 6 and above 8 are all either certainly in or certainly not in coma

To illustrate this, a graph (Fig. 1) of the probability of a patient being in coma with sums derived from any compatible combination of GCS subscores confirms that we can neither claim that all patients below a certain coma scale sum can be deemed to be in coma nor all those above that threshold be considered to be not in coma.

3. Comparative Studies

When comparing the management of one group of head injuries with that of another, it is important that the patients in each group have comparable initial conscious levels. The presumption in Birmingham that there were only 9 possible levels proved adequate for the unambitious comparative study of outcomes of head injury survivors with and without early hypoxia and hypotension[10]. Jennett and Teasdale rightly presume that more levels were needed[13]. Unfortunately, group allocation requires subscore summation and this inevitably results in discrepancies particularly for patients not in coma. (For those not in coma the number of possible subscore combinations is twice that of those in coma.) The Glasgow Coma Scale has been carefully designed and its sensitivity and fidelity are entirely appropriate for its original purpose as a tool for comparing the original conscious level and its subsequent course on groups of head injuries[14]. Its international acceptance enhances its value further provided we are not tempted to indiscriminately sum the subscores. It will undoubtedly continue unrivalled for

several further decades as a valuable tool for research workers. It has failed to overcome the problem of patients intubated, dysphasic or with periorbital hematoma and this may be one of the reasons why verbal and eye scores prove to be relatively poor predictors of outcome as compared with motor scores[5].

4. Trend Monitoring

A. *Patients already in Coma.* The term "Coma Scale" infers an ability to quantify varying grades of coma. The need to monitor minor changes in the degree of coma is less critical than the need for trend recognition of patients with less severe impairment of consciousness. All patients rendered comatosed as a result of a head injury qualify for an immediate CT scan as the hematoma risk is so high[8].

In many neurosurgical units, those in deep coma are routinely paralysed and ventilated and this then destroys all ability to measure changes in levels of coma. For those not ventilated, the 1978 modification of the GCS[6] has adequate sensitivity for monitoring these patients and any improvement in this would only require the inclusion of some simple information concerning the ability to maintain ventilation. This addition would increase the chances of an inexperienced nurse being alerted to dangerous risks of a patient developing hypoxia. From the already discussed definition of coma, the total eye and verbal scores remain below 4 and the number of possible combinations of all three subscores to produce sums up to 7 cannot exceed 10.

B. *Patients not in Coma.* For the monitoring of patients not in coma (and perhaps representing some 95% of the total number of head injuries in Europe), I believe that the Glasgow Coma Scale is totally inadequate as it is far too insensitive and does not allow for recognition of the early signs of an expanding hematoma or other complications. This hazard is accentuated if the patient is observed in a primary surgical ward with no CT or neurosurgical operative facilities immediately at hand. To safeguard against such potential tragedies, the nurses in a neurosurgical ward in Yorkshire devised in 1973 a 50-point scale using 12 subscores[3]. Minor changes were subsequently made in response to the introduction of the Glasgow Coma Scale a year later as we considered it essential to allow translation of that scale for comparative studies. Although in constant use in several general hospitals since that time, the medical staff (but not nursing) initially considered its apparent complexity might jeopardize acceptance.

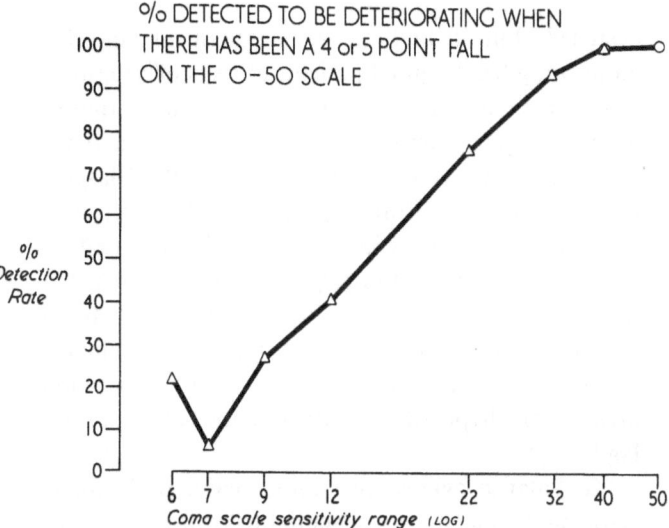

Fig. 2. The relationship between the sensitivity range of the coma scale used and the chance of detecting deterioration. Detection is defined as a one or more point fall on the cruder scales when a 4 or 5 point fall has been recorded on the 50 point scale

Several coma scales had been rigorously tested for inter-observer variability, robustness and data redundancy but no scale can be tested against itself for sensitivity without a "gold standard" scale with a higher acuity to compare it with. It is ironical that the GCS has been carefully developed and tested for one purpose and then more widely used for a completely different purpose without any attempts to challenge its capability or safety for the demands of a very different function—that of trend detection at the bedside. We had, however, a perfect opportunity to test various other scales in use against that of the 0–50 scale (Fig. 2). The subscores of a group of patients with deteriorating conscious level were translated by a computer programme to other scales. To our amazement, we found that if a patient has a 4 or 5 point fall on the 50 point scale, there is only a 40% chance of it being demonstrated on the GCS scale by just one point. This figure compared with 90% for a then newly designed 0–34 scale (Fig. 3)[9]. The 4 or 5 point fall more than compensated for the demonstrated intrinsic "noise" of observer variability of a sensitive scale (shown to be plus or minus 2 points). The 34 point scale with its 7 subscores seemed to have the optimum safe sensitivity and was introduced to Accident and Emergency Departments in Yorkshire who were anxious to have

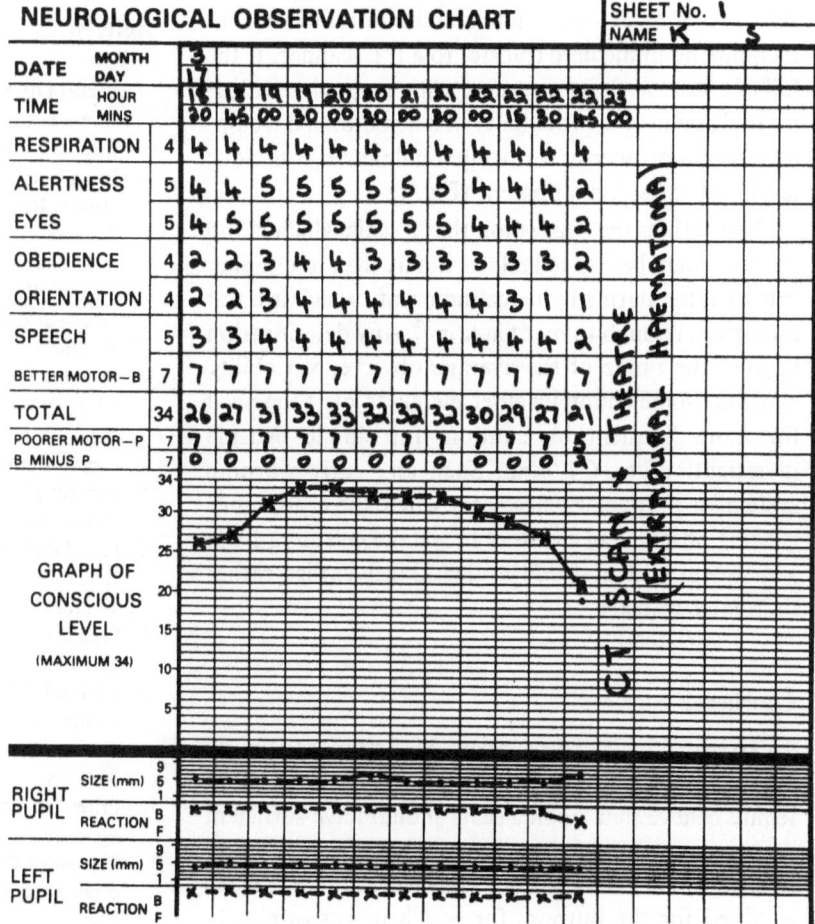

Fig. 3. A head injury observation chart using the 0–34 scale. The patient initially improved and then deteriorated slightly. The nurses responded by observing more frequently allowing earlier recognition of the subsequent significant fall in consciousness

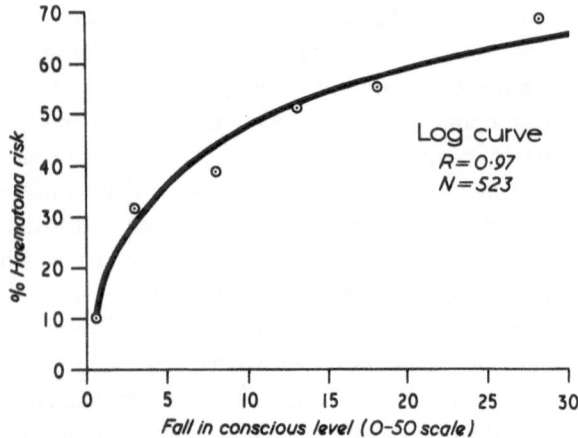

Fig. 4. From a study of 523 patients transferred to a neurosurgical unit, the probability of harbouring a hematoma is related to the preceding magnitude of conscious level fall

the advantages of a single "see at a glance" graph over to the 3 graph data presentation of subscores of the GCS (Fig. 3). It soon became apparent that a 1 point fall should initiate more frequent observations and a 2 point fall to alert a doctor who would consider an ultrasound examination for measurement of midline shift. A 3 or 4 point fall should be sufficient to recommend immediate transfer to a CT scanner. If the fall of conscious level measured with a sensitive scale is plotted against the probability of a hematoma developing, the importance of relatively small falls in conscious levels becomes very apparent (Fig. 4).

This refutes the suggestion that a scale which is too sensitive may be less reliable as it may lead to a higher rate of false alarms by detecting events which are not important enough to merit action[12]. Any deterioration beyond the range of the average observer variability warrants some action whether merely to alert the need for more frequent observation, for simple bedside investigations or CT scan. Such an "early warning system" is particularly necessary where the head injury is being observed in a district hospital some miles from a neurosurgical unit and it encourages earlier rather than later transfer.

Conclusion

To a practicing neurosurgeon, his first responsibility is to the safety of his patients. It is for this reason that I firmly believe that a coma scale should have sufficient sensitivity to be used at the bedside to allow early recognition of deterioration. The Glasgow Coma Scale is suited for the purpose for which it was originally

designed, but if used as a measurement tool for monitoring head injured patients at risks of deterioration, some alternative is required. Such an alternative does not require international agreement and standardization but must be easily translatable to the Glasgow Coma Scale for research purposes. More sensitive scales do not compete with the GCS as they are used for entirely different functions. It has been suggested that to ask our nurses to use the GCS for early trend recognition of patients vulnerable after a head injury is as insulting as asking them to measure the blood pressure of a hypovolemic patient to the nearest 25 mm Hg.!

To balance against this rather naive and almost arrogant statement, it is essential to review conscious level changes within the context of all other information about that patient as the other indicants may well have over-riding predictive powers of a complication. It is particularly important not to consider a patient as unlikely to have a hematoma just because there is no fall or even if there is a rise in carefully measured conscious level.

References

1. Becker DP, Miller JD, Ward JD, et al. (1977) The outcome from severe head injury with early diagnosis and intensive management. J Neurosurg 47: 491–502
2. Brihaye J, Frowein RA, Lindgren S, Loew F, Stroobandt G (1978) Report on the Meeting of the W.F.N.S. Neuro-Traumatology Committee, Brussels, 19–23 September 1976. Acta Neurochir (Wien) 40: 181–186
3. Cranswick T, Smith LJ, Cowell NM (1979) Recherche d'une echelle de coma de sensibilite optimale. J l'Infirm Neurochir 23: 16–20
4. Frowein RA (1976) Classification of coma. Acta Neurochir (Wien) 35: 5–10
5. Jagger J, Jane JA, Rimel R (1983) The Glasgow Coma Scale: To sum or not to sum? Lancet 2: 97
6. Langfitt TW (1978) Measuring the outcome from head injuries. J Neurosurg 48: 673–678
7. Price DJ (1976) Analogue to digital conversion of consciousness. In: Proceedings of Society of British Neurological Surgeons. J Neurol Neurosurg Psychiatry 39: 919
8. Price DJ (1985) Principles of managing intracranial injuries. Care Crit Ill 1: (5) 3–5
9. Price DJ, Marsden AK (1982) A gap practical coma scale for monitoring head injuries. In: Wilson DH, Marsden AK (eds) Care of the acutely ill and injured. John Wiley & Sons Ltd, pp 353–358
10. Price DJ, Murray A (1972) The influence of hypoxia and hypotension on recovery from head injury. Injury 3: 218–224
11. Symonds CP (1928) The differential diagnosis and treatment of cerebral states consequent upon head injuries. Br Med J 4: 829–832

12. Teasdale G, Gentleman D (1982) The description of "conscious level": A case for the Glasgow Coma Scale. Scot Med J 27: 7–9

13. Teasdale G, Jennet B (1974) Assessment of coma and impaired consciousness. Lancet 2: 81–84

14. Teasdale G, Knill-Jones R, Van Der Sande J (1978) Observer variability in assessing impaired consciousness and coma. J Neurol Neurosurg Psychiatry 41: 603–610

15. Teasdale G, Murray G, Parker L, *et al.* (1979) Adding up the Glasgow Coma Scale. Acta Neurochir. (Wien) [Suppl] 28: 13–16

Author's address: D. J. Price, F.R.C.S., Department of Neurosurgery, The General Infirmary, Leeds, Great Britain.

Acta Neurochirurgica, Suppl. 36, 112–117 (1986)
© by Springer-Verlag 1986

Prognosis and Prediction of Outcome in Comatose Head Injured Patients

R. Braakman[1], **J. D. F. Habbema**[2], and **G. J. Gelpke**[2]

[1] Departments of Neurosurgery and [2] Public Health and Social Medicine, Erasmus University Rotterdam, University Hospital Rotterdam "Dijkzigt", Rotterdam, The Netherlands

Summary

Recent studies on the prognosis of comatose head injured patients have identified single powerful prognostic features at various time points during the first month after onset of coma. Using appropriate statistical methods even more powerful combinations of prognostic features can be selected. At each time point, optimal prediction requires sets of only 3 to 5 features. These features include depth and duration of coma as assessed by the Glasgow Coma Scale, pupil reactivity to light, age in decades, and spontaneous and reflex eye movements. In individual new patients, bedside predictions are now possible, e.g. using a booklet with prognosis tables like the one used in Rotterdam. Doctors actually learn by using these tables as they retain some of the information. However, the main application is that these tables permit one to evaluate whether differences in survival rates in different centres with different management regimes are due to a difference in management efficacy or to a difference in initial severity of injury.

Keywords: Comatose head injuries; outcome head injury; prognostic features.

Introduction

In the last 15 years various research groups have identified prognostic features in groups of patients with severe head injury[2, 3, 5, 9, 16, 18–20, 24, 30–32]. Jennett et al.[18–20] were the first to explore the possibility of predicting outcome in individual patients. They emphasized that this is only possible, if population, potential predictive criteria, outcome categories, and the time points when predictive features are scored and outcome is assessed, are sharply defined[18, 20]. Moreover, a homogeneous population of a large number of severely head injured patients had to be studied and their outcome established.

Databanks of comatose head injured patients, prospectively studied and scored, were established. The International Databank, containing data on head injured patients in coma for at least 6 hours, with Rotterdam as one of the five participating centres, was established in 1972[5, 20, 21]. The American National Traumatic Coma Databank followed in 1979[15, 26]. Smaller studies were based on populations of individual centres[4, 9, 16, 28, 30–32, 43].

In this review, the results of analysis of the International Databank will be presented with special reference to the analysis of the Rotterdam population.

Single Prognostic Features

Individual features of prognostic value can be identified by comparing the scores of these features, attained at (or before) a certain time point after onset of traumatic coma with mortality and/or morbidity, e.g. after 6 months or a year[5, 9, 16, 20, 29, 30, 40].

Important clinical prognostic features are the level and duration of unconsciousness and the degree of dysfunction of the brainstem[3, 5, 20, 28].

In comatose patients the sumscore of two or three of the aspects of the Glasgow Coma Scale[18, 37] is one of the three most powerful predictive variables at every time point during the first month after onset of traumatic coma: not only on admission, but also after 1, 3, 7, 14, and 28 days[3, 5, 11, 19, 20, 38, 39].

In the first week, motor response is the most powerful predictor of death or survival. In survivors, after 2 and 4 weeks, verbal response is an important predictor of the degree of remaining disability.

As an example, the relationship between coma sumscore on admission and mortality after 6 months for 305 Rotterdam patients in the IDB is given in Table 1.

A very powerful individual prognostic feature is age[3, 5, 8, 9, 16, 20, 24, 28, 30, 32, 40]. We can confirm the

Table 1. *Relationship Between the Coma Scale Sumscore Observed on Admission and Mortality After 6 Months*

Coma scale sumscore	No. patients	Mortality rate (%)
3	28	90
4	49	77
5	26	61
6	82	46
7	54	40
8	26	33
9–10	3	67
11–15	18	67

In 19 cases, the sumscore could not be established because one of the three aspects of the scale could not be scored due to, *e.g.* edema of eyelids, intubation, etc.

Table 2. *Relationship Between Age and Mortality After 6 Months*

Age (years)	No. patients	Mortality rate (%)
0– 9	47	38
10–19	72	38
20–29	39	44
30–39	34	65
40–49	33	67
50–59	31	81
60–69	27	78
70 +	22	91
Total	305	56

Table 3. *Relationship Between Best Pupil Reaction to Light After Onset of Coma During the First 24 Hours and Mortality After 6 Months*

Pupil reaction	No. patients	Mortality rate (%)
Both reacting	150	37
One reacting	37	57
Both nonreacting	105	83
Unknown*	13	61

* In 13 cases the pupil reactions could not be assessed because of orbital hematoma or severe edema of the eyelids.

relationship between increasing age and mortality (Table 2). Older patients are more likely to develop extracranial medical complications more than 24 hours after injury[22], complications such as respiratory failure and infection, and those often prove fatal.

Another very important prognostic feature related to mortality, which has been known for many years, is pupil reactivity to light, negative pupil reactions indicating dysfunction in the rostral brainstem[1–3, 5, 19, 20, 28]. The relationship between mortality after 6 months and pupil reactivity to light on admission for the 305 Rotterdam patients is presented in Table 3.

Other brainstem responses with great predictive power during the first week are eye movements, either spontaneous or reflex, like vestibulo-ocular and cephalo-ocular responses[5, 20, 44].

Born *et al.*[3] recently drew attention to the prognostic value of five brainstem reflexes: fronto-orbicular, vertical oculo-vestibular, pupillary light, horizontal oculo-vestibular and oculo-cardiac, disappearing in this order during rostro-caudal deterioration. These authors added the sumscore of the brainstem responses to the Glasgow Coma Sumscore thus producing a Glasgow Liège Score (GLS), and claimed improvement of precision of prognosis.

In addition to certain clinical features, other characteristics also proved to very powerful predictors: assessing evoked potentials[13, 14], evaluating computer tomograms[12, 25, 29, 42, 45], electro-encephalograms[6, 36], levels of intracranial pressure[12, 27–29] and laboratory values, such as blood gases, serum osmolality and blood sugar levels[1, 10, 33].

Prediction of Outcome

Prediction of outcome always involves the time at which prediction is made, the time of outcome, and the outcome categories.

For the purposes of this study, we made predictions on admission and after 1, 3, 7, 14, and 28 days. Outcome was assessed 6 months after injury and was classified according to the five categories of the Glasgow Outcome Scale[17, 23]. Shortly after injury it may be possible to predict with a reasonable degree of accuracy whether the patient will survive or die, but not whether a surviving patient will be severely or moderately disabled or will recover. Therefore, for predictions on admission and after 24 hours, two outcome categories are distinguished: dead and alive; after 3, 7, and 14 days, three categories: dead, poor (vegetative and severely disabled) and good (moderately disabled and recovery). After 28 days, in survivors, it is possible to classify predictions into four categories.

For reliable prediction of outcome in individual patients we cannot depend upon the prognostic value of one feature only. Patients may have conflicting scores of individual features; for example, a patient of 20 years of age (indicating relatively favourable prognosis), with bilateral nonreacting pupils (forecasting poor prognosis). Predictions prove to have a higher degree of accuracy and reliability of they are based on the combined scores of two or even more powerful predictive features [5, 29, 34]. For the systematic selection of powerful combinations of features, various statistical models are available, which take into account combined scores of three or more features [5, 7, 29, 35]. The use of different models may result in a different level of significance of the various predictive features. The really important ones, however, will be apparent with all models. A comparative study of several statistical models [41] reveals that the independent multivariate multinomial model performs quite well with the data of the International Databank. We use the common stepwise forward method for selection of features [5]. The object of the selection procedure is to select from the excess of information available in the databank, a small subset of features containing nearly all of the prognostic information, as measured by the quality of the corresponding probabilistic prognosis rule. We have developed a computer programme that performs this selection by the stepwise forward method [5]. The patient's prognosis was assessed using a rule that excludes his own information as a reference patient. A measure of the quality of the rule was obtained by comparing the prediction with actual outcome. The exact composition of the selected features is determined from the 305 reference patients available. It proved to be possible to identify at each time point after injury just such a small "subset" of features which contains nearly all prognostic information. The number of these features, which in combination gives the best forecast of outcome, proves to be small: at each time point 3 to 5.

Addition of another feature does not improve prediction quality. The most powerful combinations at 1, 3, 7, 14, and 28 days of onset of coma, predicting 6 months outcome in Rotterdam, on the basis of the results of the previous 305 Rotterdam patients, is given in Table 4.

Comparable analyses, sometimes using another statistical model, have been carried out in other populations of comatose head injured patients [9, 16, 24, 28–31]. A slightly different set of features may be selected, but in all series thus far reported, there is little change in the composition of the most powerful predictive clinical features. Such a combination commonly contains: age, a combination of the three aspects of the Glasgow Coma Scale, pupil reactivity to light, eye movements— either spontaneous or elicited, the presence of improve-

Table 4. *Most Powerful Combinations of Variables Predicting 6 Months Outcome in the 305 Rotterdam Patients, Selected by the Stepwise Forward Method, at Various Time Points After Onset of Coma*

Time point	Most powerful combination of features
24 hours	age worst motor response of the best arm during first 24 hours best pupil reaction during first 24 hours
Day 3	age best E + M sumscore of the GCS during days 2–3 best pupil reaction during days 2–3
Day 7	age best E + M + V sumscore of the GCS during days 4–7 best pupil reaction during days 4–7
Day 14	age best E + M + V sumscore during days 8–14 best pupil reaction during days 8–14
Day 28	age best verbal response during days 15–28 best motor response of the best arm during days 15–28

ment or deterioration in conscious level, and the presence of a surgical mass.

Prediction in Practice

The predictions are probabilistic: a probability value is assigned to each of the possible outcome categories. These probabilities add up to 1. In Table 5 an example is given of predictions in two patients A and B. The probability of death in patient A (39%) means that four out of every ten patients with the same scores as patient A are going to die and six are going to survive. In patient B, however, the probability of death (94%) means that more than nine out of ten patients in this clinical condition have died. Such a prediction, with a

Table 5. *Example of Predictions in Two Patients, A and B*

	Patient A	Patient B
Probability of		
— death	0.39	0.94
— poor survival*	0.40	0.05
— good survival*	0.21	0.01

* Poor survival is vegetative and severely disabled, good survival is moderately disabled and good recovery.

probability over the threshold of *e.g.* 90% allocated to one outcome category is called "sharp prediction". The percentage of sharp predictions depends upon the number of outcome categories used and on the threshold value (80%, 90% or 95%, etc). If a threshold value of 90% is chosen, at least 90% of these predictions should be correct.

Increase in the level of the threshold and in the number of outcome categories results in a decreased percentage of sharp predictions. The percentage increases with time elapsed since onset of coma. On admission, *e.g.*, a few hours after the accident, it is only possible to make sharp predictions of death in very elderly patients. After 24 hours and 3 days, sharp predictions are possible only when two outcome categories are used: death and survival. On day 28 sharp predictions are possible using five outcome categories.

Prediction Aid

The aim of a prediction aid is to have an easily applicable bedside tool. The fact that only a limited number of features is selected at each time point allows one to use various types of tools at the bedside to estimate the patient's chances of survival and degree of recovery at each time point.

a) A pocket calculator with a simple computer programme, which is used in Glasgow.

b) A chart, like the one published by the Richmond group[7].

c) A booklet with tables, like the one used in Rotterdam (Table 6).

Tables are easy, generally available and understandable. The booklet used in Rotterdam, contains tables for various moments after onset of coma, using the subset of the most powerful combination of three predictive features at that moment. Table 6 contains an example of a prediction table 3 days after onset of coma. *E.g.* a patient aged 42 years, with a best eye and motor sumscore of 6 and one reacting pupil, has a probability of 44% of 6 months' survival. It is very easy to check how the prediction will change for a patient who differs with regard to the score of one of the indicators.

Clinical judgement without such a prediction aid varies greatly, even when the clinicians are considerably experienced. Using the tables has an instructive function, as the doctors actually retain some of the information. The tables provide information on whether the patient's chances of survival during his posttraumatic course are improving or deteriorating.

Table 6. *Time of Prediction: 3 Days After Onset of Coma. Probabilities of 6 months' Survival*

Age	Eyes + motor score (best state during days 2–3)	Pupil reaction (best state during days 2–3)		
		neither reacts	one reacts	both react
0–19	2, 3	0.03	0.07	0.42
	4, 5	0.26	0.50	0.86
	6	0.47	0.74	0.94
	7, 8, 9	0.73	0.89	0.97
	10	0.69	0.85	0.98
20–29	2, 3	0.02	0.07	0.28
	4, 5	0.15	0.39	0.70
	6	0.27	0.61	0.85
	7, 8, 9	0.51	0.79	0.92
	10	0.58	0.83	0.96
30–49	2, 3	0.01	0.04	0.17
	4, 5	0.10	0.28	0.61
	6	0.15	0.44	0.76
	7, 8, 9	0.40	0.71	0.89
	10	0.41	0.73	0.93
50–69	2, 3	0.00	0.01	0.07
	4, 5	0.03	0.10	0.34
	6	0.08	0.23	0.57
	7, 8, 9	0.18	0.43	0.73
	10	0.20	0.44	0.82
70 +	2, 3	0.00	0.01	0.03
	4, 5	0.02	0.07	0.24
	6	0.03	0.11	0.35
	7, 8, 9	0.12	0.34	0.65
	10	0.09	0.29	0.68

Example of a page of the probability tables used as an aid in the prediction of outcome for comatose head injury patients in Rotterdam.

This allows more rational management decisions. The information is also extremely valuable when dealing with the family, who is not so interested in what we are doing, but in improvement or deterioration and in the ultimate outcome. In this respect, a high rate of sharp predictions, predictions with a low degree of doubt, is desirable. Prediction aids permit one to evaluate whether differences in survival rates in different centres with different management regimes are due to the difference in management efficacy or to differences in initial severity of injury. Of the 18% difference in survival rate between two series of head injured patients in the Netherlands, 10.5% of this proved to be due to differences in injury severity on admission[11].

References

1. Auer L, Gell G, Richling B, Oberbauer R (1979) Predicting outcome after severe head injury—a computer-assisted analysis of neurological symptoms and laboratory values. Acta Neurochir (Wien) [Suppl] 28: 171–173

2. Becker DP, Miller JD, Ward JD, Greenberg RP, Young HF, Sakalas R (1977) The outcome from severe head injury with early diagnosis and intensive management. J Neurosurg 47: 491–502

3. Born JD, Albert A, Hans P, Bonnal J (1985) Relative prognosis value of best motor response and brain stem reflexes in patients with severe head injury. Neurosurgery 16: 595–601

4. Bowers SA, Marshall LF (1980) Outcome in 200 consecutive cases of severe head injury treated in San Diego County: a prospective analysis. Neurosurgery 6: 237–242

5. Braakman R, Gelpke GJ, Habbema JDF, Maas AIR, Minderhoud JM (1980) Systematic selection of prognostic features in patients with severe head injury. Neurosurgery 6: 362–370

6. Bricolo A, Turazzi S, Facciolo F (1979) Combined clinical and EEG examinations for assessment of severity of acute head injuries. Acta Neurochir (Wien) [Suppl] 28: 35–39

7. Choi SC, Ward JD, Becker DP (1983) Chart for outcome prediction in severe head injury. J Neurosurg 59: 294–298

8. Frowein RA (1979) Prognostic assessment of coma in relation to age. Acta Neurochir (Wien) [Suppl] 28: 3–11

9. Frowein RA, Haar K auf der, Terhaar D (1980) Assessment of coma reliability of prognosis. Neurosurg Rev 3: 67–74

10. Gaab M, Trost HA, Pflughaupt KW (1979) The prognostic value of osmolality within the first week of sustaining head injury. Acta Neurochir (Wien) [Suppl] 28: 115–119

11. Gelpke GJ, Braakman R, Habbema JDF, Hilden J (1983) Comparison of outcome in two series of patients with severe head injuries. J Neurosurg 59: 745–750

12. Gennarelli TA, Spielman GM, Langfitt TW, Gildenberg PL, Harrington T, Jane JA, Marshall LF, Miller JD, Pitts LH (1982) Influence of the type of intracranial lesion on outcome from severe head injury. J Neurosurg 56: 26–32

13. Greenberg RP, Becker DP, Miller JD, Mayer DJ (1977) Evaluation of brain function in severe human head trauma with multimodality evoked potentials: Part II. Localization of brain dysfunction and correlation with posttraumatic neurological conditions. J Neurosurg 47: 163–177

14. Greenberg RP, Mayer DJ, Becker DP, Miller JD (1977) Evaluation of brain function in severe human head trauma with multimodality evoked potentials: Part I. Evoked brain-injury potentials, methods, and analysis. J Neurosurg 47: 150–162

15. Gross CR, Wolf C, Kunitz SC, Jane JA (1985) Pilot traumatic coma data bank: a profile of head injuries in children. In: Dacey RG et al. (eds) Trauma of the central nervous system. Raven Press, New York, pp 19–26

16. Heiskanen O, Sipponen P (1970) Prognosis of severe brain injury. Acta Neurol Scand 46: 343–348

17. Jennett B, Bond M (1975) Assessment of outcome after severe brain damage: A practical scale. Lancet 1: 480–484

18. Jennett B, Teasdale GM, Knill-Jones RP (1975) Predicting outcome after head injury. J R Coll Physicians Lond 9: 231–237

19. Jennett B, Teasdale G, Braakman R, Minderhoud J, Knill-Jones R (1976) Predicting outcome in individual patients after severe head injury. Lancet 1: 1031–1034

20. Jennett B, Teasdale G, Braakman R, Minderhoud J, Heiden J, Kurze T (1979) Prognosis of patients with severe head injury. Neurosurgery 4: 283–289

21. Jennett B, Teasdale G, Galbraith S, Pickard J, Grant H, Braakman R, Avezaat C, Maas A, Minderhoud J, Vecht CJ, Heiden J, Small R, Caton W, Kurze T (1977) Severe head injuries in three countries. J Neurol Neurosurg Psychiatr 40: 291–298

22. Kraus J, Conroy C, Cox P, Ramstein K, Fife D (1985) Survival times and case fatality rates of brain-injured persons. J Neurosurg 63: 537–544

23. Langfitt TW (1978) Measuring the outcome from head injuries. J Neurosurg 48: 673–678

24. Lewin W, Roberts AH (1979) Long-term prognosis after severe head injury. Acta Neurochir (Wien) [Suppl] 28: 128–133

25. Lobato RD, Cordobes F, Rivas JJ, de la Fuente M, Montero A, Barcena A, Perez C, Carbrera A, Lamas E (1983) Outcome from severe head injury related to the type of intracranial lesion: a computerized tomography study. J Neurosurg 59: 762–774

26. Marshall LF, Becker DP, Bowers SA, Cayard C, Eisenberg H, Gross CR, Grossman RG, Jane JA, Kunitz SC, Rimel R, Tabaddor K, Warren J (1983) The national traumatic coma data bank. Part 1: Design, purpose, goals, and results. J Neurosurg 59: 276–285

27. Miller JD, Becker DP, Ward JD, Sullivan HG, Adams WE, Rosner MJ (1977) Significance of intracranial hypertension in severe head injury. J Neurosurg 47: 503–516

28. Miller JD, Butterworth JF, Gudeman SK, Faulkner JE, Choi SC, Selhorst JB, Habison JW, Lutz HA, Young HF, Becker DP (1981) Further experience in the management of severe head injury. J Neurosurg 54: 289–299

29. Narayan RK, Greenberg RP, Miller JD, Enas GG, Choi SC, Kishore PRS, Selhorst JB, Lutz HA, Becker DP (1981) Improved confidence of outcome prediction in severe head injury. J Neurosurg 54: 751–762

30. Overgaard J, Hvid-Hansen O, Land AM, Pedersen KK. Christensen S, Haase J, Hein O, Tweed WA (1973) Prognosis after head injury based on early clinical examination. Lancet 2: 631–635

31. Pagni CA (1973) The prognosis of head-injured patients in a state of coma with decerebrated posture: analysis of 471 cases. J Neurosurg Sci 17: 289–295

32. Pazzaglia P, Frank G, Frank F, Gaist G (1975) Clinical course and prognosis of acute post-traumatic coma. J Neurol Neurosurg Psychiatry 38: 149–154

33. Pentelényi T, Kammerer L, Péter F, Fekete M, Korányi L, Stützel M, Veress G, Bezzegh A (1979) Prognostic significance of the changes in the carbohydrate metabolism in severe head injury. Acta Neurochir (Wien) [Suppl] 28: 103–107

34. Price DJ, Knill-Jones R (1979) The prediction of outcome of patients admitted following head injury in coma with bilateral fixed pupils. Acta Neurochir (Wien) [Suppl] 28: 179–182

35. Stablein DM, Miller JD, Choi SC, Becker DP (1980) Statistical methods for determining prognosis in severe head injury. Neurosurgery 6: 243–248

36. Steudel WI, Krüger J (1979) Using the spectra analysis of the EEG for prognosis of severe brain injuries in the first post-traumatic week. Acta Neurochir (Wien) [Suppl] 28: 40–42

37. Teasdale G, Jennett B (1974) Assessment of coma and impaired consciousness: A practical scale. Lancet 2: 81–84

38. Teasdale G, Murray G, Parker L, Jennett B (1979) Adding up the Glasgow coma score. Acta Neurochir (Wien) [Suppl] 28: 13–16

39. Teasdale G, Parker L, Murray G, Knill-Jones R, Jennett B (1979) Predicting the outcome of individual patients in the first week after severe head injury. Acta Neurochir (Wien) [Suppl] 28: 161–164

40. Teasdale G, Skene A, Parker L, Jennett B (1979) Age and outcome of severe head injury. Acta Neurochir (Wien) [Suppl] 28: 140–143

41. Titterington DM, Murray GD, Murray LS, Spiegelhalter DJ, Skene AM, Habbema JDF, Gelpke GJ (1981) Comparison of discrimination techniques applied to a complex data set of head injured patients. J Statist Soc A 144: 145–175

42. Toutant SM, Klauber MR, Marshall LF, Toole BM, Bowers SA, Seelig JM, Varnell JB (1984) Absent or compressed basal cisterns on first CT scan: ominous predictors of outcome in severe head injury. J Neurosurg 61: 691–694

43. Turazzi S, Bricolo A, Pasut ML (1984) Review of 1,000 consecutive cases of severe head injury treated before the advent of CT scanning. Acta Neurochir (Wien) 72: 167–195

44. Van den Berge JH (1985) Horizontal eye-movements in severe, traumatic brain damage. Thesis, Erasmus University Rotterdam

45. Van Dongen KJ, Braakman R, Gelpke GJ (1983) The prognostic value of computerized tomography in comatose head injured patients. J Neurosurg 59: 951–957

Authors' address: Prof. Dr. R. Braakman, Department of Neurosurgery, University Hospital Rotterdam "Dijkzigt", NL-3015 GD Rotterdam, The Netherlands.

Acta Neurochirurgica, Suppl. 36, 118–120 (1986)

Dizziness and Vertigo in the Posttraumatic Syndrome

A Physiological Background

S. Lund

Department of Neurology, Sahlgren's Hospital, University of Göteborg, Sweden

Summary

Some important physiologic mechanisms involved in equilibrium control are briefly reviewed and a new method to study clinically the integration of vestibular and proprioceptive functions is presented.

Keywords: Posture; dizziness; vestibular; proprioception.

Dizziness and vertigo are common symptoms in the posttraumatic syndrome as well as in other diseases of different etiology. This reflects the fact that the equilibrium control systems of the central nervous system (CNS) are complex and morphologically widespread. To maintain equilibrium control the CNS has access to information mainly from three different sensory systems:

1. Vision.

2. The vestibular apparatus, informing CNS on how the head is related to the surrounding gravitational forces, *i.e.* the horizon.

3. The proprioceptive system with mechanoreceptors in joints, ligaments and muscles. This system is the source for information on how different body segments (eye, head, limbs, trunk) are positioned or moved in relation to each other.

The deep neck muscles are richly supplied with such mechanoreceptors (muscle spindles) contributing together with the vestibular apparatus to the powerful postural reflexes well known from animal experimental physiology. The equillibrium control centres also to some extent trust on information from other sources, *e.g.* hearing.

A. The word "movement" can have two meanings. Either the body, or a part of the body, moves in a stationary environment, self movement. This is illustrated by a simple saccad or pursuit eye movement or by a complex combination of eye-head-trunk movement which during naturally occurring conditions rapidly changes its static and dynamic characteristics. Movement can also mean that something in the environment is moving relative the stationary body or the eye. This is illustrated by a wasp or a snow ball approaching the eye, or if you are standing on the deck of a boat at sea and by proprioceptive input from the ankle joints are experiencing the changing supporting area under your feet, that is the rolling of the boat. However, exactly the same proprioceptive input can be activated by self movement if the body is swaying when standing on a stationary supporting surface. The visual and the proprioceptive systems cannot, as receptors, differentiate between self movement and environmental movement. The vestibular system can monitor only self movement since the gravitational forces are constant and accordingly a change in the vestibular input always means that a self movement is being performed.

It follows from this that for maintained equilibrium control there is need for a physiological nervous mechanism capable of differentiating self movement from environmental movement when visual or proprioceptive input is to be analysed by the CNS. The lecture will discuss one such possible mechanism in some details, the reafference principle Dysfunction in this differentiating mechanism may well explain symptoms of dizziness and vertigo.

B. This differentiating mechanism is, however, not enough to ensure equilibrium control. There is also need for an integrating function between the three main sensory systems. Two examples will now be given.

The first example concerns coordination of eye-head movements. Eye movements are frequently during natural movements smoothly combined with head and sometimes also trunk movements. This calls for an integration of, on the first hand, visual and vestibular inputs. This integration is subserved by the vestibulo-ocular reflex (VOR). Disturbed function in the VOR may well explain dizziness and vertigo.

The second example concerns coordination of head-trunk-limb movements. The head can be freely moved on will, yet it provides accomodation for the vestibular apparatus which can evoke powerful postural protective reflex movements in the limbs and the trunk as well as imperative eye movements (nystagmus) when it is activated by—head movements. Why are we not thrown to the ground by these reflexes simply by shaking the head or nodding? The answer is that the vestibular input evoked by the shaking of the head is exactly counteracted by a proprioceptive input from neck mechanoreceptors, thus suppressing the postural reflexes and the nystagmus. If, on the other hand, the same vestibular input occurs alone (*i.e.* the whole body is moving or tumbling over) this complete counter-action does not occur and the postural reflexes necessary for equilibrium control are immediately elicited.

This integration of vestibular and proprioceptive functions can be studied in man[1] and the method (VERTIGOMETRI) will be described in the lecture. Disturbed integration may well explain symptoms of dizziness and vertigo.

C. Even if all the functions and mechanisms so far mentioned are operating smoothly and well-coordinated this is not enough to fulfill the demands we put on the equilibrium control centres. Dynamic motor

acts like running, grasping and climbing to mention a few, all voluntary to some degree, are performed under constantly changing equilibrium control programs. This necessitates linking of the equilibrium and for instance the locomotor functions. Disturbed linking may explain dizziness and vertigo when these symptoms occur during voluntary movements.

D. Many equilibrium control functions are learned and trained at an unconscious level as well as executed at an unconscious level. This explains why the patient hampered by dizziness and vertigo meets with great difficulties when trying to verbalize his experiences. There is simply not enough words for it in the language. It is hard to describe defects in a complex sensory control system which you knew almost nothing about when it was working and you were healthy. This calls for an open ear when we face a patient complaining of dizziness or vertigo.

The doctor on the other hand, needs more diagnostic tools aimed at measuring defects in strictly defined partial functions within the complex equilibrium control system.

Integration of Proprioceptive and Vestibular Functions in Human Equilibrium Control

Method

The subject is standing under an infrared opto-electronic camera (IROS) with light-emitting diodes attached to the head and shoulders. A computer program calculates the position of the head and

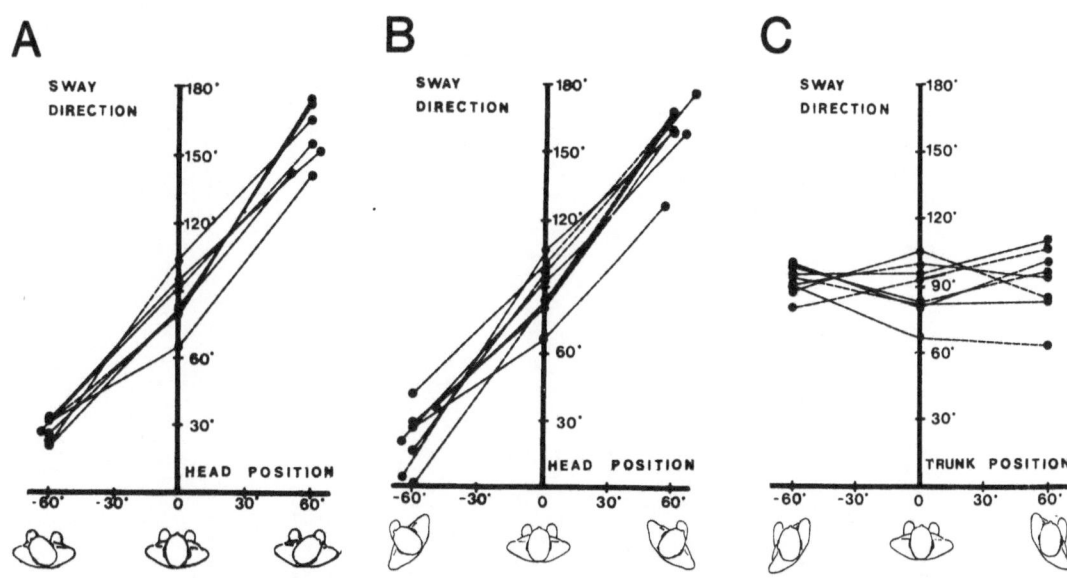

Fig. 1

shoulders as well as the resting sway and the sway induced by a short direct current pulse between electrodes on the mastoid processes behind the ears. This pulse is used as a reproducible vestibular error signal. The subjects take different head positions by turning the head or trunk alone or in combination. The feet are not moved. Since the head is in the horizontal plane in all positions and the galvanic vestibular error signal is also the same, the vestibular afferent input is the same in all the experimental situations. A change in output, the direction of the induced sway response, must reflect the altered proprioceptive input in the different potions.

Results

Fig. 1 shows the results from eight normal subjects. These results were obtained by force plate recordings. In A the head alone is turned to different positions, inducing a changed proprioceptive input from the neck joints. The direction of the induced sway response is also changed. In B the position of the head is changed

by inducing a different proprioceptive input in the trunk joints. Still, the direction of the induced sway response is altered in the same way as in A. In C the subjects induce neck and trunk proprioceptive inputs that should cancel each other. And they do. In this figure the position of the head is not changed, neither is the direction of the induced sway response.

Conclusion

The effect of proprioceptive input from different spinal segmental levels on human equilibrium control can now be measured and defects can be related to symptoms of vertigo and dizziness.

Reference

1. Lund S, Broberg C (1983) Effects of different head positions on postural sway in man induced by a reproducible vestibular error signal. Acta Physiol Scand 117: 307–309

Author's address: S. Lund, M.D., Department of Neurology, Sahlgren's Hospital, University of Göteborg, S-413 45 Göteborg, Sweden.

Acta Neurochirurgica, Suppl. 36, 121–122 (1986)

Possible Mechanisms of "Vegetative State"

J. E. Starmark and **S. Lindgren**

Department of Psychiatry III, Lillhagens sjukhus, and Department of Neurosurgery, Sahlgrenska sjukhuset, Göteborg, Sweden

Summary

A scaling of severity degrees of the vegetative state must perhaps consider the remaining as well as the deficient integrating functions from the arousal and cortical systems to an automatically working but partly disconnected part of the "central brain" with no awareness but some wakefulness.

Keywords: Arousal; awareness; automatic CNS generator; vegetative state.

Pathoanatomical changes found after death from disease or injury are often held more responsible for previous clinical pictures and abnormal symptoms than the remaining ("normal") structures.

The "vegetative state" (1972[3]) after head trauma is generally assumed to occur after mechanical damage to the white matter or after hypoxia-ischemia in the acute or later s.c. "secondary" stage.

The absence of cortical function and the presence of neocortical necrosis have been pointed out. It is also assumed that spontaneous actions such as eye opening, movements of eyes and movements of postural character, some autonomic functions and some other responses are elicited from a subcortical level. Many of these "actions" do not occur in the same patient in the acute stage of the posttraumatic coma and in fact are ranked among signs with "less severity" in most "coma scales".

However, such scales consider the acute posttraumatic impaired responses due to a generally depressed activity of arousal mechanisms and lower brainstem reticular formation (and the locus coeruleus)[2] as well as of awareness—with integration of the "upper reticular formation" (diencephalon)—limbic and posterior hypothalamic systems and of cortical function.

The "improvement dissociation" in the arousal/awareness in Glasgow Coma Scales, applied to "vegetative patients", may, however, not be due to improvement of the whole system. It may be the result of the earlier disconnection of the "upper reticular formation". This may 2–4 weeks after trauma start an automatic generation of "subcortical" symptoms, sometimes perhaps with help of remaining descending parts of reticular formations.

The course is not similar to the partial but often rapid improvement seen after diaschisis in the acute stage of a unilateral brain infarction. It is rather a combination of partly "recovered" but distorted wakefulness and no awareness (cognition). The emotional-autonomic (transmitter) systems may be partially involved. Similar aspects of pathophysiology of arousal partly related to anatomical structures have recently been discussed by Plum and Saper[4].

Thus, the actions in the "vegetative state" may not be influenced by ordinary stimuli used in "coma scaling". Bricolo[1] observed somewhat varying symptoms and time course in patients in similar "states". However, they found that these patients had a higher incidence of mesencephalic and diencephalic syndromes.

Acknowledgement

This study is supported by Swedish Medical Research Council proj no B86-27X-6613-03B and the Folksam Insurance Company.

References

1. Bricolo A, Turazzi S, Feriotti G (1980) Prolonged posttraumatic unconsciousness. Therapeutic assets and liabilities. J Neurosurg 52: 625–634

2. Elam J, On the physiological regulation of brain norepinephrine neurons in rat locus coeruleus. Thesis 1985, university of Gothenburg. (To be published in "Brain Research")
3. Jennett B, Plum F (1972) Persistent vegetative state after brain damage. Lancet 1: 734–737
4. Plum F, Saper CB (1983) Abnormal physiology in relation to arousal; newer concepts of autonomic projections. In: Papo, Giovanelli, Gaini, Tomei (eds) Advances in neurotraumatology. Internat Congr Ser no 612, Elsevier

Authors' address: J. E. Starmark, M.D., Department of psychiatry III, Lillhagens sjukhus, S-42203 Hisings Backa 3, Sweden.

Acta Neurochirurgica, Suppl. 36, 123–124 (1986)

Abnormalities of Sympathetic Regulation After Cervical Cord Lesions

G. Wallin

Department of Clinical Neurophysiology, Sahlgren's Hospital, University of Göteborg, Sweden

Summary

Microneurographic recordings suggest that hypertensive reactions in patients with cervical spinal cord lesions usually are due, not to exaggerated sympathetic nerve reactions, but rather to the combination of more diffuse sympathetic nerve activation than normally, exaggerated vascular reactions and absence of blood pressure restraining reflexes.

Keywords: Cervical cord lesions; sympathetic outflow; sympathetic activity in skin; muscle.

After cervical spinal cord lesions spinal sympathetic neurones become deprived of regulatory influence from supraspinal structures which seriously disturb control of blood pressure and temperature. The main clinical effects of defective blood pressure regulation are orthostatic reactions and hypertensive responses to visceral and other stimuli applied distal to the lesion. The reason for the blood pressure increases is thought to be exaggerated sympathetic nervous reactions.

With the introduction of the microneurographic technique direct recordings of sympathetic action potentials can be made in human extremity nerves. In intact man such recordings have revealed that sympathetic outflow to muscles contributes to homeostatic blood pressure regulation whereas outflow to skin is important for thermoregulation and also participates in emotional reactions. In agreement with this the two types of sympathetic activity have different characteristics and are controlled by different reflex mechanisms. Muscle sympathetic activity is composed of bursts of vasoconstrictor impulses which are discharged with the cardiac rhythm, predominantly during transient blood pressure reductions. Skin sympathetic activity contains a mixture of sudomotor and vasoconstrictor impulses which occur in bursts of varying duration and with no obvious cardiac rhythmicity. Variations of afferent inflow from arterial or cardiopulmonary baroreceptors lead to reciprocal changes of muscles sysmpathetic activity. Skin sympathetic activity on the other hand, is influenced by thermal and respiratory stimuli and in addition by arousal and emotional reactions.

In patients with complete traumatic spinal cord lesions sympathetic outflow below the level of the lesion differs from the normal in several respects: a) both in skin and muscle nerves spontaneus sympathetic activity is much lower in the patients, b) in muscle nerves no evidence of baroreflex modulation of sympathetic activity is present in the patients, c) in skin nerves sympathetic activity in the patients is not influenced by changes of temperature, d) much stronger cutaneous stimuli are necessary to evoke sympathetic reflex discharges in the patients than in intact subjects. In patients such reflexes occurred synchronously in skin and muscle nerve branches, whereas in normal subjects they occur only in skin nerves, e) in the patients sympathetic reflex discharges were followed by cutaneous vasoconstriction of longer duration than in normal subjects, f) bladder stimuli induced only weak or moderate increases of sympathetic outflow to muscles and nevertheless marked hypertensive reactions occurred.

The results suggest that excitability of decentralized spinal sympathetic neurones is decreased rather than increased whereas cutaneous blood vessels show exaggerated reactions to sympathetic nerve impulses. Furthermore, spinal sympathetic outflow is less differentiated than when supraspinal connections are intact. Both abnormalities probably contribute to episodes of hypertension in patients with spinal cord injuries.

References

Stjernberg L, Blumberg H, Wallin BG (1986) Sympathetic activity in man after spinal cord injury. Outflow to muscle below the lesion. Brain in Press

Wallin BG, Stjernberg L (1984) Sympathetic activity in man after spinal cord injury. Outflow to skin below the lesion. Brain 107: 183–198

Author's address: G. Wallin, M.D., Department of Clinical Neurophysiology, Sahlgren's Hospital, University of Göteborg, S-413 45 Göteborg, Sweden.

Acta Neurochirurgica, Suppl. 36, 125–128 (1986)

Molecular Mechanisms for Ischemic Brain Damage and Aspects on Protection

St. Rehncrona

The Department of Neurosurgery, University of Lund, Sweden

Summary

Multiple factors are responsible for the development of irreversible cell damage in the ischemic brain. Different molecular mechanisms may operate alone or may influence each other to create a vicious circle leading to a point of no-return. Tissue energy failure, disruption of ionic homeostasis, and severe tissue lactic acidosis can be regarded as major basic mechanisms that provoke a sequence of events finally leading to degradation and death of brain cells. Accumulation of calcium, liberation of free fatty acids, and pathologic free radical reactions during the postischemic phase may have additional pathogenetic significance.

Possibilities to protect the ischemic brain are discussed with respect to the different pathogenetic mechanisms. Primarily, these include measures taken to decrease the cerebral energy demands and to prevent the development of severe tissue lactic acidosis.

Keywords: Brain ischemia; cell damage; molecular mechanisms; lactic acidosis; brain protection.

Brain Energy Metabolism and Critical Levels of Ischemia

Relative to other organs the brain has unusually high energy demands. During resting conditions the cerebral blood flow (CBF) accounts for about 15% of the cardiac output and the cerebral oxygen consumption is close to 20% of the total oxygen utilized by the body. Since the stores of oxygen in the tissue are virtually nil and the stores of high energy phosphates are small, the brain is constantly dependent on an adequate blood supply providing oxygen and substrates for energy production. While hypoxia restricts the oxygen supply to the tissue, ischemia decreases both oxygen and substrate availability. In both cases the cerebral energy state, *i.e.* the balance between production and utilization of energy, may be seriously menaced. Therefore it is mandatory first to discuss some features of brain energy metabolism before discussing mechanisms of damage. (For details and literature see 19.)

Normally brain tissue extracts 6 times as much oxygen as glucose from the blood and the production of CO_2 is roughly equivalent to the amount of oxygen consumed. Therefore it can be concluded that the energy demands normally are satisfied by the complete oxidation of glucose according to:

$$glucose + 6\ O_2 \rightarrow energy + 6\ CO_2 + 6\ H_2O$$

The energy formed is stored in high energy phosphate compounds: ATP (adenosine triphosphate) and PCr (phosphocreatine). Glycolysis, *i.e.* the first steps in the break down of glucose, is a cytoplasmic event and does not require oxygen:

$$glucose + 2\ NAD^+ + 2\ ADP +$$
$$2\ Pi \rightarrow 2\ pyruvate + 2\ NADH + 2\ H^+ + 2\ ATP$$

In the presence of oxygen puryvate is further oxidized by the mitochondrial metabolism to produce *36 ATP*. Thus provided that tissue oxygen availability is adequate, the total energy yield from 1 mole of glucose is 38 moles of ATP, which is 19 times the energy yield of anaerobic glycolysis. If tissue oxygenation is critically depressed, the rate of glycolysis will increase but the energy yield from anaerobic glycolysis is far from being sufficient and may imply a disturbance of cellular pH homeostasis (see below).

Principally the energy produced is utilized for three purposes. First, it is used for transmission of nerve impulses, including the synthesis of transmitter substances and synaptic events. Second, energy is consumed by active pumping of ions across the cell membranes to maintain intra- extracellular ionic homeostasis and gradients. Third, energy is constantly required for resynthesis of cellular constituents (including those of membranes) for maintaining structural integrity.

The brain may tolerate a certain fall in perfusion pressure. When autoregulatory mechanisms are exhausted some decrease in CBF can be compensated for by increased oxygen extraction. In man integrated neuronal functions will be the first to suffer a further reduction in blood flow. Obvious EEG changes can be detected if CBF is reduced to around $0.2 \, ml \times g^{-1} \times min^{-1}$ (around 30% of normal) and a decrease in CBF to around $0.15 \, ml \times g^{-1}$ causes flattening of EEG (the level of transmission failure)[20]. Animal experiments have shown changes in the cerebral energy state when CBF is reduced to about 45% of normal[7, 10], but first when CBF falls to below 10% of normal there is a total energy failure and release of intracellular potassium ions (often termed as membrane failure)[1]. This last ischemic level is assumed to be critical for cellular viability.

From this reasoning we also conclude that there may exist an ischemic CBF range between transmission failure and membrane failure, usually termed "ischemic penumbra", in which neuronal electrical function is totally abolished but the cells remain viable.

Effects of Energy Depletion

It is true that ischemic brain cell damage relates to tissue energy failure. Thus all experimental models in which ischemia results in irreversible cell damage seem to be complicated by cerebral energy failure. Furthermore, restitution of energy production and the energetic balance in the tissue certainly is a prerequisite for neurologic recovery. However, even if energy failure is a common denominator in situations leading to irreversible injury it cannot alone be decisive. Thus complete ischemia (at normothermia) results in a total depletion of ATP and PCr with 2–3 min but still the brain can tolerate considerably more prolonged ischemic periods with full restitution. Nevertheless it is important to consider the immediate effects of energy depletion.

Since no energy is available for maintaining normal ionic gradients, in the severely ischemic brain, the cells are depolarized and the ion homeostasis severely disturbed. The energy dependent Na^+/k^+ pump is halted and there is a massive efflux of k^+ to extracellular fluids. By the same token intracellular concentrations of Na^+ and Cl^- will increase causing an influx of water from the extracellular space. Furthermore, the deterioration of ionic homeostasis includes an influx of Ca^{2+} to the intracellular compartment. The intra-

cellular increase in free calcium is a triggering factor for increased phospholipase activity causing a massive release and accumulation of free fatty acids (FFA). Thus the content of FFA in the tissue increases by more than 5 times during 5 min and by about 12 times the normal during 30 min of severe incomplete or complete ischemia[18]. The source of the released FFA is mainly membrane phospholipids and, therefore, the change in FFA may indicate structural membrane alterations, even if the corresponding decrease in phospholipid content may be too small to detect. Furthermore, the increase in FFA per se may have pathophysiologic relevance by causing tissue edema[2, 3] and by a deleterious influence on mitochondrial respiratory functions. With respect to the latter, increased concentrations of FFA are known to uncouple mitochondrial oxidative phosphorylation, *i.e.* consumption of oxygen without ATP-production, an effect that also may be the result of increased cytosolic Ca^{2+} concentration[8].

Free Radicals and Lipid Peroxidation

During the last few years the hypothesis that pathologic free radical reactions cause peroxidative damage in brain ischemia[6] has attracted great interest. This may seem a bit paradoxical since these oxidative reactions require molecular oxygen. However, at least theoretically such reactions may operate during incomplete ischemia or in the postischemic/ reoxygenation phase. Free radicals are molecules with an unpaired electron in an outer shell rendering them highly reactive, especially for attacking polyenoic fatty acids (in membrane lipids). Free radicals may be formed by univalent reduction of oxygen, with the subsequent formation of superoxide radicals, hydrogen peroxide and hydroxyl radicals. In fact oxygen free radicals can be formed in the mitochondrial respiratory chain. It was, therefore, speculated that free radical production may be pathologically enhanced by a reduction (but not abolishment) of oxygen availability at the terminus of the respiratory chain. The hypothesis of free radical damage in ischemia was originally based on findings of a decreased content of ascorbic acid and cholesterol in ischemic brain tissue and protection of barbiturates with scavenging properties[5]. Moreover, results showing that incomplete ischemia may be more harmful than complete ischemia supported the hypothesis[11, 15]. However, most of the later and, more extensive investigations have given nonconformative results[4, 13, 18]. In addition a much more plausible explanation to the harmful effect of a trickling blood flow during ischemia has been established (see below).

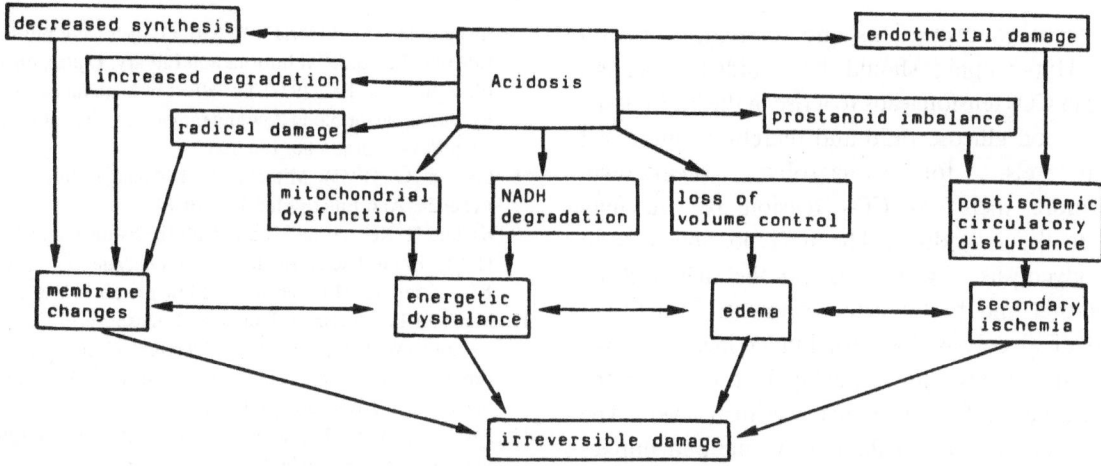

Fig. 1. Some possible deleterious effects of intracellular acidosis in brain ischemia. (Modified from Rehncrona S, Ann Emerg Med 1985[12]

Even if pathologic free radical mechanisms do not seem to have a major importance during the ischemic period their existence in a circumscribed tissue compartment, *e.g.* like mitochondrial membranes, can hardly be excluded. Currently peroxidative reactions are discussed as a possible factor aggravating injury during the recirculation/reoxygenation phase[21, 22] but solid evidences are still lacking.

Brain Lactic Acidosis

As mentioned above severe incomplete ischemia and hypoxia may be more harmful than complete ischemia. It was recently shown that this fact is explained by the more excessive brain tissue lactic acidosis in the former situations[9, 12, 14, 16, 17]. When ischemia is complete, lactic acid is produced by anaerobic glycolysis to a maximal level, which depends on the preischemic tissue stores of glucose and glycogen. If ischemia is incomplete (or in severe hypoxia) oxygen delivery is insufficient for oxidative metabolism but the remaining blood flow allows a continued supply of glucose for anaerobic breakdown. Therefore lactic acid is continuously produced causing tissue lactate concentration to reach excessive levels. Thus complete ischemia, when induced in normoglycemic animals, causes lactate to accumulate in the tissue to around $12 \mu mol \times g^{-1}$ (corresponding to a decrease in intracellular pH to around 6.5) while lactate concentration during severe incomplete ischemia or tissue hypoxia may well increase to above $20–25 \mu mol \times g^{-1}$ (intracellular pH around or below 6.0). In fact a tissue lactate concentration of $20–25 \mu mol \times g^{-1}$ was shown to be critical for cellular viability and for the possibility for neurologic recovery.

The level to which lactate accumulates during incomplete ischemia, which is the more clinically relevant situation, is dependent on: 1) the rate of the residual blood flow, 2) the length of the ischemic period and 3) the blood glucose concentration. Several experimental studies on rats, monkeys and rabbits as well as two clinical investigations have now been able to correlate morphologic brain damage, deficient recovery of energy metabolism, deficient recovery of neurophysiological and functional variables to either severe tissue lactic acidosis and/or to hyperglycemia during the ischemic period. The deleterious effect of lactic acidosis most probably is related to a severe fall in intracellular pH affecting almost all enzyme systems and the biophysiological homeostasis of the cell (see Fig. 1).

Aspects on Protection at the Molecular Level

Clearly a multifold of factors and mechanisms operating alone or in concert either during or after ischemia may influence the possibility for restitution. This complexity combined with the fact that ischemia usually is a heterogeneous event explains why brain protection in terms of cell biochemistry must be somewhat speculative and that protective effects may be difficult to prove in clinical situations (for ref see[23]).

Two major mechanisms aggravating ischemic brain damage are however established. The first is energy depletion and, therefore, measures taken to decrease cellular energy demands (*i.e.* decrease $CMRO_2$) may in certain situations have beneficial effects. Such therapy includes the use of hypothermia and barbiturates. The second factor is severe tissue lactic acidosis, which should either be prevented or treated. Thus measures should be taken to avoid hyperglycemia in patients with a critically reduced cerebral perfusion pressure[12, 14]. Such measures include: a) the avoidance of, or treatment of stress, which increase blood glucose levels; b) the avoidance of infusion-solutions with unnecessarily high glucose concentrations and, c) treatment with insulin. Hypercapnia should be avoided, since an increase in CO_2 tension leads to a rise in the brain tissue glucose/blood glucose ratio and thereby to increased substrate-levels for anaerobic breakdown. Furthermore increased CO_2 tension per se may aggravate tissue acidosis. The next possibility is to inhibit glycolysis. Again, this can be achieved by hypothermia and barbiturate treatment. Even if inhibition of glycolysis does not hinder lactic acidosis from occurring, it will at least delay the time period for lactic acid concentration to reach critical levels. The third possibility is still a theoretical one and implies measures to increase intracellular buffer capacity. However, since no suitable buffers yet are available and adequate data are lacking, this possibility may be most convenient for future research.

With respect to pathological free radical mechanisms and to the assumed deleterious effect of increased intracellular Ca^{2+} concentration, their exact relationship, if any, to brain cell damages is obscure and data on protective effects of free radical scavengers and calcium entry blockers are contradictory.

Conclusions

Recent experimental research has substantially increased our knowledge on the pathophysiology of ischemic brain cell damage. However, relatively little of this knowledge is yet applicable to clinical situations even if some hints to protection can be given. It should be thoroughly emphasized that none of the protective measures suggested should be used as an alternative to surgical intervention aiming at the removal of a life-threatening focal expansivity, but rather as adjuvant therapy.

References

1. Astrup J (1982) Energy-requiring cell functions in the ischemic brain. J Neurosurg 56: 482–497
2. Chan PH, Fishman RA (1978) Brain edema: Induction in cortical slices by polyunsaturated fatty acids. Science 201: 358–360
3. Chan PH, Fishman RA, Caronna J, Schmidley JW, Prioleau G, Lee J (1983) Induction of brain edema following intracerebral injection of arachidonic acid. Ann Neurol 13: 625–632
4. Cooper AJL, Pulsinelli WA, Duffy TE, Glutathione and ascorbate during ischemia and post-ischemic reperfusion in rat brain. J. Neurochem 35: 1242–1245
5. Demopoulos HB, Flamm ES, Pietronigro DD, Seligman ML (1980) The free radical pathology and the microcirculation in the major central nervous system disorders. Acta Physiol Scand [Suppl] 491: 91–119
6. Demopoulos H, Flamm E, Seligman M, Power R, Pietronigro D, Ransohoff J (1977) Molecular pathology of lipids in CNS

membranes. In: Göbsis FF (ed) Oxygen and physiological function. Professional Information Library, Dallas, pp 491–508
7. Eklöf B, Siesjö BK (1972) The effect of bilateral carotid artery ligation upon the blood flow and the energy state of the rat brain. Acta Physiol Scand 86: 155–165
8. Fiskum G (1985) Mitochondrial damage during cerebral ischemia. Ann Emerg Med 14: 810–815
9. Kalimo H, Rehncrona S, Söderfeldt B, Olsson Y and Siesjö BK (1981) Brain Lactic Acidosis and ischemic cell damage: 2. Histopathology. J Cereb Blood Flow Metab 1: 313–327
10. Marshall LF, Welsh F, Durity F, Lounsbury F, Graham DJ, Langfitt TW (1975) Experimental cerebral oligemia and ischemia produced by intracraniell hypertension. Part 3: Brain energy metabolism. J Neurosurg 43: 323–328
11. Nordström C-H, Rehncrona S, Siesjö BK (1978) Effects of phenobarbital in cerebral ischemia. Part two: Restitution of cerebral energy state, as well as glycolytic metabolites, citric acid cykle intermediates and associated amino acids after pronounced incomplete ischemia. Stroke 9: 335–343
12. Rehncrona S (1985) Brain Acidosis. Ann Emerg Med 14: 770–776
13. Rehncrona S, Folbergrová J, Smith DS, Siesjö BK (1980) Influence of complete and pronounced incomplete cerebral ischemia and subsequent recirculation and cortical concentrations of oxidized and reduced gluthione in the rat. J Neurochem 34: 477–486
14. Rehncrona S, Kågström E (1983) Tissue lactic acidosis and ischemic brain damage. Am J Emerg Med 1: 168–174
15. Rehncrona S, Mela L, Siesjö BK (1979) Recovery of brain mitochondrial function in the rat after complete and incomplete cerebral ischemia. Stroke 10: 437–446
16. Rehncrona S, Rosén I, Siesjö BK (1981) Brain lactic acidosis and ischemic cell damage: 1. Biochemistry and Neurophysiology. J Cereb Blood Flow Metab 1: 297–311
17. Rehncrona S, Rosen I, Smith M-L (1985) Effect of different degrees of brain ischemia and tissue lactic acidosis on the short-term recovery of neurophysiologic and metabolic variables. Exp Neurol 87: 458–473
18. Rehncrona S, Westerberg E, Åkesson B, Siesjö BK (1982) Brain cortical fatty acids and phospholipids during and following complete and severe incomplete ischemia. J Neurochem 38: 84–93
19. Siesjö BK (1978) Brain energy metabolism. J Wiley and Sons, Chichester New York Brisbane Toronto.
20. Trojaborg W, Boysen G (1973) Relation between EEG regional cerebral blood flow and internal carotid artery pressure during carotid endarterectomy. Electroencephalogr Clin Neurophysiol 34: 61–69
21. White BC, Krause GS, Aust SD, Eyster G (1985) Postischemic tissue injury by iron-mediated free radical lipid peroxidation. Ann Emerg Med 14, 804–809
22. Yoshida S, Inoh S, Asano T, Sano K, Kubota M, Shimazaki H, Ueta N (1980) Effect of transient ischemia on free fatty acids and phospholipids in the gerbil brain. Lipid peroxidation as a possible cause of postischemic injury. J Neurosurg 53: 323–331
23. Wiedemann K, Hoyer S (eds) (1983) Brain protection. Morphological, pathological and clinical aspects. Springer, Berlin Heidelberg New York Tokyo

Author's address: St. Rehncrona, M.D., The Department of Neurosurgery, University of Lund, Sölvegatan 25, S-223 62 Lund, Sweden.

Acta Neurochirurgica, Suppl. 36, 129–132 (1986)

Structural Aspects of Ischemic Brain Damage

H. Kalimo and **M.-L. Smith**

Department of Pathology I, University of Göteborg, Sweden, and Laboratory for Experimental Brain Research, University of Lund, Sweden

Summary

The structural changes during cerebal ischemia are reviewed. In the acute phase the neurons may show either pale or dark type of ischemic injury. The former is usually associated with complete ischemia and the structural alterations are fairly inconspicious, while the latter is seen in incomplete ischemia or ischemia with recirculation and is characterized by shrinkage of neurons with extensive mitochondrial swelling and astrocytic edema. Both types of injury may be irreversible, but long post-ischemic period is usually necessary to see the final outcome of the insult, all the more since the neurons may not die until after a free postischemic interval (even with resumed function) of several hours to days. The delayed death is preceded by peculiar proliferation of cytoplasmic membranes before the doomed neurons become shrunken and disintegrate. This "maturation phenomenon" or "delayed neuronal death" is understandably important since it suggests that a longer postischemic interval for therapeutic interventions may exist.

Several factors both during and after the ischemic insult can modify the changes and affect the severity of the damager Among the most important ones are the degree of lactic acidosis during the ischemic period, as well as the characteristics of the neurons, since excitoxic damage by transmitter substances released by the ischemic insult has been suggested to be responsible for the delayed neuronal death.

Keywords: Cerebral ischemia; nerve cell injury; structure.

Critical Thresholds

Combined neurophysiological and regional blood flow studies on experimental brain ischemia have demonstrated two critical thresholds of impaired blood flow (Astrup[2]). At the first threshold of energy shortage the electrical activity of the neurons ceases, *i.e.* transmission failure occurs, while the neurons still maintain their intracellular ion homeostasis. Even though direct proof is lacking it is very likely that these electrically silent neurons do not show structural abnormalities, not even at the electron microscopic (EM) level. When the second threshold, *i.e.* membrane failure is reached, the basic ion pumps of the plasma membrane also fail in the absence of energy. Massive outflow of potassium ions and influx of sodium and calcium ions as well as of water into the cells ensue. Besides, intracellular shifts between different membrane-bound compartments occur. These ion and fluid shifts cause changes in the volume and "composition" of the brain cells, which are also visible microscopically (Kalimo *et al.*[13]).

Acute Phase

Depending on the type of ischemia, whether it is complete (with no remaining flow; Kalimo *et al.*[11], Jenkins *et al.*[8]) or incomplete (with trickling insufficient flow; Garcia *et al.*[5]) the acute change is either of the *(1) pale or (2) dark type of ischemic nerve cell injury* (Garcia *et al.*[5], Kalimo *et al.*[11, 13]). Furthermore, the pale type may turn to the dark type if the circulation is re-established (Arsenio-Nunes *et al.*[1], Jenkins *et al.*[9], Paljärvi *et al.*[20]).

In the *pale type of nerve cell injury* major volume changes of the neurons or their organelles do not occur. The structural alterations in this injury are actually quite discrete, not easily detectable in routine light microscopic (LM) preparations. It is characterized by increased electron lucency of the cytoplasm in neuron (as well as in other brain cells), clumping of nuclear chromatin (a very sensitive indicator of ischemia with acidosis) and of cell sap, as well as slight dilatation of RER cisternae and mitochondria (Kalimo *et al.*[11], Jenkins *et al.*[8]). No drastic changes in the volume of the cells or their organelles are seen. This may be explained by the fact that in the complete absence of circulation only the small volume of extracellular fluid is available for redistribution across the leaky cell membranes.

In the *dark type of nerve cell injury* the nerve cells shrink, their cytoplasm becomes markedly condensed and electron dense. Characteristically the mitochondria undergo extensive swelling which in LM preparations appear as cytoplasmic microvacuolation. Simultaneously the neighbouring astrocytes show marked swelling with watery appearance of the cytoplasm indicating both transfer of fluid from neurons to astrocytes and increase in the total tissue water, *i.e.* cytotoxic edema. Such major transfers of ions and water across the leaking membranes are possible, since the dark type of injury is usually seen either in incomplete ischemia or during the recirculation period. In the former case there is a trickling (yet insufficient) blood flow to carry extra fluid into the ischemic brain, in the latter the restored blood flow (often even postischemic hyperperfusion) does the same.

Thus, some of the dark type of changes are related to the edema and may be reversed, if energy production and thereby fluid homeostasis can be restored, whereas some other irreversibly damaged dark neurons continue to disintegrate. The exact mechanism for the acute irreversible damage is not known and several possibilities have been suggested (Siesjö *et al.*[24]). The influx of calcium ions into the cytoplasm with consequent activation of degradative enzymes is considered one of the critical events. Such excessive accumulation of calcium has been demonstrated also structurally with electron microscope (van Reempts *et al.*[28]). The critical time of irreversibility has not been established: estimations from a few minutes (Suzuki *et al.*[26], Smith *et al.*[25]) to up to 60 min (Hossmann and Kleihues *et al.*[6]) have been presented. Certainly that time varies in different regions of the brain (selective vulnerability; Brierley and Graham *et al.*[3]) and, furthermore, the final outcome obviously depends on several factors both during and after the ischemic insult.

One of the most important adverse factors during the ischemic insult seems to be the degree of tissue lactic acidosis (for the biochemical aspects see Rehncrona in this symposium). Experimentally it has been shown that high tissue lactate concentrations does definitely worsen the prognosis of the ischemic insult (*e.g.* Myers *et al.*[19], Rehncrona *et al.*[23]) and clinical studies also strongly allude that the same applies to human beings (Pulsinelli *et al.*[22], Longstreth and Inui *et al.*[18]). Structurally the deleterious effect of high lactate concentration during ischemia manifests itself as a very severe pale type of ischemic nerve cell injury (Kalimo *et al.*[12]). In all brain cells the nuclear chromatin and cell sap are severely clumped with fluffy condensations, whereas mitochondria are only slightly to moderately swollen. These changes are most likely related to the very low intracellular pH-values (around or below pH 6.0) which cause denaturation. It may be pointed out that even though these pale type of ischemically injured neurons are irreversibly damaged, their outlook is not as dramatically striking as that of the neurons expressing

the dark type of ischemic injury, and thus, their detection in light microscopic sections is difficult or even impossible. Therefore, the determination of the irreversibility as well as quantification of the nerve cell damage in LM tissue sections can require long survival periods to allow the lysis of the dead cells to occur (Smith *et al.*[25]).

Late Phase

It has also been demonstrated that nerve cells exposed to ischemia may succumb fairly late, after a post-ischemic free interval from several hours to a couple of days (Figs. 1 and 2), during which the neurons show a temporary restoration of their energy production and electrical activity (Diemer and Siemkowicz *et al.*[4], Suzuki *et al.*[27]). This "maturation phenomenon" or "delayed neuronal death" is proportional to the intensity of the ischemic insult, *i.e.* the neurons die sooner after a more severe insult (Klatzo *et al.*[17]). It is best seen in the CA 1 (Sommer's) sector of hippocampus (Kirino *et al.*[14]) but it seems to occur also elsewhere in the brain (Pulsinelli *et al.*[21]).

The structural changes in neurons dying in the delayed manner after an ischemic insult have been described in detail only in the CA 1 region of hippocampus of gerbil (Ito *et al.*[7], Suzuki *et al.*[26], Kirino and Sano *et al.*[15, 16]) and rat (Kirino *et al.*[14]). They seem to follow the same sequence in both species. During the first day after five minutes of ischemia the CA 1 neurons do not show any significant light microscopic changes, which is understandable since the neurons have been shown to be functionally intact, actually hyperactive (Suzuki *et al.*[27]). Neither during the second postischemic day, when the CA 1 neurons have already become silent, are there any marked structural changes: only clumping of the chromatin and small cytoplasmic slits. Not until three days after the insult did marked nerve cell destruction, *i.e.* shrinkage, dark staining and finally disintegration occur (Suzuki *et al.*[26]). In the same gerbil model electron microscopy has revealed during the first two postischemic peculiar accumulation of membrane cisternae and dark granular material in the cytoplasm of the CA 1 neurons destined to die. Finally shrunken dark-stained neurons (similar to the acute dark type of injury except for lack of mitochondrial ballooning) appear (Kirino and Sano *et al.*[16]).

The definite cause of this delayed neuronal death is not known. Excitotoxic damage has been suggested, *i.e.* the delayed neuronal death is due to excessive, "toxic" stimulation by excitatory transmitters (glutamate being the most suspected one) which are released in high

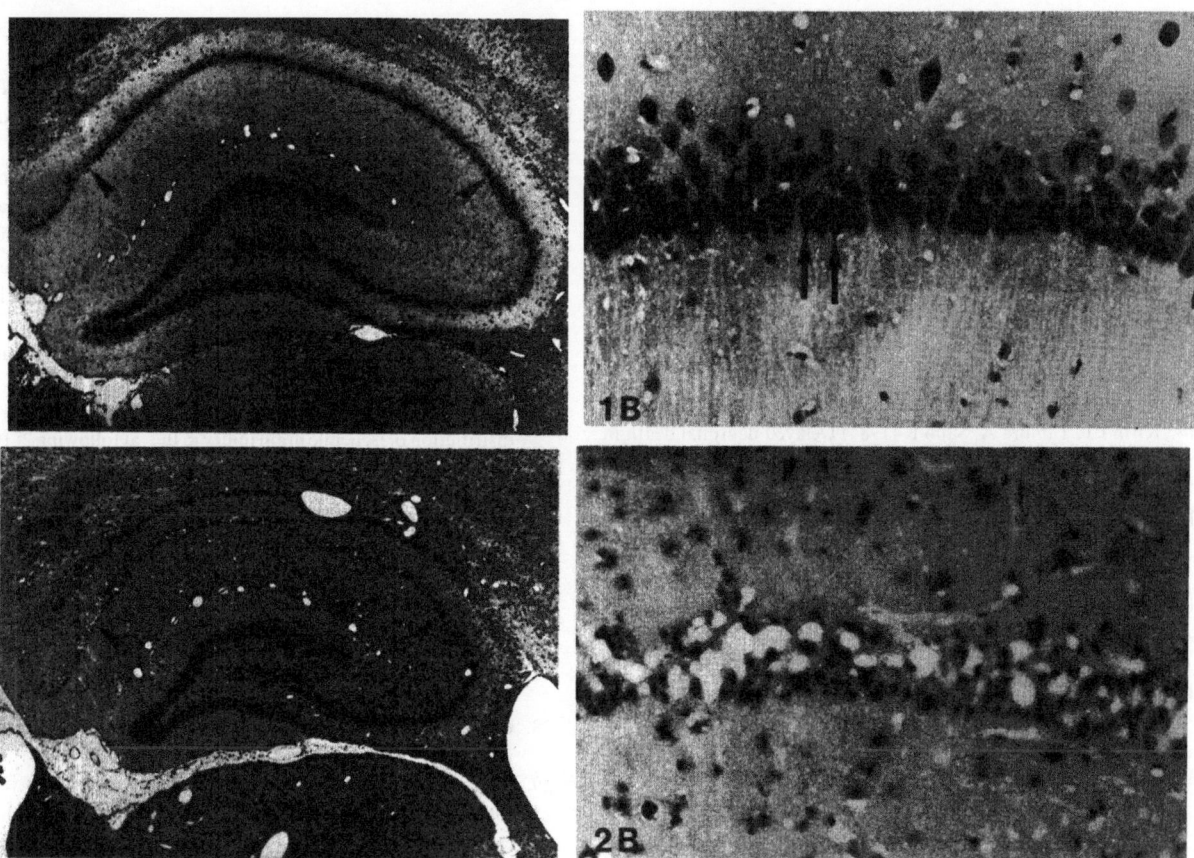

The pictures show the appearance of so-called "maturation phenomenon" or "delayed neuronal death" in the rat hippocampus after an ischemic insult of 10 min (Smith *et al.* 1984)

Fig. 1 A. Following recirculation for 2 days nearly all of the CA 1 neurons (between the arrows) are still preserved

Fig. 1 B. Shows at a higher magnification the nearly normal looking CA 1 neurons. Only a couple of them (arrows) are condensed being the forerunners of the pending cell death

Fig. 2 A. After recirculation for 4 days nearly all CA 1 neurons are destroyed

Fig. 2 B. A higher magnification to show the loss of neurons and vacuolation in the CA 1 region

concentrations to the extracellular space by the ischemic insult (Jørgensen and Diemer *et al.*[10], Wieloch *et al.*[29]). Understandably, this phenomenon of delayed damage is clinically very important, since the long postinsult period may provide an interval for therapeutic intervention.

References

1. Arsenio-Nunes ML, Hossmann KA, Farkas-Bargeton E (1973) Ultrastructural and histochemical investigation of the cerebral cortex of cat during and after complete ischemia. Acta Neuropathol 26: 329–344

2. Astrup J, Siesjö BK, Symon L (1981) Thresholds in cerebral ischemia—the ischemic penumbra. Stroke 12: 723–725

3. Brierley and Graham (1984) In: Hume Adams J, Corsellis J, Duchen LW (eds) Greenfield's neuropathology. E Arnold Ltd, pp 152–155

4. Diemer NH, Siemkowicz E (1980) Increased 2-deoxyglucose uptake in hippocampus, globus pallidus and substantia nigra after cerebral ischemia. Acta Neurol Scand 61: 56–63

5. Garcia JH, Kalimo H, Kamijyo Y, Trump BF (1977) Cellular events during partial cerebral ischemia. I. Electron microscopy of feline cerebral cortex after middle-cerebral artery occlusion. Virchows Arch Cell Pathol 25: 191–206

6. Hossmann K-A, Kleihues P (1973) Reversibility of ischemic brain damage. Arch Neurol 29: 375–382

7. Ito U, Spatz M, Walker JT, Klatzo I (1975) Experimental cerebral ischemia in Mongolian gerbils. I. Light microscopic observations. Acta Neuropathol (Berl) 32: 209–223

8. Jenkins LW, Povlishock JT, Becker DP, Miller JD, Sullivan HG (1979) Complete cerebral ischemia. An ultrastructural study. Acta Neuropathol (Berl) 48: 113–125

9. Jenkins LW, Povlishock JT, Lewelt W, Miller JD, Becker DP (1981) The role of postischemic recirculation in the development of ischemic neuronal injury following complete cerebral ischemia. Acta Neuropathol (Berl) 55: 205–220

10. Jørgensen MB, Diemer NH (1982) Selective neuron loss after cerebral ischemia in the rat: Possible role of transmitter glutamate. Acta Neurol Scand 66: 536–546

11. Kalimo H, Garcia JH, Kamijyo Y, Tanaka J, Trump BF (1977) The ultrastructure of "brain death". II. Electron microscopy of feline cortex after complete ischemia. Virchows Archiv Cell Pathol 25: 207–220

12. Kalimo H, Rehncrona S, Söderfeldt B, Olsson Y, Siesjö BK (1981) Brain lactic acidosis and ischemic cell damage: 2. Histopathology. J Cereb Blood Flow Metabol 1: 313–327

13. Kalimo H, Paljärvi L, Olsson Y, Siesjö BK (1983) Structural aspects of energy failure states in the brain. In: Wiedemann K, Hoyer S (eds) Problems and perspectives of brain protection. Springer, Berlin Heidelberg New York, pp 1–11

14. Kirino T, Tamura A, Sano K (1984) Delayed neuronal death in the rat hippocampus following transient forebrain ischemia. Acta Neuropathol (Berl) 64: 139–147

15. Kirino T, Sano (1984 a) Selective vulnerability in the gerbil hippocampus following transient ischemia. Acta Neuropathol (Berl) 62: 201–208

16. Kirino T, Sano K (1984 b) Fine structural nature of delayed neuronal death following ischemia in the gerbil hippocampus. Acta Neuropathol (Berl) 62: 209–218

17. Klatzo I (1975) Pathophysiologic aspects of cerebral ischemia. In: Tower DB (ed) The nervous system, vol 1. Raven Press, New York, pp 313–322

18. Longstreth WT, Inui TS (1984) High blood glucose level on hospital admission and poor neurological recovery after cardiac arrest. Ann Neurol 15: 59–63

19. Myers RE (1979) A unitary theory of causation of anoxic and hypoxic brain pathology. In: Fahn S, Davis JN, Rowland LP (eds) Advances in neurology, vol 26: Cerebral hypoxia and its consequences. Raven Press, New York, pp. 195–213

20. Paljärvi L, Alihanka J, Kalimo H (1984) Significance of fluid flow for morphology of acute hypoxic-ischaemic brain cell injury. Neuropath Appl Neurobiol 10: 43–52

21. Pulsinelli WA, Brierley JB, Plum F (1982) Temporal profile of neuronal damage in a model of transient forebrain ischemia. Ann Neurol 11: 491–498

22. Pulsinelli WA, Levy DE, Sigsbee B, et al. (1983) Increased damage after ischemic stroke in patients with hyperglycemia with or without established diabetes mellitus. Am J Med 74: 540–544

23. Rehncrona S, Rosén I, Siesjö BK (1980) Excessive cellular acidosis: An important mechanism of neuronal damage in the brain? Acta Physiol Scand 110: 435–437

24. Siesjö BK (1981) Cell damage in the brain: A speculative synthesis. J Cereb Blood Flow Metabol 1: 155–185

25. Smith ML, Auer RN, Siesjö BK (1984) The density and distribution of ischemic brain injury in the rat following 2–10 min of forebrain ischemia. Acta Neuropathol (Berl) 64: 319–332

26. Suzuki R, Yamaguchi T, Kirino F, Orzi F, Klatzo I (1983) The effects of 5-minute ischemia in Mongolian gerbils: I. Blood-Brain barrier, cerebral blood flow, and local cerebral glucose utilization changes. Acta Neuropathol 60: 207–216

27. Suzuki R, Yamaguchi T, Li C-L, Klatzo I (1983 b) The effects of 5-minute ischemia in Mongolian gerbils: II. Changes of spontaneous neuronal activity in cerebral cortex and CA 1 sector of hippocampus. Acta Neuropathol (Berl) 60: 217–222

28. van Reempts J (1984) The hypoxic brain: histological and ultrastructural aspects. Behav Brain Res 14: 99–108

29. Wieloch T, Lindvall O, Blomqvist P, Gage FH (1985) Evidence for amelioration of ischaemic neuronal damage in the hippocampal formation by lesions of the perforant path. Neurol Res 7: 24–26

Author's address: H. Kalimo, M.D., Department of Pathology I, University of Göteborg, S-413 45 Göteborg, Sweden.

Acta Neurochirurgica, Suppl. 36, 133–136 (1986)

CBF in Head Injury

Erna Enevoldsen

Neurological Department, University Hospital, Odense, Denmark

Summary

In the last few years the possibility of measuring CBF by means of intravenous isotop injection technique and portable monitor has made the use of measuring CBF in the clinical setting of the brain injured patient of current interest. However, knowledge about the hemodynamics of the head trauma is inevitable for the interpretation of the CBF results. In this communication a short outline of the results obtained during the last decades studies about the hemodynamic of the damaged brain is given. The essence of these studies seems to be:

The local level of CBF do not indicate the severity of the brain injury, as low as well as high flow may be seen initially in severely injured brain tissue. The oxygen uptake ($CMRO_2$) is related to the severety of the brain trauma, as low $CMRO_2$ correlate to poor clinical condition. In severely damaged brain tissue the autoregulation may appear normal (false autoregulation) whereas the autoregulation in moderately damaged tissue may appear impaired for weeks. The carbon dioxide response (CO_2) is only impaired if the brain tissue is severely damaged. Thus, low $CMRO_2$ and dissociation between apparently normal autoregulation and impaired CO_2 response seem to predict poor outcome.

Keywords: Head injury; regional cerebral blood flow; autoregulation; hyperventilation; non-invasive methods of CBF measurements.

Introduction

A major problem in the treatment of the brain injured patient is to maintain cerebral blood flow sufficiently to avoid ischemia. During the acute phase of brain injury the blood flow varies individually depending on several factors as blood pressure, intraventricular pressure, tissue acidosis and the ability of the brain vessels to respond to blood pressure and CO_2 changes. To disclose brain ischemia, measurements of CBF are suggested as a valuable tool in the observation of the brain injured patient in line with measurements of intracranial pressure. As non-invasive, non-risk and non-expensive methods are available, daily CBF observations in the individual patients are possible[14].

Methods of CBF Studies

CBF may be determined by means of measuring the rate of the clearance from the brain of a radioactive tracer, usually the inert gas 133-Xenon, which is soluble and readily diffusible between blood and brain tissue. Previously the Xenon had to be administrated intra-arterially, but at the present time inhalation and intravenous techniques are available making repeated measurements possible without any risk[14, 28]. Thus, a time course of the CBF may be studied. In the future advanced methods such as PET and NMR probably will be more common in spite of the great costs of these methods.

Results

CBF Measuring in Head Injury

Several studies have shown that in the individual patient suffering from a head trauma, the overall as well as the focal CBF may be normal (45–55 ml/100 g/min), decreased or increased[1, 3, 6, 9, 23, 24]. In the first days after injury subnormal flow is most commonly seen, but no correlations exist between the degree of the flow decrease and the severity of the trauma or the clinical condition. Focally the CBF is often increased corresponding to the injured areas[6, 7, 16, 24]. This uncoupling between CBF and the severity of the trauma may not be incomprehensible when we consider that regional CBF (rCBF) is determined by several factors, such as CPP (systemic arterial blood pressure [SAP] minus local tissue pressure), $PaCO_2$ and the degree of tissue acidosis. If the tissue is severely injured, acidosis will develop causing dilatation of the vessels (vasoparalysis) resulting in hyperemia[4]. Secondarily developed brain edema increases the ICP, with fall in perfusion pressure and CBF decrease. When the injured patient recovers the CBF approaches normal values, but usually the flow values are subnormal at the time the consciousness is regained[6—8].

CBF and Oxygen Uptake of the Brain Tissue

The cerebral metabolic rate for oxygen ($CMRO_2$) may be calculated by multiplying the arteriovenous difference of oxygen and the CBF. The normal value of $CMRO_2$ is about 3 ml/100 g/min. In injured brain tissue the $CMRO_2$ is decreased and, unlike the CBF, the $CMRO_2$ is related to the clinical state of the acute comatose patient[2, 3, 5, 10, 30]. Severe decrease in $CMRO_2$ can be seen in spite of normal CBF, *i.e.,* the luxury perfusion syndrome[20]. The brain tissue cannot use the offered oxygen, the arteriovenous oxygen difference is small and the venous blood colour is red, approaching the arterial blood colour[17]. These red veins may be seen during craniotomy. A critical low limit of $CMRO_2$ has still not been found in head trauma[5].

Autoregulation

The ability of the brain to maintain the CBF constant, independent of changes in CPP, may be tested by raising or lowering the blood pressure. Usually angiotensin is used for the raising and arfonad for the lowering of the blood pressure. The injured brain tissue may have lost its capacity of autoregulation, and thus lost its protection against blood pressure fluctuations. When the autoregulation is impaired, then increasing blood pressure will not, as normally, be compensated by constriction of the arterioles. So a blood pressure rise will be transmitted to the capillaries and veins, where the high SAP causes high pressure gradient in the capillaries, resulting in leak out of water, electrolytes and plasma proteins to the brain tissue, and vasogenic edema develops. Initially most unconscious head trauma patients have disturbed autoregulation diffusely or locally, and it is lost in all comatose patients with lesion at the bulbar level[3, 7, 9, 24]. In more severely injured brain tissue the autoregulation may be impaired for weeks, but in severely injured brain tissue (lacerated tissue) the autoregulation can appear as normal (false autoregulation) in the sense that CBF remains constant in spite of change in SAP[7]. False autoregulation is usually seen focally in areas with pronounced edema, and may be caused by simultaneous changes in SAP and tissue pressure leaving the CPP unchanged. The

autoregulation recovers parallelly to the clinical condition, the false autoregulation through a period with impaired autoregulation[7].

Response of CBF to Carbon Dioxide

A sudden change in $PaCO_2$ normally changes CBF 2–6% for every mmHg change in PCO_2. In injured brain tissue the CO_2 responsiveness may be impaired in varying degrees[7, 9, 11, 24] but only in very severely injured brain tissue is the responsiveness totally lost. Actually impaired and lost responsiveness correlate with poor clinical condition and predict poor prognosis[7, 9, 24]. The responsiveness may improve with recovery of the clinical condition and deteriorate with deterioration of the clinical condition. It is known from experimental studies and from brain injured patients that the autoregulation suffers before the CO_2 responsiveness[7, 9, 20]. Thus, some patients may present impaired autoregulation simultaneously with normal CO_2 responsiveness[7, 29]. This dissociation is seen in moderately injured brain tissue. The opposite possibility, *i.e.,* impaired CO_2 responsiveness associated with true normal cortical autoregulation is only seen in brain stem injuries, whereas false autoregulation in combination with impaired CO_2 response suggest severely damaged tissue[7].

Intracranial Pressure and CBF

Most studies concerning the relation between ICP and CBF indicate that there is no consistent correlation if ICP is normal or slightly increased unless space-occupying lesions are present intracranially. However, high ICP (40–60 mmHg) seems to be correlated to low CBF and poor prognosis[3, 6, 8, 9, 15, 18, 24, 33].

CBF and Outcome

The CBF level cannot predict the outcome of the brain injured patient[3, 7, 9]. Very low CBF as well as high CBF may indicate poor prognosis. Thus, in some patients evoked electrocortical activity may be absent even though the CBF is high[12]. This probably illustrates the uncoupling between CBF and metabolism, the luxury perfusion syndrome[20]. However, the course of the CBF may give a hint about prognosis as early normalization of CBF predicts good outcome[6, 7].

Treatment of the Brain Ischemic/Hyperemic Patient

Maintaining a sufficient CBF and avoiding complications as brain edema may be a goal in the treatment of the brain injured patient[8, 21, 22]. Unfortunately no drugs have been found having a beneficial effect on CBF. In the literature papaverine and acetazolamide are known to have dilating effect on the brain vessels[31, 32]. However, they seem only to dilate normal vessels, and not the vessels in the injured areas. This dilatation of the normal vessels may increase the ICP and so be disadvantageous. In contrast to this, drugs with vasoconstrictive effect on the brain vessels such as aminophylline may have a beneficial effect. As they constrict the normal vessels, they decrease the blood volume and thus the ICP, resulting in increased CPP in the injured non reacting brain tissue.

As increase in SAP may provoke development of vasogenic edema, factors which increase the blood pressure must be avoided. The brain injured patient should be kept sedated; pain, a filled bladder, cumbersome manipulation and noise should be avoided. The CPP must be kept at a sufficient level by maintaining the ICP at an acceptable level (< 20 mmHg?) by means of hyperventilation[11, 13, 21, 22] and ventricular drainage[8, 21, 22, 33]. The oxygen supply must be sufficient. In addition low hemoglobin concentration, high body temperature, and coincident illness such as heart diseases and diabetes must be treated optimally.

Future Research

At the present time measurements of CBF seem not to have any practical importance, neither in the estimate of the clinical condition of the head trauma patient nor in the estimate of the effect of the treatments. The reason for performing the CBF measurements could be the unique clinical course in each patient, resulting in a missing knowledge about the prognosis of the injury in the individual patient, and about the consequences of the treatment used. If repeated CBF measurements could be done in every patient during the acute phase, the course of the brain damage could be followed and if necessary an adequate intervention be possible. Thus, it is obvious that a patient with cerebral hyperemia may be treated differently from a patient with ischemia. However, if the CBF measurements may be used in the daily observation of the patients, the method must be easy to carry out, without risks for the patient and the staff, non-expensive, and it has to be carried out in the ward without moving the patient[8, 21, 22].

A mobile detector using intravenous 133-Xenon technique may possibly be suitable for this purpose[14]. The method implies the possibility of repeated measurements, with a mobile equipment which can be handled without risk by one person, a nurse or a laboratory worker. More sophisticated and expensive methods as PET, NMR, and dynamic computer-assisted tomography may hardly be of practical importance in the daily observation of the patient but may still in the future be devoted the study of selected groups and problems.

References

1. Baldy-Moulinier M, Frerebeau Ph (1969) Cerebral blood flow in cases of coma following severe head injury. In: Brock M, Fieschi C, Ingvar D *et al* (eds) Cerebral blood flow. Springer, Berlin Heidelberg New York, pp 216–218
2. Baldy-Moulinier M, Roquefeuil B, Escuret E, Viguie E, Frerebeau Ph (1975) Hemodynamic and metabolic modifications into the brain following short lasting and prolonged changes of arterial pressure and PaO_2 in comatose patients. In: Harper M *et al* (eds) Blood flow and metabolism in the brain. 13.34–13.37
3. Bruce DA, Langfitt TW, Miller JD *et al* (1973) Regional cerebral blood flow, intracranial pressure and brain metabolism in comatose patients. J Neurosurg 38: 131–144
4. Bruce DA, Schut L, Bruno LA *et al* (1978) Outcome following severe head injuries in children. J Neurosurg 48: 679–688
5. Cold GE (1978) Cerebral metabolic rate of oxygen ($CMRO_2$) in the acute phase of brain injury. Acta Anaesthesiol Scand 22: 249–256
6. Enevoldsen EM, Cold G, Jensen FT *et al* (1976) Dynamic changes in regional CBF, intraventricular pressure, CSF pH and lactate levels during the acute phase of head injury. J Neurosurg 44: 191–214
7. Enevoldsen EM, Jensen FT (1978) Autoregulation and CO_2 responses of cerebral blood flow in patients with acute severe head injury. J Neurosurg 48: 689–703
8. Enevoldsen EM (1981) Dynamic changes in regional cerebral blood flow, cerebral ventricular pressure, cerebrospinal pH and lactate during the acute phase of severe head injury. FADL's forlag, København, Århus, Odense
9. Fieschi C, Battistini N, Beduschi A *et al* (1974) Regional cerebral blood flow and intraventricular pressure in acute head injuries. J Neurol Neurosurg Psychiatry 37: 1378–1388
10. Genarelli TA, Obrist WD, Langfitt TW *et al* (1979) Vascular and metabolic reactivity to changes in PCO_2 in head injured patients. In: Popp, Bourke, Nelson *et al* (eds) (1979) Seminars in Neurological Surgery: Neural Trauma. Raven Press, New York, pp 1–8
11. Gordon E, Bergvall U (1973) The effect of controlled hyperventilation on cerebral blood flow and oxygen uptake in patients with brain lesions. Acta Anaesthesiol Scand 17: 63–69
12. Greenberg RP, Sakalas R, Miller JD *et al* (1977) Multimodality evoked potentials and CBF in patients with severe head injury. In: Ingvar, Lassen (eds) (1977) Cerebral Function, Metabolism and Circulation. Munksgaard, Copenhagen, pp 498–499
13. Hoppe E, Christensen L, Christensen KN (1981) The clinical outcome of patients with severe head injuries, treated with high dose dexamethasone, hyperventilation and barbiturate. Neurochirurgia 24: 17–20

14. Jabre A, Simone L, Redmond S (1985) A comparative study of the portable regional CBF monitor and the portable mean hemispheral CBF monitor: Advantages and Disadvantages in Clinical Practice. Acta Neurochir 77: 142–145

15. Johnston IH, Johnston JA, Jennet WB (1970) Intracranial pressure changes following head injury. Lancet 2: 433–436

16. Kasoff SS, Zingesser LH, Shulman K (1972) Compartmental abnormalities of regional cerebral blood flow in children with head trauma. J Neurosurg 36: 463–470

17. Lanfitt TW (1971) The microcirculation in mechanical brain injury. In: Head Injuries. Proceedings of an International Symposium in Edinburgh and Madrid. Edinburgh/London, Churchill Livingstone, pp 221–223

18. Langfitt TW (1976) Incidence and importance of intracranial hypertension in head injured patients. In: Beks JWF, Bosch DA, Brock M (eds) Intracranial Pressure Ill. Springer, Berlin Heidelberg New York, pp 67–72

19. Langfitt TW, Obrist WD, Gennarelli TA et al (1977) Correlation of cerebral blood flow with outcome in head injured patients. Ann Surg 186: 411–414

20. Lassen NA (1966) The luxury perfusion syndrome and its possible relation to acute metabolic acidosis localized within the brain. Lancet 2: 1113–1115

21. Marshall LF, Smith RW, Shapiro HM (1979) The outcome with aggressive treatment in severe head injury. Part 1. The significance of intracranial pressure monitoring. J Neurosurg 50: 20–25

22. Marshall LF, Smith RW, Shapiro HM (1979) The outcome with aggressive treatment in severe head injuries. Part 2. Acute and chronic barbiturateadministration in the management of head injuries. J Neurosurg 50: 26–30

23. Obrist WD, Dolinskas CA, Gennarelli TA et al (1979) Relation of blood flow to CT scan in acute head injury. In: Popp, Bourke, Nelson et al (eds) Seminars in Neurological Surgery: Neural Trauma. Raven Press, New York, pp 41–50

24. Overgaard J, Tweed WA (1974) Cerebral circulation after head injury. I. Cerebral blood journal and its regulation after closed head injury with emphasis on clinical correlation. J Neurosurg 41: 531–541

25. Overgaard J, Tweed WA (1976) Cerebral circulation after head injury. II. The effects of traumatic brain edema. J Neurosurg 45: 292–300

26. Overgaard, Mosdal C, Tweed WA (1981) Cerebral circulation after head injury. III. Does reduces regional cerebral blood flow determine recovery of brain function after blunt head injury? J Neurosurg 55: 63–74

27. Overgaard J (1976) Reflections on prognostic determinants in acute severe head injury. Proceedings of the Chicago Neural Trauma Conference, March 1975. Ransohoff J, McLaurin. Grune & Stratton, New York, pp 11–21

28. Risberg J, Prohovnik I (1981) rCBF measurements by 133-Xe inhalation: Recent methological advances. Prog Nucl Med 7: 70–81

29. Shalit MN, Reinmuth OM, Shimojyo Sodo et al (1967) Carbon dioxide cerebral circulatory control. III. The effects of brainstem lesions. Artch Neurol 17: 342–353

30. Shalit MN, Beller AJ, Feinsod M (1972) Clinical equivalents of cerebral oxygen consumption in coma. Neurology (Minneap) 22: 155–160

31. Sokoloff L (1959) The action of drugs on cerebral circulation. Pharmacol Rev 11: 1

32. Sokoloff L, Keyy SS (1971) To-days dDrugs: Cerebral vasodilators. Brit Med J 2: 702

33. Vapalathi M (1970) Intracranial pressure, acid-base status of blood and cerebrospinal fluid, and pulmonary function in the prognosis of severe brain injury: a prospective study in 51 brain-injured patients. Thesis, Helsinki

Author's address: E. Enevoldsen, Neurological Department, University Hospital, Odense, Denmark.

Acta Neurochirurgica, Suppl. 36, 137–141 (1986)

Brain Edema

B. B. Johansson

Department of Neurology, University Hospital, Lund, Sweden

Summary

Current concepts on the development of brain edema are briefly reviewed. The common classification into vasogenic and cytotoxic edema is a simplification and does not cover all types of edema. Alternative routes of edema resolution are discussed. More basic data on the mechanisms of development and regression of brain edema are needed before more successful treatments are likely to be found.

Keywords: Brain edema; blood-brain barrier; edema resolution; brain-CF pathways; brain-lymphatic pathways.

Definition

Brain edema is an increase in brain volume caused by an accumulation of water. Brain edema should be separated from brain enlargement due to increased blood volume.

Classification

Various classifications have been proposed for brain edema. The currently most used classification into vasogenic and cytotoxic edema was introduced by Klatzo[15]. In vasogenic edema, a damage to the blood brain barrier (BBB) enables plasma proteins and electrolytes to enter the brain. The edema fluid spreads predominantly in the extracellular spaces of the white matter via low resistance pathways and may reach the other hemisphere via corpus callosum. Figure 2 illustrates this kind of edema, which in clinical practice is most typically seen around brain tumors.

No dysfunction of the BBB is present in cytotoxic edema, characterized by intracellular swelling indicating disturbed osmoregulation. Any failure of the energy-dependent pump mechanisms responsible for uphelding the ion concentration gradients across cell membranes will result in ion and fluid shifts between the intra- and extracellular compartments[35] and changes in the extracellular ion content will lead to fluid shifts between brain and blood. Experimentally, trietyltin and hexachlorophene have been extensively used as models for cytotoxic edema. The term "cytotoxic" seems less suitable to cover the intracellular swelling in hypoxia and hypoosmolarity but is used also for these conditions[15].

The complex types of edema that are seen in ischemic and traumatic lesions are not easily classified into the two groups discussed above (see below). Furthermore, the paraventricular interstitial edema in hydrocephalus, thought to be caused by the entry of cerebrospinal fluid from the ventricles, is not covered by the classification.

The importance of the extravasated plasma proteins for formation of vasogenic edema has been stressed[16, 20]. A time correlation between protein leakage and brain water content has been established in some experimental models, however, other factors such as whether or not the BBB opening is associated with tissue necrosis seems to influence the degree of edema formation[13]. Various "brain edema factors" have been proposed[1].

Altering the extracellular homeostasis is likely to influence the cell function and pure models of vasogenic edema do probably not exist. Even in the classical model of vasogenic edema, cold lesion, there is evidence for intracellular axonal transport of exogenous proteins[34]. In fat embolism, a model with BBB opening and severe, rapidly developing brain edema, the edema is to a large extent intracellular in gray as well as in white matter (Johansson, Li and Olsson, unpublished observation). In the analysis of edema, it seems essential to consider whether edema is

— intra and/or extracellular

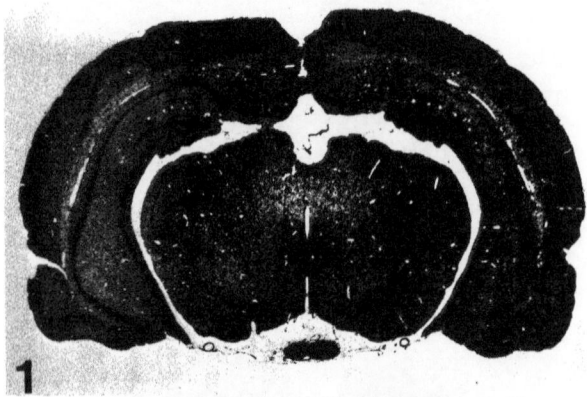

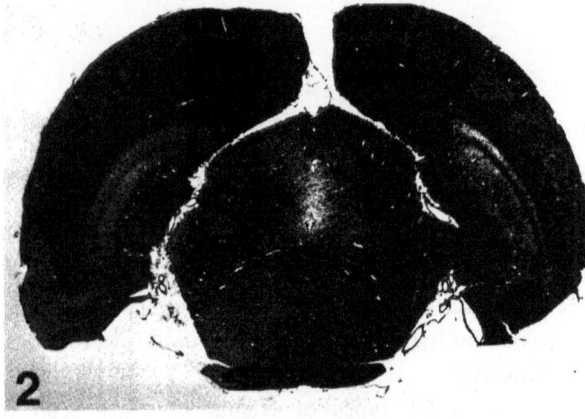

Figs. 1 and 2. Brain sections from stroke-prone hypertensive rats. Fig. 1 shows a rat with no BBB dysfunction. When these rats develop BBB dysfunction, indicated by extravasation of fibrinogen in the cortex on the left hemisphere in Fig. 2, the high blood pressure leads to extensive spread of plasma constituents in the white matter, illustrated by positive staining for antifibrinogen in the entire white matter on both sides (antifibrinogen + hematoxylin counterstain). From Fredriksson *et al.* 1985[7], by permission

— occurring in gray and/or white matter
— combined with BBB opening
— combined with tissue necrosis

Blood-Brain Barrier

Some knowledge of the blood brain barrier (BBB) is needed for the discussion of brain edema.

The brain endothelial cells are joined together by tight junctions and have a low pinocytotic activity[29]. The entry of a substance will mainly depend on its lipid solubility and whether or not it has access to any of the specific carriers in the endothelial cells[3, 25].

The brain endothelial cells have a high metabolic activity as indicated by a very high content of mitochondriae. Thus, 10–11% of the cytoplasma is made up of mitochondria compared to 2.7% in other blood

vessels and 4% in proximal renal tubules[26]. The electrical resistance of microvessels at the brain surface corresponds to that of a tight epithelium[5]. The luminal and abluminal surfaces of the cell membrane are not identical. The enzymes alkaline phosphatase and gamma-glutamyl transpeptidase are found on both sides whereas Na, K -ATPase and 5′-nucleotidase are found only on the abluminal side[2] which is likely to be relevant for the carrier mechanisms. Specific transport carriers have been identified for hexosis, short-chained monocarboxylic acids, amino acids (separate carriers for neutral, basic and acidic proteins), nucleic acid precursors, purines, choline, T-3 and T-4[25]. The carriers are stereo specific and are subject to competition and inhibition. They can adapt or readjust under various circumstances such as fasting and hyperglycemia. Fluoro-deoxyglucose and 2-deoxyglucose have affinity for the hexose carrier used by d-glucose; hence these substances can be used to estimate brain glucose metabolism. The presence of enzymatic barriers is another unique feature of brain vessels[9].

The endothelial cells are not freely permeable to water as previously thought[28]. The BBB is functionally similar to membranes known to regulate water permeability. The regulation of water permeability over the BBB is under neurogenic and endocrine influences[27, 28]. What significance these observations may have for the net uptake of water and the regulation of brain water volume is a matter of controversy.

Clinical Conditions

An intracellular edema occurs in hypoxia, acute water intoxication and other conditions with rapidly developing hypoosmolarity in the serum.

Cytotoxic edema due to exogenous substances has been observed in babies intoxicated by the use of hexachlorophene in the bath-water or, accidentally, in too high concentration in baby powder. A few cases of triethyltin intoxication have been reported.

Alterations in the BBB of importance for the discussion of brain edema are present in brain-tumors, trauma, embolism, cardiovascular disorders, chemical influences and radiation. An increase in blood pressure will greatly enhance the edema formation in the presence of a BBB opening[17, 19] and may also in itself alter the BBB, particularly when the blood pressure elevation is combined with vasodilatation such as during epileptic seizures and hypercapnia[11].

Whether the plasma constituents enter the brain via a transendothelial or interendothelial route is controversial and may differ in the various models of BBB opening[11, 12].

In ischemia, an initial shift of water from the extracellular to the intracellular department occurs due to increased intracellular osmolarity[10]. There is a close correlation between the degree of edema, pH and lactate in the tissue[24]. The accumulation of lactic acid is influenced by preischemic blood glucose levels. As is well known from clinical medicine, the early phase of edema, which may be severe and associated with a midline shift in hemispheric lesions, may show no contrast enhancement on CT. After various times, depending, *e.g.* on whether the ischemia is complete, partial or transitory, a blood-brain barrier dysfunction will allow leakage of plasma proteins; a leakage that may last longer than the clinically apparent edema.

Brain bulk enlargement after acute head injury may be due to acute brain edema or to an increase of the cerebral blood volume. It has been suggested that the presence of brain edema has been overestimated and that swelling due to vasoparalysis is initially a much larger problem than edema[23]. According to a recent report, dynamic CT scans in nonfatally injured patients suggested a hyperemic state. On the other hand, in 17 of 25 fatally injured patients, CT scans, mostly done with 2 hours after the impact, revealed a brain edema. It was concluded that acute brain edema occurs more rapidly than is usually thought and is the more common cause of brain bulk enlargement in cases of fatal head injury[39]. In traumatic brain damage, an increase in blood pressure may aggravate the condition by increasing the brain edema and/or enhancing blood volume due to defect autoregulation in the traumatic tissue[17, 19, 33].

The introduction of computer tomography has greatly enhanced our possibility to diagnose brain edema in patients, for a review see Greenberg[8].

Resolution of Brain Edema

There is evidence for several clearing routes. The relative importance of the various possible clearing mechanisms discussed below is unclear.

1. Clearance of edema fluid by "bulk flow", that is, essentially independent of molecular sizes, to the ventricular CSF. This mechanism seems to be operative predominantly in the presence of a driving pressure and sustained egress of plasma constituents from the BBB lesion. Bulk flow is generally considered to be a main route under conditions with vasogenic edema. The driving force is able to carry the fluid to the opposite hemisphere via the corpus callosum which indicate a low resistance pathway[30, 31].

2. Clearance via diffusion to the cerebrospinal fluid is probably of minor importance for resolution of edema.

3. Clearance by uptake and degradation of extravasated plasma proteins into astrocytes and microglia[16, 20].

4. Degradation of plasma constituents by other, so far unknown ways in the brain parenchyma. It should be observed that the degradation of proteins may increase the osmolarity and hence temporarily enhance the edema.

5. A transvascular route of protein removal in arterioles and venules has been suggested in cold lesion edema[38]. Passage back to the blood over the brain microvessels might be of particular importance in hydrocephalic edema.

6. Increasing evidence supports the possibility that a significant fraction of CSF drains into the lymphatic system[4, 21], predominantly via the cribriform plate to deep cervical lymph.

The possible role of this route in the pathophysiology of hydrocephalus as well as in clearance of edema fluid is debated. Blockade of CSF access to the dorsal surface of the hemisphere did not produce hydrocephalus unless the olfactory route of CSF drainage into the lymphatic system was obstructed as well according to one study[32]. In experiments with infusion of artificial CSF into the ventricular system or the cisterna magna, an increased concentration of labeled albumin was present in the optic nerves, olphactory bulbs, episcleral tissue and deep cervical lymph nodes when the ICP was raised[21]. Drainage of CSF was similar irrespective of whether the infusion site was the ventricles or cisterna magna. Transcortical bulk transfer of CSF was not evident with raised ICP. It was concluded that, with elevated ICP, CSF drained via pathways that are less evident under normal pressure. In contrast, in another study the recovery of albumin in lymph was reduced from 14.8% in the controls to 6.9% at the highest infusion rate indicating that the proportion of CSF draining through this route relative to others was reduced at high ICP[4]. Nevertheless, the total flow through the cribriform plate might be elevated. The main resistance to drainage is likely to be the channels through the cribriforme plate, a resistance that will be fixed because of the rigidity of the bone. Marmarou[32], failed to show a significant passage to the lymph nodes in infusion edema. However, it is not clear from their study which lymph nodes where investigated. As stressed by Widner[32] only the deep cervical lymph nodes seem to receive a significant drainage from the brain. The pathway from the brain to the lymph is of functional significance as indicated by an immunological reaction in the lymph nodes after antigen deposit into the brain[37].

7. A further pathway has been described in stroke-prone spontaneously hypertensive rats with multifocal damage of the blood-brain barrier. Extravasated protein was observed to spread from leakage sites in deeper layers of the cortex upwards mainly along the perivascular space of penetrating vessels and then spread laterally within the subpial zone[14].

The *long term effects of brain edema* have not been well evaluated. Feigin has stressed the importance of edema fluid for permanent changes in the white matter[5]. There is experimental evidence that plasma might damage myelin[18]. Alteration of the extracellular environment is likely to have an effect on the function and metabolism of brain cell. BBB transport mechanisms are bidirectional and the disturbances of the barrier may affect not only the entry but also the removal of substances from the brain parenchyma. Faulty out-transport of metabolites and removal of toxic waste products may contribute to tissue damage. The significance of compression of microvasculature by edema fluid or of the increase of intercapillary diffusion distance for the production of tissue hypoxia is controversial.

Treatment

A treatment may be effective by a direct effect on the water content, by tightening the blood-brain barrier, by enhancing the resolution of brain edema, or by decreasing the intracranial pressure. A full account of the various treatment tried is outside the scope of the present paper. Basic care includes monitoring of blood gases, blood pressure and temperature.

Hyperosmolar solutions have been widely used and is of value particularly to gain time, *e.g.* before an operation. However, in the presence of a BBB disturbance the agents used (mainly urea and mannitol) will pass over into the brain and therefore no long-lasting effect can be expected. The fact that urea enters the cells makes this drug particularly prone to a rebound effect. The effect of nonosmotic diuretics such as furosemide and acetazolamide on the water content and CSF production in edema is debated.

Dexamethasone is of undisputable value in the treatment of the brain edema surrounding brain tumors. The mechanism is not clear; membrane stabili-

zation, effect on ion fluxes and a direct effect on tumor cells are a few of the suggested mechanisms. There is no hard evidence that steroids, even in high doses, have any favorable effect on the edema in connection with trauma and ischemia.

The possible effect of barbiturate treatment is controversial. The initial optimism has by and large been replaced by a critical attitude. Barbiturate may be of some value in carefully selected patients[22].

Several drugs that stabilize membranes and reduce pinocytotic activity have been found to effectively reduce BBB opening during hypertension and epileptic seizures[12]. So far, they have not been shown to prevent or reduce brain edema.

Acknowledgement

Studies from the authors own laboratory were supported by the Swedish Medical Research Council (14X-4968).

References

1. Baethmann A, Oettinger, W, Rothenfusser W, Kempski O, Unterberg A, Geiger R (1980) Brain edema factors: current state with particular references to plasma constituents and glutamate. Adv Neurol 28: 171–195
2. Betz AL, Firth JA, Goldstein GW (1980) Polarity of the blood-brain barrier: distribution of enzymes between the luminal and antiluminal membranes of brain capillary endothelial cells. Brain Res 192: 17–28
3. Bradbury MBW (1979) The concept of a blood-brain barrier. J Wiley & Sons, New York
4. Bradbury MWB, Westrup RJ (1984) Lymphatics and the drainage of cerebrospinal fluid. In: Shapiro K *et al.* (eds) Hydrocephalus. Raven Press, New York, pp 69–81
5. Crone C, Olesen SP (1982) Electrical resistance of brain microvascular endothelium. Brain Res 242: 49–55
6. Feigin I, Popoff N (1962) Neuropathological observations on cerebral edema. Arch Neurol 6: 151–160
7. Fredriksson K, Auer RN, Kalimo H, Nordborg C, Olsson Y, Johansson BB (1985) Cerebrovascular lesions in stroke-prone spontaneously hypertensive rats. Acta Neuropathol (Berl) 68: 284–294
8. Greenberg JO (1984) Neuroimaging in brain swelling. Neurologic clinics 2: 677–694
9. Hardebo JE, Owman Ch (1980) Barrier mechanisms for neurotransmitter monoamines and their precursors at the blood-brain interface. Ann Neurol 8: 1–10
10. Hossmann KA (1976) Development and resolution if ischemic brain swelling. In: Pappius H, Feindel W (eds) Dynamics of brain edema. Springer, Berlin Heidelberg New York, pp 219–227
11. Johansson, BB, The blood-brain barrier in acute and chronic hypertension. In: Eisenberg HM, Suddith RL (eds) The cerebral microvasculature. Adv Exp Med Biol 131: 211–226. Plenum, New York
12. Johansson BB (1981) Pharmacological modification of hypertensive blood-brain barrier opening. Acta Pharmacol Toxicol 48: 242–247

13. Johansson BB, Linder L-E (1981) Hypertension and brain edema—An experimental study on acute and chronic hypertension in the rat. J Neurol Neurosurg Psychiatry 44: 402–406

14. Kalimo H, Fredriksson K, Nordborg C, Auer RN, Olsson Y, Johansson BB, The spread of brain edema in hypertensive encephalopathy. Medical Biology, Vol 64, 1986 in press

15. Klatzo I (1967) Presidential address: Neuropathological aspects of brain edema. J Neuropathol Exp Neurol 26: 1–13

16. Klatzo I, Chui E, Fujiwara K, Spatz M (1980) Resolution of vasogenic brain edema. Adv Neurol 28: 359–373

17. Klatzo I, Wisniewski H, Steinwall O, Streicher E (1976) Dynamics of cold injury edema. In: Klatzo I, Seitelberger F (eds) Brain edema. Springer, Berlin Heidelberg New York, pp 554–563

18. Konat G, Offner H (1982) Effect of serum on the isolated CNS myelin membrane. Neurochemistry International 4: 143–147

19. Langfitt TW, Weinstein JD, Kassell NF, Jackson JLF (1967) Contributions of trauma, anoxia, and arterial hypertension to experimental acute brain swelling. Trans Am Neurol Ass 92: 257–259

20. Marmarou A, Nakamura T, Tanaka K, Hochwald GM (1984) The time course and distribution of water in the resolution phase of infusion edema. In: Go KG, Baethmann A (eds) Brain edema. Plenum, New York, pp 37–44

21. McComb JG, Davson H, Hyman S, Weiss MG (1982) Cerebrospinal fluid drainage as influenced by ventricular pressure in the rabbit. J Neurosurg 56: 790–797

22. Messeter K, Nordström CH, Sundbärg G, Algotsson L, Ryding E (1986) Cerebral hemodynamics in patients with acute severe head trauma. J Neurosurg, in press

23. Miller DM, Corales RL (1981) Brain edema as a result of head injury: fact of fallacy? In: de Vlieger M et al. (eds) Brain edema. Wiley & Sons, New York, pp 99–115

24. Myers RE (1979) Lactic acid accumulation as a cause of brain edema and cerebral necrosis resulting from oxygen deprivation. In: Korobkin R, Guilleminault G (eds) Advances in perinatal neurology. Spectrum, Jamaica NY, pp 85–114

25. Oldendorf WH (1977) The blood-brain barrier. Exp Eye Res [Suppl] 177–190

26. Oldendorf WH, Cornford ME, Brown WJ (1977) The large apparent work capability of the blood-brain barrier: a study of the mitochondrial content of capillary endothelial cells in brain and other tissues of the rat. Ann Neurol 1: 409–417

27. Raichle ME, Grupp RL (1978) Regulation of brain water permeability by centrally released vasopressin. Brain Res 143: 191–194

28. Raichle ME, Hartman BK, Eichling JO, Sharpe LG (1975) Central noradrenergic regulation of cerebral blood flow and vascular permeability. Proc Natl Acad Sci (Wash) 72: 3726–3730

29. Reese TS, Karnovsky MJ (1967) Fine structural localization of a blood to brain barrier to exogenous peroxidase. J Cell Biol 34: 207–217

30. Reulen HJ, Graham R, Spatz M, Klatzo I (1977) Role of pressure gradients and bulkflow in dynamics of vasogenic brain edema. J Neurosurg 46: 24–35

31. Reulen HJ, Tsuyumu M (1981) Pathophysiology of formation and natural resolution of vasogenic brain edema. In: de Vlieger M et al. (eds) Brain edema. J Wiley & Sons, New York, pp 31–48

32. Schurr, PH, Mc Laurin RL, Ingraham FD (1953) Experimental studies on the circulation of the cerebrospinal fluid and methods of producing hydrocephalus in the dog. J Neurosurg 10: 515–525

33. Schutta HS, Kassel NF, Langfitt TW (1968) Brain swelling produced by injury and aggravated by arterial hypertension. Brain 91: 281–294

34. Tengvar Ch, Olsson Y (1982) Uptake of macromolecules into neurons from a focal vasogenic cerebral edema and subsequent axonal spread to other brain regions. Acta Neuropathol (Berl) 57: 233–235

35. van Harreveld A (1966) Brain tissue electrolytes. Butterworths, London

36. Widner H, Jönsson BA, Strand SE, Johansson BB (1984) In vivo demonstration of passage from the brain parenchyma into the deep cervical lymph nodes in the rat. Intern J Microcirc 3/4: 451

37. Widner H, Johansson BB, Möller B (1985) Qualitative demonstration of a link between brain parenchyma and the lymphatic system. J Cereb Blood Flow Metabol 5: [Suppl] 1: 87–88

38. Vorbrodt AW, Lossinsky AS, Wisniewski HM, Suzuki R, Yamaguchi T, Masaoka H, Klatzo I (1985) Ultrastructural observations on the transvascular route of protein removal in vasogenic brain edema. Acta Neuropathol (Berl) 66: 265–273

39. Yoshino E, Yamaki T, Higuchi T, Horikawa Y, Hirikawa K (1985) Acute brain edema in fatal head injury: analysis by dynamic CT scanning. J Neurosurg 63: 830–839

Author's address: B. B. Johansson, M.D., Department of Neurology, University Hospital, S-221 85 Lund, Sweden.

Acta Neurochirurgica, Suppl. 36, 142 (1986)

Possible Evaluation of Treatment and Prognosis in Brain Contusions by Means of the Isoenzyme Creatine Kinase (CK-BB) in the Blood

H. K. Nordby, P. Urdal, and **R. Nesbakken**

Department of Neurosurgery, Ullevål sygehus, Oslo, Norge

We have measured blood CK-BB in 36 consecutive patients suffering from brain contusions. These 36 patients were divided into 2 prognostic groups on the basis of the Glasgow Coma Score (GCS). A GCS of 6 or less was found in 17 of the patients. They were chosen for intracranial pressure (ICP)-guided intensive care. The remaining 19 patients who had a GCS of 7 or higher were treated on the basis of their clinical signs only, without the use of invasive monitoring.

All patients had brain contusions, and all of them had elevated levels of CK-BB in the blood samples that were drawn within 6 hours of accident. The highest levels were found in patients with the lowest GCS. The blood CK-BB levels decreased rapidly during the first day. Early brain tamponade resulted in a very rapid decrease in blood CK-BB, most probably due to cessation of circulatory wash-out of enzymes from the damaged brain[1].

Normalization of blood CK-BB within 36 hours in nontamponade patients seems to be an indication of treatment efficacy as it signalizes an acceptable outcome as far as our patients are concerned.

Rapid normalization occurred more often in patients subjected to ICP-guided intensive care than in those treated without ICP guidance even if the former patients belonged to a poorer prognostic group according to their GCSs.

In 9 additional patients simultaneous samples of blood and lumbar cerebrospinal fluid (CSF) were available. The CK-BB levels were generally higher in the CSF and sustained high levels were found in patients with secondary brain injuries. Lumbar taps are usually contraindicated after head injury, thus valuable information from CK-BB levels in lumbar CSF cannot be obtained. The measurement of CK-BB in blood may give information on prognosis without subjecting the patients to unnecessary risks.

Keywords: Head injury, prognostic enzyme indication; neurosurgical intensive care.

Reference

1. Nordby KH, Urdal P (1985) Creatinine kinase BB in blood as index of prognosis and effect of treatment after severe head injury. Acta Neurochir (Wien) 76: 131–136

Acta Neurochirurgica, Suppl. 36, 143–144 (1986)

Posttraumatic Monitoring of Intracranial Pressure

U. Pontén

Department of Neurosurgery, University Hospital, Uppsala, Sweden

Summary

ICP-monitoring is a good guide for surgical and nonsurgical treatment of unconscious patients with severe traumatic brain injuries. Intraventricular and extradural recordings usually are reliable but have systematic differences. Subdural screws tend to underestimate ICP > 20 mm Hg. High ICP correlates with poor outcome. Plateau-waves induced by external stimulation indicate a tight brain situation requiring treatment. In critical situations monitoring of the cerebral perfusion pressure is recommended. ICP recordings can never substitute personal supervision of the patient.

Keywords: Traumatic brain injuries; intracranial pressure monitoring; neurosurgical intensive care.

Indications

Intracranial pressure (ICP) monitoring is indicated to guide surgical or nonsurgical treatment when clinical signs and symptoms are difficult to evaluate and when the physiological and anatomical volume compensatory mechanisms are used to a considerable extent which means that deterioration may occur rapidly. These patients are in coma, usually reaction level ≥ 6 (RLS). Operable hematomas are removed, multiple small contusions or diffuse brain swelling may still remain. The CT scan usually shows narrow cisterns and ventricles.

Methods

Ventricular fluid pressure (VFP) recording through an indwelling catheter usually in the right frontal horn is the most reliable method since it can be calibrated against external pressures at any time. If the ventricle is punctured during isovolumetric pressure recording even small slit-like ventricles can easily be found and cannulated. If the ventricles are very small drainage of CSF may cause ventricular collapse and loss of pressure recording. This can be prevented by setting the outflow resistance to a level that is higher than normal (25–30 mm Hg)[2, 3].

Extradural pressure (EDP) transducers usually can be calibrated only before and after the implantation which requires a very stable system. Some available equipments seem to be reasonably stable in this respect. Systematic differences may occur between the mounted EDP and the VFP[7]. This is usually of no clinical significance. The main advantage of EDP recordings is less risk for meningitis.

Subdural screws of different types have a tendency to underestimate pressures above 20 mm Hg[4].

Complications

With a standardized protocol for the ICP recordings it is possible to keep the rate of established clinical infections (*i.e.* meningitis) around 2%[3]. Expansive hematomas are extremely rare both for VFP and EDP, unless the patient has a coagulopathy.

Observations

True spontaneous reversible plateau-waves as those originally described by Lundberg[2] mostly in connection with brain-tumors are seldom seen nowadays. The reason is that patients are usually treated before pressure recording is instituted since it is now generally realized that these waves represent the final dangerous part on the evolution of intracranial hypertension. When plateau-waves occur, they usually indicate a large focal expansive lesion. Prolonged (> 5 minutes) pressure elevations after manipulations with the patient, like suction of the air-ways or neurological examination, will indicate "a tight brain", *i.e.* a high resistance (or low compliance) of the intracranial space. These pressure responses may be regarded as induced plateau-waves. They may, as the spontaneous plateau-waves do, correlate with reversible or irreversible deterioration of the patient mainly with increased brain stem symptoms, respiratory stand-still being the final sign of brain-stem ischemia. These induced plateau-waves usually rise from a moderately increased base-level of the ICP, but may occur also from base-levels that are within the normal range (≤ 15 mm Hg). The tendency for induced plateau-waves depends upon to what extent the volume compensatory mechanisms are used, *i.e.* how far out to the right on the volume pressure curve the patient has reached. However, this tendency can also be controlled by for instance heavy sedation.

An increased base level of ICP is generally accepted as a bad prognostic sign. Pressures above 60 mmHg is connected with more than 90% mortality[1]. A level between 20 and 30 mm Hg is usually given as an indication for active surgical treatment or nonsurgical ICP controlling treatment[5,6].

The ICP level itself is not the relevant parameter since pressures between 50 and 100 mm Hg may be well tolerated if the pressures are induced by infusion of liquid in the lumbar CSF space. The ICP in the course after head injury is, however, an indication of the degree of brain swelling and brain herniation that is prevailing. Furthermore, a raised ICP tends to decrease the cerebral blood-flow (CBF). The cerebral perfusion pressure (PP), that is the difference between the mean arterial pressure (MAP) and the mean ICP, is a more relevant parameter. Normal values for PP are 60 mm Hg or more and the critical level is around 30 mm Hg. However, in some cases the patient may deteriorate with ischemic symptoms and die even with a fairly normal ICP and normal PP. This is then explained by an increased cerebral vascular resistance due to generalized brain edema or vaso-spasm. In these cases CBF, or the cerebral oxygen consumption, are the relevant parameters to determine.

Implications for Treatment

The ICP recording should be used for guiding the nonsurgical treateatment of increased intracranial pressure and sometimes also the indications for surgery. The ICP recording should be combined with arterial pressure recording, preferably continuous. A cerebral perfusion pressure of 50 mm Hg or more should be kept by increasing the arterial pressure or lowering the ICP. ICP reducing treatment should start at an VFP of > 20 mm Hg. If the ICP is recorded with a ventricular catheter, drainage of CSF may be used unless the ventricles are very small. The outflow pressure, however, should not be lower than 20–25 mm Hg in these cases.

It must be realized that continuous recording of ICP and PP by no means can replace a close supervision of the clinical state of the patient. Continuous recording of ICP has a strong educational value for all categories of the personnel since the effects on the pressure of all manipulations with the patient are readily shown in the ICP recording.

References

1. Langfitt TW (1976) The incidence and importance of intracranial hypertension in head-injured patients. In: Beks JWF *et al* (eds) Intracranial pressure III. Springer, Berlin Heidelberg New York, pp 67–72
2. Lundberg N (1960) Continuous recording and control of ventricular fluid pressure in neurosurgical practice. Acta Psychiat Neurol Scand 36: [Suppl] 149
3. Lundberg N, Kjällquist Å, Kullberg G, Pontén U, Sundbärg, G (1974) Nonoperative management of intracranial hypertension. In: Krayenbühl H (ed) Advances and technical standards in neurosurgery, vol 1. Springer, Wien New York, pp 1–59
4. Mendelow AD, Rowan JO, Murray L, Kerr AE (1983) A clinical comparison of subdural screw pressure measurements with ventricular pressure. J Neurosurg 58: 45–50
5. Miller JD, Becker DP, Wards JD, Sullivan HG, Adams WE, Rosner MJ (1977) Significance of intracranial hypertension in severe head injury. J Neurosurg 47: 503–516
6. Narayan RK, Kishore PRS, Becker DP, Ward JD, Enas GG, Greenberg RP, Da Silva AD, Lipper MH, Choi SC, Mayhall CG, Lutz HA, Young HF (1982) Intracranial pressure: to monitor or not to monitor? A review of our experience with severe head injury. J Neurosurg 56: 650–659
7. Sundbärg G, Nornes H (1972) Simultaneous recording of the epidural and ventricular fluid pressure. In: Brock M, Dietz H (eds) Intracranial pressure. Springer, Berlin Heidelberg New York, pp 46–50

Author's address: U. Pontén, M.D., Department of Neurosurgery, University Hospital, S-751 85 Uppsala, Sweden.

Acta Neurochirurgica, Suppl. 36, 145 (1986)

Prognosis as the Basis for Selection to Treatment After Severe Head Injury

H. K. Nordby and **R. Nesbakken**

Department of Neurosurgery, Ullevål sygehus, Oslo, Norge

After severe head injury intensive care is sometimes given to patients who turn out to be fatally injured or who never regain mental activity. Large scale prognostic work has been performed in many centres in order to administer treatment and give advice on the basis of previous clinical experience. Jennet et al. were able to predict confidently (more than 0.97 probability) death or survival after severe head injury in no more than 61% of their patients when clinical data for up to 3 days was available[1]. In addition to this type of clinical data, Narayan et al. used CT scan, ICP monitoring (ventricular catheter or a subarachnoid screw) and multi-modality evoked potentials[2]. They achieved 64% confident predictions (90% confidence level) by a combination of clinical and evoked potentials data from the first day after accident. Their statistical methods were, however, different from those of Jennett[2].

We made a study of 64 patients selected from a series of 130 with very severe head injury classified according to the Glasgow Coma Score (GCS of 6 or below). The clinical examination of brain pathology was often impossible in these patients because few motor responses were left and medication often obscured those which remained. Epidural intracranial pressure (ICP) monitoring was used to disclose risk of secondary brain injury and guide a treatment protocol. After 6–12 months the Glasgow Outcome Scale (GOS) was used for final assessment of outcome. We found that long term monitoring of the ICP during the period of intensive care treatment revealed important but clinically silent brain injury. Both the initial and the maximum level of ICP were prognostically significant[3]. In order to guide intensive care prevention of secondary brain injuries, continuous monitoring of the epidural ICP was superior to clinical examination or CT scan. Patients with a GCS of 3 (24 hours best GCS), bilaterally dilated fixed pupils which did not respond to treatment, and those having long-lasting uncontrollable ICP increase to more then 40 mm Hg did not survive with an acceptable recovery[4].

In our experience, treatment effect is clinically undetectable both when the prognosis is poor and when it is good. Therefore, a prognostic selection of patients is necessary. Furthermore, many therapeutic interventions are potentially dangerous in themselves (pharmacological paralysis, hypothermia, heavy osmotherapy). No patient should be subjected to maximum efforts to prevent secondary brain injury unless there is a positive indication, i.e. that the patient may make a reasonable recovery. A policy comprising the use of all available means should not be advocated, neither long term intensive care, unless such a recovery is indicated. The level of treatment should be matched to the prognosis and the actual type of pathology disclosed by the diagnostic tools during the intensive care.

Keywords: Head injury prognosis; ICP-treatment selection; GCS-ICP.

References

1. Jennet B, Teasdale G, Braakman R, Minderhoud J, Knill-Jones R (1976) Predicting outcome in individual patients after severe head injury. Lancet I: 1031–1034
2. Narayan RK, Greenberg RP, Miller JD, Enas GG, Choi SC, Kishore PRS, Selhorst JB, Lutz HA, Becker DP (1981) Improved confidence of outcome prediction in severe head injury. J Neurosurg 54: 751–762
3. Nordby HK, Gunnerød N (1985) Epidural monitoring of the intracranial pressure in severe head injury characterized by non-localizing motor response. Acta Neurochir (Wien) 74: 21–26.
4. Nordby HK, Nesbakken R (1984) The effect of high dose barbiturate de-compression after severe head injury: a controlled clinical trial. Acta Neurochir (Wien) 72: 157–166.

Author's address: H. K. Nordby, M.D. Department of Neurosurgery, Ullevål sygehus, Oslo, Norge.

Acta Neurochirurgica, Suppl. 36, 146 (1986)

Comments on Nonoperative Treatment of Severe Brain Injuries

Importance of Controlled Ventilation and Hyperventilation

E. Gordon

Karolinska Hospital, Stockholm, Sweden

All patients unconscious from brain injury should be intubated and hyperventilated in a ventilator. There are obvious advantages to intubate and ventilate all patients with a specified degree of impairment of consciousness. It is more dangerous to await the development of abnormalities and complications, when the institution of this treatment may come too late[2, 7].

The control of the neurological state of the patient during ventilator treatment is by no means jeopardized as muscle relaxants are not necessary. With intermittent doses of small amounts of phenoperidine the patient is calm and without pain, and conscious level is not affected.

In cases of moderate and severe brain injuries, patients will often remain unconscious because of elevated ICP. These patients should remain intubated and hyperventilated until their level of consciousness improves and certain primitive means of communication can be established. This level corresponds to a score of 9–10 on the GCS. During this period it is very useful to follow ICP with direct measurement. Fluctuations in this parameter and reactions to specific treatment can provide useful guidelines for further management[1, 4, 6]. Lowering of high ICP is one of the ways to improve the intracranial conditions as pointed out by Barbro Johansson in this supplement.

Many clinicans have expressed opinions that the ICP-lowering effect of controlled hyperventilation is rather shortlasting. This is contrary to our experience as we have seen good effect also after 2–3 weeks. The pathophysiological explanation for this phenomenon is clear enough: in the severely damaged brain with foci of ischemia and hypoxia acid metabolites are generated as long as these lesions prevail. The acidosis causes vasodilatation and hyperemia in areas of the brain where cerebral vessels have preserved CO_2-reactivity. In a recent article[3] Messeter et al. stresses the importance of considering this reactivity for successful lowering of high ICP during barbiturate treatment of brain injured comatous patients.

Controlled hyperventilation should be continued as indicated above, and compose the basis of all other treatment offered to the severely head injured patient[2, 5].

References

1. Becker DP, Vries JK, Young HF, et al (1975) Controlled cerebral perfusion pressure and ventilation in human mechanical brain injury: Prevention of progressive brain swelling. In: Lundberg N, et al. (ed) Intracranial pressure II. Springer, Berlin Heidelberg New York, pp 480–484
2. Gordon E (1971) Controlled respiration in the management of patients with traumatic brain injuries. Acta Anaesthesiol Scand 15: 193–208
3. Messeter K, Nordström CH, Sundbärg G, Algotsson L, Ryding E (1986) Cerebral hemodynamics in patients with acute severe head trauma. J Neurosurg, in press
4. Paulson OB (1971) Restoration of autoregulation by hypocapnia. In: Ross Russell RW (ed) Brain and blood flow. Pitman, London, pp 313–321
5. Rossanda M (1968) Prolonged hyperventilation in treatment of unconscious patients with severe brain injuries. Scand J Clin Lab Invest 22: [Suppl] 102, XIII: E
6. Rossanda M, Collice M, Porta M, et al (1975) Intracranial hypertension in head injury: Clinical significance and relation to respiration. In: Lundberg N et al (eds) Intracranial pressure II. Springer, Berlin Heidelberg New York, pp 475–479
7. Rossanda M, Di Giugno G, Corona S et al (1966) Oxygen supply to the brain and respirator treatment in severe comatose status. Acta Anaesthesiol Scand 3 [Suppl] 23: 766–774

Author's address: E. Gordon, M.D., Karolinska Hospital, Stockholm, Sweden.

Acta Neurochirurgica, Suppl. 36, 147–150 (1986)

Craniofacial Surgery for Trauma

C. Lauritzen, B. Vällfors, and J. Lilja

Departments of Plastic Surgery and Neurosurgery, Sahlgrenska Hospital, University of Göteborg, Sweden

Summary

Craniofacial surgical techniques have yielded as an important spin-off better methods of treating severe craniofacial trauma.

In this paper surgical techniques are discussed.

It was concluded that the most important factors for successful reconstruction after craniofacial trauma is to do as much as possible the first time, to obtain wide exposure, ensure rigid fixation of bone pieces and grafts and to make use of a work bench procedure where bone fragments are assembled on a side table for subsequent reattachment to the head.

Keyword: Craniofacial trauma.

Elective craniofacial surgery for malformations has brought neurosurgeons and plastic surgeons into a close relationship which has entailed important progress in the emergency treatment of severe craniofacial trauma.

Craniofacial surgery, originated by the French wizard surgeon Paul Tessier, is characterized by accuracy, made possible by the new techniques to obtain exceptional anatomical access to the area of surgery.

Another striking feature of craniofacial surgery is the notorious breaking of established surgical rules. Thus hair is never shaven off heads despite an anticipated intracranial operation. Intraoral surgery is frequently carried out at the same time as the dura is exposed. Old rules about antiseptics have been defied with the help of modern broad spectrum antibiotics. In addition, all time low records of hypotension anesthesia have been set with the help of skilled anesthesiologists yielding to the demands from the craniofacial surgeons.

It is the aim of this paper to present our current treatment for craniofacially injured patients and to exemplify by one case report some of the surgical techniques that we use.

Preoperative Care and Investigations

When a severe injury to the head and face has occurred emergency treatment is instituted as soon as the patient reaches the hospital unless paramedics have not started already in the ambulance. Adequate airways are ensured, anti-shock treatment started and the neurosurgeon makes his initial examination. When the patient is stable skull X-rays and skull CAT scans are taken. Ophthalmology examination is usually also included. The patient's head is not shaven and only a narrow strip for a coronal incision is cut. A tracheostomy is performed when indicated. If other fractures are present an orthopedic surgeon will be called in to work on those along with the craniofacial team.

Surgical Techniques

A bicoronal skin incision is made by cutting cautery attached to the surgical scalpel. This will minimize bleeding and seem not to prevent healing. The forehead scalp is peeled down anteriorly in an extra-pericranial plane thus leaving the periosteum attached to the bone until the first fractures are reached. From this point the dissection will be subperiosteal and brought as far down as past the zygomatic arches when indicated and subperiosteally also into the orbits. When the upper jaw is fractured, an upper buccal sulcus incision is carried out to meet with the dissection coming from above so that the whole face can be stripped off its soft tissue cover. When facial lacerations are present these will be used to facilitate access, but can usually not replace the coronal incision.

All bone fragments are dissected free and put on a separate tray. Fractures and dural tears at the skull base behind an intact orbit are seen after lateral or localized midface blows. To get easy access for dural repair in this

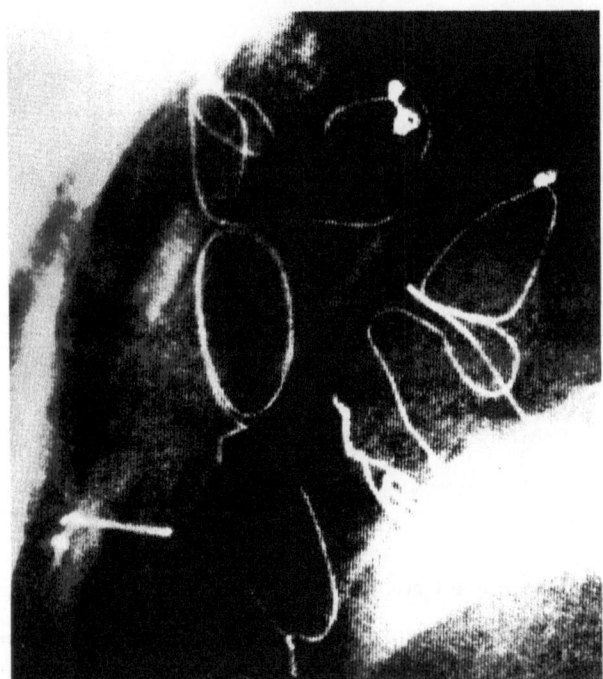

Fig. 1. X-ray demonstrating rib grafts linked together in a modified chain-link fence manner. The wires are encompassing the whole rib and joined together without drill holes in the rib

situation the orbit can be disassembled as far as is needed.

While the neurosurgeon tends to brain lacerations and dural tears the plastic surgeon on a side-table at the same time reassembles all the bony pieces and wire them together so as to make them into one and bigger piece that can be wired back with only a few wires when the neurosurgeon has finished.

When bone is missing primary bone grafts are used taken from ribs or split skull bone. These too have to be tightly wired. For ribs a modified chain-link fence[6] procedure is used (Fig. 1) to obtain stability.

Orbit

The bony architecture of the orbic is inspected and restored. If necessary, an operating microscope is used for dissecting the optic nerve to make sure there is no compression.

If torn the medial canthal ligaments are reattached. The orbital floor is inspected and bone grafted if missing. Also, if there is a fracture with herniation of orbital contents, a bone graft will be inserted.

The Lacrimal Drainage System

Injuries in the vicinity of the medial canthal region demand probing of both puncta and irrigation of the lacrimal system to ascertain its patency. Dye can be

injected through the canaliculi and be made to stain a Q-tip inserted beneath the inferior turbinate. When the tear ducts at any level is intercepted it is repaired at once according to the technique appropriate for the level of injury[4].

The Jaws

Jaw fractures are handled in cooperation with oral surgeons of the team. Jaw suspension wires are brought down when needed from the lateral orbital rims or from wherever stable bone is otherwise present. These have to be used cautiously, however, as a severely fractured face can be forshortened by too vigourous tightening of such wires.

Soft tissue repair is undertaken according to classical plastic surgical principles. Missing soft tissue is skin grafted. No flaps are used at this stage. Stensen's duct is probed and repaired if necessary, leaving a silastic catheter in for 2 weeks.

Postoperative care. If swelling has not developed at the end of surgery a full face plaster is applied and left in place for 2–3 days. This will limit postoperative swelling and stabilize injured tissues. The hair is washed after 3 days and the patient is gradually mobilized. If present intermaxillary fixation will be maintained for 7–8 weeks and removed by the oral surgeons under local anaesthesia.

Case Report

A 21-year-old male was brought to the craniofacial centre after a car accident. Skull X-rays revealed on AP-views frontal bone fractures, a right orbital roof displacement and fractures of the mandible. Profile views revealed a dislocated nose (Fig. 2 a). The full extent of the facial fractures could, however, only be seen on CAT scans where a total fronto-naso-ethmoidal posterior oblique disjunction could be seen (Fig. 2 b). There was also a left-sided diaphyseal femur fracture.

The patient was brought to the operating room where a tracheostomy was performed an during which time an orthopedic surgeon put the left femur under traction and performed a fasciotomy.

By a coronal approach and removal of bone pieces exploration of the anterior fossa was undertaken and a dural tear was sewn after which the whole fronto-naso-ethmoidal complex was replaced en bloque.

The fasciotomy was skin grafted. The patient underwent an uneventful recovery with a few scars as his only sequelae (Fig. 3).

Discussion

Fractures of the facial skeleton unless perfectly reduced, will leave severe sequelae that can totally change the life situation for the victim. A disfigured face

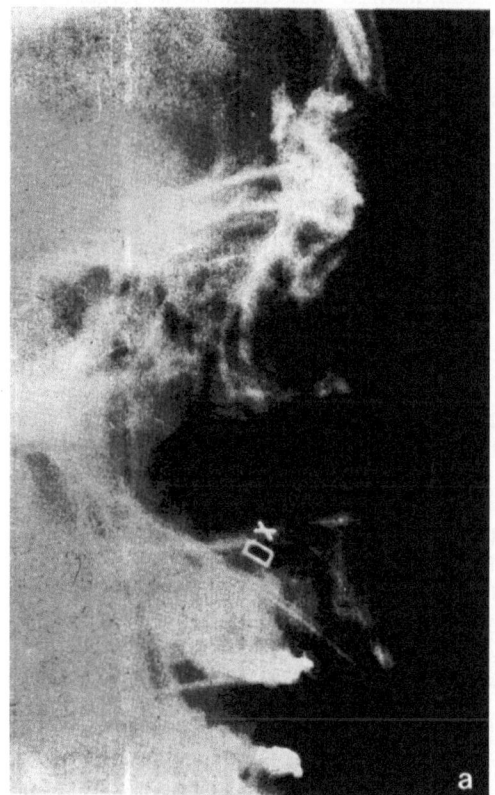

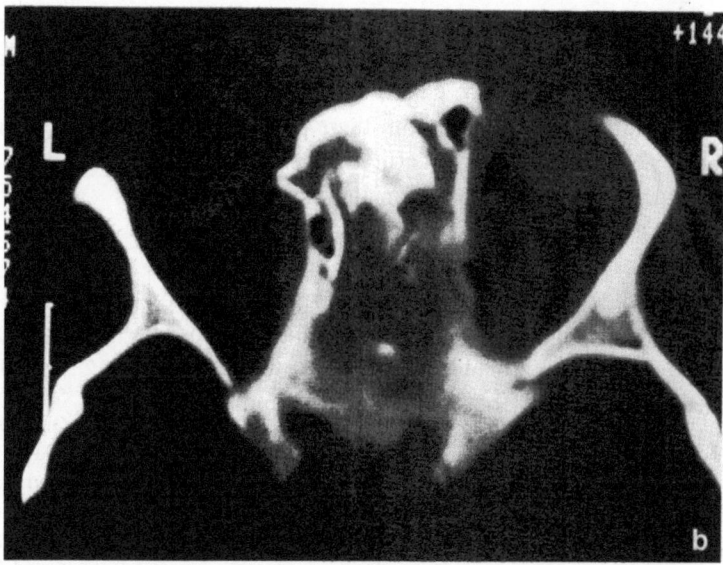

Fig. 2. Skull X-ray of 21-year-old man. a) Lateral view disclosing a severely displaced nose. b) CAT scan demonstrating the full extent of fronto-nasal-ethmoidal posterior oblique disjunction

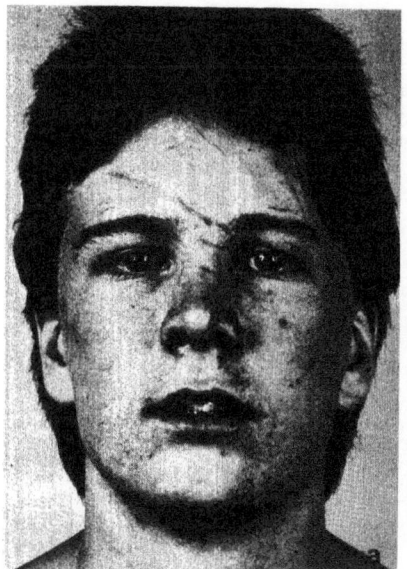

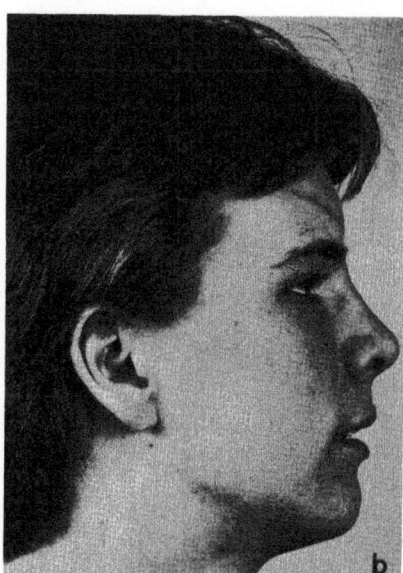

Fig. 3. 21-year-old boy 3 months after severe midface and mandibular fracture. a) Frontal view. b) Profile view

is a most severe social handicap and a functional handicap such as diplopia is almost intolerable.

Before the development of craniofacial surgery facial fractures were treated through the existing skin lacerations if present and otherwise through small incisions placed in the eyebrows, eyelids, side-burns or within the hair-bearing scalp or sometime through an intraoral approach. All these incisions had to be made small and stay within the area of relative concealment and were seldom ideally located for fracture reduction and fixation. This often meant inadequate reductions and inadequate stabilization or even altogether overlooking fractures deeper inside or further away. As the surgeon could seldom see the whole injured area the perfect anatomical understanding of the interrelationship between the pieces of bone could rarely be obtained. With craniofacial surgical techniques this has changed for the better and no fracture of the face or skull needs to pass with less than a perfect reduction.

Merville and others[5, 2, 1] have stressed that the reconstruction of the face has to start from wherever there is stable bone and go from there piece by piece. Our way of removing every fractured bone fragment for subsequent assembly away from the patient brings 3 distinct advantages. First, the neurosurgeon gets a better access for inspection and dural repairs. Second, considerable time is saved by letting the plastic surgeon repair the fractures at the same time that the neurosurgeon does his work. In addition it is easier to place drill holes and wires and obtain perfect fitting and stability when the pieces of bone are held in the hand.

CAT scan, which was developed during the same period of time as Tessier developed cranio-facial surgery has proven to be most valuable in connection with craniofacial trauma. Some fronto-ethmoidal fractures, such as the one in our case report, would be difficult to interpret correctly on ordinary skull films. Without CAT scan and CF surgery such fractures would be almost untreatable.

It can be summarized that craniofacial surgery has much improved the means by which facial trauma can be treated. We are in agreement with Gruss that only one time is optimal for facial trauma treatment—the first time[3]. Exposure should be wide for easy access. Bone fragments and grafts must be tightly wired. Stability is a major prerequisite for graft take[6, 3]. Work bench surgery saves time and improves the results.

References

1. Adams WN (1942) Internal wiring fixation of facial fractures. Surgery 12: 523
2. Gruss JS (1982) Fronto-naso-orbital trauma. Clin Plast Surg 9: 577
3. Gruss JS (1985) Naso-ethmoid-orbital fractures: Classification and role of primary bone grafting. Plast Reconstr Surg 75: 303
4. Lauritzen C, Lilja J (1985) Nasolacrimal obstruction in craniofacial surgery. Scand J Plast Reconstr Surg 19: 269
5. Merville LC, Real JP (1981) Fronto-orbito-nasal dislocations. Scand J Plast Reconstr Surg 15: 287
6. Munro IR, Chen YR (1981) Radical treatment for fronto-orbital dysplasia: The chain-link fence. Plast Reconstr Surg 67: 719

Author's address: C. Lauritzen, M.D., Ph.D., Department of Plastic Surgery, Sahlgren's Hospital, S-413 45 Göteborg, Sweden.

Acta Neurochirurgica, Suppl. 36, 151–154 (1986)

Traumatic Intracranial Hematomas:
Pathophysiological Aspects on Their Course and Treatment

J. Löfgren

Department of Neurosurgery, Sahlgren's Hospital, University of Göteborg, Sweden

Summary

Hematomas in head injuries as a general rule reach their definite size within minutes after the trauma, the bleeding being effectively checked by an interaction of an increased intracranial pressure and the natural hemostatic processes. In epidural hemorrhage the development of arteriovenous shunting in the epidural space may result in continuing bleeding. In special circumstances vascular injury may produce delayed hemorrhage related to increased transmural pressure in the vascular bed and the development of a hyperfibrinolysis syndrome. The clinical effect of a hematoma is quantitatively related to its volume, but modified to a considerable degree in the particular case by the size of the extraaxial space and the arterial blood pressure. Some implications for treatment are commented upon.

Keywords: Delayed intracerebral hemorrhage; epidural hematoma; intracranial pressure; subdural hematoma.

Mechanical trauma to the head may result in bleeding in intracranial tissue planes or disruptive hemorrhage in the brain parenchyma. The accumulation of hematomas of surgical significance is a low probability even, however, occurring only in a few percent of the cases entering an emergency service with a head injury. If one considers the most severe cases with prolonged unconsciousness, the probability of a hematoma increases to about ⅓. The various types of hemorrhagic lesions differ considerably in their pathogenesis and development. A knowledge of the mechanisms involved may enhance the understanding of clinical management problems. In this survey the characteristic evolution of some specific types of traumatic hematomas will be discussed after a description of the course of an intracranial bleeding in general.

General Course of an Intracranial Hemorrhage

There are fundamental differences between the course of a bleeding in the intracranial cavity and that in other body cavities. For example, a hemorrhage into the abdomen may cease after a considerable period of time when blood loss has resulted in arterial hypotension and a reduction in the bleeding pressure, permitting the formation of a hemostatic clot. In major bleeding in the skull cavity the intracranial pressure (ICP) rapidly rises due to the accumulation of blood and may reach the level of the arterial pressure within 20–30 seconds[14, 20, 21]. The initial rapid bleeding is converted by the decrease in the bleeding pressure into a slow oozing. Clot formation can take place and the bleeding may thus stop within a few minutes from its beginning provided the hemostatic mechanisms are intact. In small children arterial hypotension may contribute to the hemostasis due to the large ratio between the volume of the hematoma and the total blood volume. During the period of high ICP the cerebral blood flow is compromised. Within minutes after the bleeding has stopped ICP is reduced, however, to a more tolerable level because of a transitory increase in the outflow of cerebrospinal fluid (CSF), a simple mechanical effect of the elevated hydrostatic pressure. Due to an increase in the CSF outflow resistance caused by blood in the subarachnoid space or by a mass effect, the ICP may not resume its initial steady state value, but settle at a higher level. If a prior coagulopathy exists the bleeding may continue at a slow rate maintaining the pressure in the hematoma and progressive cerebral compression.

The critical volume of an acute supratentorial

expanding mass at which a significant elevation of ICP and disturbance of vital neural functions develop seems to be about 4–5% of the intracranial volume. At about 10%, a definite lethal volume is reached associated with an ICP approximating the arterial blood pressure and an advanced transtentorial herniation syndrome. In most cases hemostasis is achieved before the hematoma has expanded to this extent. While these figures are based mainly on experimental studies in animals, clinical experience suggests similar relationships in patients with expanding lesions[1, 19]. Four percent of the intracranial volume corresponds to a volume of about 50 ml or to a spherical hematoma on the CT scan with a diameter of slightly more than 4 cm. A hematoma with a volume of more than 100 ml or about 8% of the intracranial volume, corresponding to a spherical hematoma with a diameter of 6 cm, constitutes a life-threatening situation. In posterior fossa hemorrhages the critical diameter is less due to the constrained space and is about 3 cm according to clinical experience with spontaneous cerebellar hemorrhage. Additive effects of multiple lesions may also be taken into account.

These volume effects are presumably closely related to the size of the extraaxial fluid space within the intracranial cavity. This space increases with increasing age and thus, with other factors being equal, augments the tolerance of the system to an expanding mass. As an example, it has been demonstrated that the volume of chronic subdural hematomas at presentation is a function of the age of the patient[3]. Conversely, it can be inferred that children with their relatively small extraaxial space will show a corresponding intolerance towards expanding lesions. In head injuries with an associated brain swelling the extraaxial volume may of course be severely reduced.

The tolerance to an expanding mass is furthermore directly related to the arterial blood pressure[16]. Thus, a reduction of mean arterial pressure from 140 mm Hg to 60 mm Hg causes a 30% decrease of the lethal volume of an acute expanding mass. This fact underlines the extreme importance of maintaining the arterial blood pressure in cases of intracranial mass lesions of critical dimensions. On the other hand, in the case of incomplete hemostasis, a rise in the arterial pressure may result in an enhanced bleeding and a worsening of the situation.

Even if many other factors modify the response to an expanding mass, volumetric considerations of this kind may provide a rational basis for the assessment of clinical situation in a patient with a hematoma and for decisions concerning operative treatment.

Epidural Hematomas

In addition to a vascular injury, an epidural hematoma presupposes an extensive detachment of the dura from the skull by local bone deformation. The hematoma develops rapidly within the potential space created. The subsequent evolution seems to be a major exception from the course outlined above due to the development of an arteriovenous shunting in the epidural space to diploic veins[2, 7, 23]. Such arteriovenous shunting may delay clotting of the hematoma and maintain bleeding for a considerable time accounting for the relatively protracted and progressive course, which is typical for these hematomas, as well as for the occasional "lucid interval". One can compare for contrast this clinical course with that in a hemorrhage into the subarachnoid space[23]. On the CT scan a specific picture of a heterogenous hematoma is seen with a relatively lucent area representing fluid blood surrounded by high-density retracting clots. This phenomenon has been called the "lucent swirl" sign[22]. It must be regarded as an ominous sign indicating active arterial bleeding in the epidural space and may be associated with rapid deterioration of the patient. The term "hyperacute hematoma" has appropriately been suggested for this variant of epidural hematoma[6].

In minor arterial or venous bleeding in the epidural compartment the shunt effect may be insignificant and the hematoma may undergo rapid clotting. In this way the occurrence of chronic epidural hematomas may be understood which have been recognized with increasing frequency in recent years. These are characteristically located distant to the temporal region and presumably have a noncritical volume. While the evacuation of a hyperacute hematoma is a surgical emergency, chronic hematomas can often be managed conservatively.

Acute Subdural Hematomas

Acute subdural hematomas occur mainly in acceleration injuries that produce short-duration, high-strain rate loading of the head that take place especially in accidents involving falls[5]. Disrupature of bridging veins ore contrecoup contusions may produce bleeding in the subdural space. This type of loading may also cause a diffuse axonal injury which has been considered the main reason for the poor prognosis in acute subdural hematomas where a mortality around 70% is commonly reported. Subdural hemorrhage may also occur without an associated diffuse injury and this may particularly be the case when the bleeding is arterial in origin. Several recent reports have demonstrated that subdural hemorrhage is in more than 50% of the cases caused by lesions of cortical arteries adherent to the dura and consequently easily torn in a comparatively slight impact trauma[17]. The hematoma may develop rapidly as described and the patient arrive at the hospital in an advanced stage of tentorial herniation and deep coma. This situation may be misinterpreted as due to a severe coexisting brain injury, while the real cause actually is the prolonged compression of the brain. This concept is supported by the report of Seelig[17] of a mortality of 30% in acute subdural hematomas operated upon within 4 hours and 90% if operated upon later on.

Ongoing hemorrhage in the subdural space may sometimes be demonstrated in acute cases[6], related presumably to a shunting phenomenon or deficient coagulation mechanisms. In either case a continuing extremely high ICP is probably the result, responsible for the dismal prognosis in this subset of acute subdural hematomas even if there is expeditious treatment.

Delayed Intracranial Hemorrhage

Serial CT scans have demonstrated that both extra-axial and intraaxial hematomas may develop hours or days after the trauma in a significant number of cases. The mechanisms of these developments are poorly understood, but a number of probable pathogenetic factors has been indentified[4, 10]. In Fig. 1 an attempt is made to summarize the interaction of these potential factors. Central in this scheme is the transmural pressure in the vascular bed, that is, the pressure causing the bleeding. A main pathogenetic factor is probably loss of the tamponading effect of a high ICP as a consequence of the removal of a mass lesion or intense hyperosmolar or other pressure-reducing therapy. Coalescing hemorrhages may evolve in areas of brain contusions presumably related to local circulatory disturbances and vasoparalysis in a mechanically damaged vascular bed. These developments may

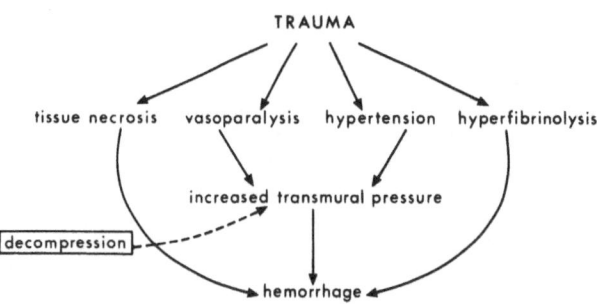

TRAUMA

tissue necrosis   vasoparalysis   hypertension   hyperfibrinolysis

increased transmural pressure

decompression

hemorrhage

Fig. 1. Outline of potential factors involved in the causation of delayed traumatic intracranial hemorrhage

be aggravated in the case of arterial hypertension acting on a unprotected vascular bed.

Another factor in the production of delayed hemorrhage might be a disseminated intravascular coagulation-fibrinolysis syndrome which may evolve in head injuries, especially in those with brain tissue destruction, even if usually of a mild degree. Hemostatic abnormalities may also occur with alcohol intake. For these reasons repeat CT scans are indicated in severe head injuries at 48 hours or earlier. While a delayed extraaxial compressive lesion is usually an indication for operation, a conservative approach may be appropriate in the often indolent parenchymal lesions.

Chronic Subdural Hematomas

Chronic subdural hematomas may be regarded as a special case of delayed hemorrhage. The mechanism of their evolution is not completely understood. They are unique hematomas in several respects. They rarely occur on the basis of acute subdural hematomas in cases of severe head injury, which are usually rapidly organized or resolved. Instead they develop after rather trivial head injury and in special categories of individuals, i.e. elderly people, alcoholics, and patients with shunt-treated hydrocephalus. A main factor in their development seems to be brain atrophy and a low ICP resulting in a low resistance to the extracerebral accumulation of fluid[11–13]. An inflammatory response is induced with ingrowth from the dura of granulation tissue containing fenestrated and fragile macrocapillaries. Plasma filtration and daily "microbleeds" from these incompetent vessels lead to the subsequent enlargement of the hematoma[9] and a clinical course typically fluctuating or even apoplectiform. Thus, the primary determinant of the evolution of these hematomas seems to be the special properties of the vascular neomembrane formed. The hemorrhagic state and expansion of the hematoma is promoted by a high fibrinolytic activity in the hematoma fluid related to the presence of fibrinogen degradation products and to an overproduction of tissue plasminogen activator in the outer membrane[8, 9].

Simultaneously with this production of hematoma fluid there is a continuing absorption in the neomembrane. With "maturation" of the membrane absorptive forces may predominate and result in a spontaneous resolution of the hematoma. There is seemingly a delicate balance between production and absorption which explains the effectiveness in most instances of simple burr hole evacuation of the hematoma[12, 13, 15].

By removal of the fibrinolytic agents in the hematoma fluid the net direction of fluid transfer is reversed and resolution may take place within days.

References

1. Aronson SM, Okazaki H (1963) A study of some factors modifying response of cerebral tissue to subdural hematoma. J Neurosurg 20: 89–93
2. Ericsson K, Håkansson S, Löfgren J, Zwetnow NN (1979) Extravasation and arteriovenous shunting after epidural bleeding. A radiological study. Neuroradiology 17: 239–244
3. Fogelholm R, Heiskanen O, Waltimo O (1975) Chronic subdural hematoma in adults. Influence of patient's age on symptoms signs and thickness of hematoma. J Neurosurg 42: 43–47
4. Fukamachi A, Nagasaki Y, Kohno K, Wakao T (1985) The incidence and developmental process of delayed traumatic intracerebral hematomas. Acta Neurochir (Wien) 74: 35–39
5. Gennarelli TA, Thibault LE (1982) Biomechanics of acute subdural hematoma. J Trauma 22: 680–685
6. Greenberg J, Coken WA, Cooper PR (1985) The "hyperacute" extraaxial intracranial hematoma: Computed tomographic findings and clinical insignificance. Neurosurgery 17: 48–56
7. Habash AH, Zwetnow NN, Ericson K, Löfgren J (1983) Arteriovenous epidural shunting in epidural bleeding. Radiological and physiological characteristics. An experimental study in dogs. Acta Neurochir (Wien) 67: 291–313
8. Ito H, Komai T, Yamamoto S (1978) Fibrinolytic enzyme in the lining walls of chronic subdural hematoma. J Neurosurg 48: 197–200
9. Ito H, Yamamoto S, Komai T, Mizukoshi H (1976) Role of local hyperfibrinolysis in the etiology of chronic subdural hematoma. J Neurosurg 45: 26–31
10. Kaufman HH, Moake JL Olson JD, et al. (1980) Delayed and recurrent intracranial hematomas related to disseminated intravascular clotting and fibrinolysis in head injury. Neurosurgery 7: 445–449
11. Loew F, Wüstner S (1960) Diagnose, Behandlung und Prognose der traumatischen Hämatome des Schädelinneren. Acta Neurochir (Wien) [Suppl] VIII, Wien, Springer
12. Loew F, Kivelitz R (1976) Chronic subdural hematomas. In: Vinken PJ, Bruyns GW (ed) Handbook of clinical neurology, vol 24, part II. North-Holland Publ Co, Amsterdam Oxford and American Elsevier Publ Co New York
13. Loew F (1982) Management of chronic subdural hematomas and hygromas. In: Krayenbühl H et al. (ed) Advances and technical standards in neurosurgery. Springer, Wien New York
14. Löfgren J, Zwetnow NN (1972) Kinetics of arterial and venous hemorrhage in the skull cavity. In: Brock M, Dietz H (eds) Intracranial pressure, experimental and clinical aspects. Springer, Berlin Heidelberg New York, pp 155–159
15. Markwalder TM, Seiler RW (1985) Chronic subdural hematomas: to drain or not to drain? Neurosurgery 16: 185–188
16. Schrader H, Löfgren J, Zwetnow NN (1985) Influence of blood pressure on tolerance to an expanding mass. Acta Neurol Scand 71: 114–126
17. Seelig JM, Becker DP, Miller JD, Greenberg RP, Ward JD, Chois SC (1981) Traumatic acute subdural hematoma. New Engl J Med 304: 1511–1518
18. Shenkin HA (1982) Acute subdural hematoma. J Neurosurg 57: 254–257
19. Steiner L, Bergvall V, Zwetnow NN (1975) Quantitative estimation of intracerebral and intraventricular hematoma by computer tomography. Acta Radiol (Stockh) [Suppl] 346: 143–154
20. Steiner L, Löfgren J, Zwetnow NN (1975) Characteristics and limits of tolerance in repeated subarachnoid hemorrhage in dogs. Acta Neurol Scand 52: 241–267
21. Steiner L, Löfgren J, Zwetnow NN (1975) Lethal mechanism in repeated subarachnoid hemorrhage in dogs. Acta Neurol Scand 52: 268–293
22. Zimmerman RA, Bilaniuk LT (1982) Computed tomographic staging of traumatic epidural bleeding. Radiology 144: 809–812
23. Zwetnow NN, Habash AH, Löfgren J, Håkansson S (1983) Comparative analysis of experimental epidural and subarachnoid bleedings in dogs. Acta Neurochir (Wien) 67: 67–101

Author's address: J. Löfgren, M.D., Department of Neurosurgery, Sahlgren's Hospital, University of Göteborg, Sweden.

Acta Neurochirurgica, Suppl. 36, 155–158 (1986)

Head Injuries in Children—Special Features

F. Gjerris

Department of Neurosurgery, Rigshospitalet, Copenhagen, Denmark

Summary

Head injury in children is very common. Mostly the trauma is slight and the child improves without defects. Even after severe injuries, which can be fatal for an adult, many children will survive in a good condition. Prediction of survival and of quality of life after severe head injuries can be difficult. Predictors of a bad outcome are: low age, initial low grade of coma, abnormal motor responses, fixed pupils, abnormal eye movements, very high ICP, presence of diffuse cerebral edema or intracranial hematoma and obliteration of basal cisters on CT scans. Many children surviving a severe diffuse head injury will be mentally retarded or show behavioural changes.

Keywords: Head injury children; anatomic and pathophysiologic traumatic features; children-adults trauma differences.

Introduction

Head injuries in children are very common. Severe head injuries are a major cause of mortality and disability in childhood. Knowledge of prophylaxis in the traffic has not yet resulted in arrangements, which can prevent these accidents.

The purpose of the present paper is to review some incidence figures, some symptoms and signs of focal or diffuse cerebral injuries and to underline predictive prognostic values in head injured children.

Incidence

The average incidence rate of head trauma in the U.S.A. is 220/100,000 for all children and the death rate is 10/100,000.—The risk of head injury in children is dependent of many factors, *i.e.* traffic prophylaxis, the factual population ratio of children and the social-, economic- and hospital organization in the different countries.

In the Scandinavian countries there is about 4 million children and from the above figures 8,800 will have a head injury and 400 will die. From official statistics it is known that 200 children will be killed in the traffic every year and about half of these will die after their head injury, *i.e.* 100 per one million (the number of children less than 15 years of age in Denmark) and thus we find exactly the same figure as mentioned above from the U.S.A.

Distribution

The type of accidents depends of the age of the child. "Battered child syndrome" is most common in pre-school children, home accidents in the age group of less than 5 years, road accidents in children of 5–9 years of age and sport, fall and road accidents in children of 10–14 years of age. In a French[4] series of 1,719 children below two years of age 80% suffered of fall accident. The distribution of head injuries is very equal in boys and girls in the age group below 15 years of age (b/g in %): Fatal 6/4, severe 5/5, moderate without skull fracture 11/9, moderate with skull fracture 30/38 and mild 47/44[5]. In another series of moderate head injuries boys were at a far greater risk than girls and had a much higher accident rate[13]. Children with head injuries are coming from highly congested and lower income areas, their fathers seem more likely to be unemployed or unskilled, the parents more likely to be divorced, separated or not officially married and there seems to be a higher incidence of premorbid behaviour problems[15].

Pathophysiology and Pathology

The *primary brain or skull lesions* occur in the moment of the accident and is a result of a direct or indirect injury (rotation, acceleration and deceleration) to the skull and the brain. *Secondary brain or skull lesions* develop after the accident, for example a

Table 1. *Skull-brain Injuries in Children Compared to Adults*

Anatomy	*Clinical picture*
Head mass rel. bigger	whiplash, "battered child" mult. lesions, subd. hem.
Bone thinner	depressed fr., indent. focal symptoms incl. ep.
Skull less rigid	impact damping (less contre-coup)
Anterior skull base less cavities	CSF-fistul. etc less freq.
Pathophysioloy	
Volume compens. (cran.)	
Circul. cond.: less stable	conscious degree and neurol. def.-vary
Reaction in temp. and respir.-greater	
Fontanel	facilit. diagn. & ther.
Future studies	
Properties of immature brain	
< 2 years	
2–10 years	influence on posttraum..
Myelination	clin. picture?
Water content (white matter)	
Vascular autoregulation	

(Modified from Lindgren S, personal comm. 1985)

growing intracranial hematoma or a brain edema. The primary lesions are irrevocable while the secondary are potentially treatable. The secondary causes of lesions can be divided in two groups: an *intracranial, i.e.* hematomas, brain congestion or edema and an *extracranial, i.e.* cerebral complications caused by hypoxia or hypotension.

The mass of the head is bigger in relation to the body, especially in infancy, the skull is thinner than in adults, the bone less rigid and the skull base is more smooth. The compliance of the intracranial space is lesser and the systemic circulation conditions less stable in children. The visco-elastic properties of the immature brain are different compared with older children and the myelinization is not complete before 2–4 years of age (Table 1).

The child brain is therefore more vulnerable to oxygen deficiency, has probably a greater tendency to brain "swelling" of edema and an increased permeability of blood brain-barrier after head injury.

Symptomatology and Clinical Findings

The symptoms and signs depend of the age of the child. In infancy and childhood the battered child

syndrome and subdural hematomas are common. The *infant concussion syndrome* has among others been described by Bruce[3]. The baby becomes sleepy, pale, with tachycardia and clammy skin, no focal signs, a soft fontanel and a varying level of consciousness. An *epidural hematoma* in an infant can be associated with anemia and shock. *Intracerebral hematomas* are rare in newborns, acute *subdural hematomas* are more common in children less than 2 years than extradural hematomas.

Traumatic cerebral congestion = hyperperfusion syndrome is seen within the first 6–24 hours. The typical clinical picture of brain edema most often develops 24 hours after a head injury in a child, who is awake[3]. Suddenly he develops progressing agitation, headache and unconsciousness. CT scan will in these cases show a diffuse bilateral swelling of the brain with a small ventricular system, no sulci and no basal cisterns. The mortality in children with diffused brain edema has been rather high, but with aggressive treatment the mortality was only 9% in a series from U.S.A.

Transient neurological dysfunction has been described clinically as transient cortical blindness, transient hemianopia or transient hemiparesis and most often seen in children after minor head injury, mostly of focal type[14] or described as convulsive and nonconvulsive cases (for review see: Snoek et al.[16]). Transient cortical blindness in children was found with an incidence of 1% in a consecutive series of head injured patients[10].

Case story: "A nine year old girl had a slight occipital head trauma by falling backwards in the schoolyard. There was no unconsciousness. On the way to the doctor at the school she claimed of blindness and there was found dilated fixed pupils and no vision. During transportation to a neurosurgical unit the vision slowly went back and at arrival she was neurologically intact. At follow-up she was normal."

Cortical traumatic blindness is alarming but all children will be completely normal within a few hours[9].

The brain injury can clinically be divided in *primary, i.e.* mild or severe commotio, diffuse or severe diffuse cerebral lesions[8] and *secondary, i.e.* hematomas, edema, ischemia, hydrocephalus and intracranial effects of extracranial complications.

Most head injuries in childhood are of the closed mild type with a short episode of unconsciousness followed by a short period of confusion, somnolence, vomiting and irritability. These children can also have focal signs (pathoanatomically most often correlated to a brain contusion). A more severe injury is seen in between 10–15% of children with head injury with either focal or more diffuse signs. They will have a longer coma and even abnormal motor signs. A coma of more than 24 hours with decerebrate rigidity is a sign of a very severe diffuse head injury correlated patho-anatomically most often to the so-called diffuse axonal brain injury[8].

The *skull injury* can be divided in *primary, i.e.* fissures, comminute fractures, depression fractures and cranial nerve lesions and *secondary* (with concomitant injury of the meninges), *i.e.* hematomas, liquorrhoea, meningitis and hydrocephalus. Growing skull fracture is a very rare fracture type and 90% occurs below the age of 3. There are four essential features: A skull fracture in infancy, a dural tear under the fracture, a brain injury beneath the fracture and an enlargement of the fracture during time.

Hematomas

The incidence of epidural hematomas is between 1–3% of head injuries in all age groups, and 3.5% in children less than 15 years of age[6]. Subdural hematomas are the most common intracranial hematomas in children. Chronic subdural hematomas are quite frequent in infants. Only 70% of children with an epidural hematoma have a skull fracture against 95% of adults.

Assessment of Grades of Coma

The primary evaluation of a head injured child requires an accurate description and definition of the level of consciousness and the use of coma scales[12]. It should be remembered that the assessment of coma grade can be difficult in smaller children. It is also necessary to estimate the spontaneous and induced motor responses, the pupillary reaction to light stimulation and the eye movements, including the ocular brain stem reflexes and the respiratory pattern[2]. Agitation can be the only sign of increasing ICP and signs of herniation may arise very suddenly.

Prognosis

The prognosis is better for children than adults, often will children survive a severe head injury which will be fatal for an adult. The prognosis after a concussive head injury is nearly always good. Even after severe diffuse brain injuries some children will survive in a good condition, but a rather great part of them will be retarded or have behavioural changes, *i.e.* "minimal brain dysfunction" or hyperactivity[15]. Post-traumatic early amnesia of less than one day nearly

never results in deficits[8]. After coma for more than one week only one-third will be functioning within normal IQ but still have behavioural disturbances. An ICP of more than 40 mm Hg during treatment with hyperventilation gives a very bad prognosis[1].

A surprisingly low mortality rate following severe head injury has been found in one series of children treated with early intensive therapy, immediate CT-diagnosis, monitoring of ICP, hyperventilation and use of sedatives[3]. Other authors find a much higher mortality rate in severe head injuries in children[1, 11, 18].

Discussion

Is serial or prospective CT-scanning necessary in children with severe head injury? A repeat CT during the first week on the third day or earlier should be obtained on head injured children with no improvement. Two-thirds of the patients deteriorating neurologically after the first 48 hours had new lesions on repeat CT-scanning. Diminished and obliterated basal cisterns on the first CT scan correlate well to the clinical state and are a bad prognostic sign, first described by Espersen and Petersen[7] and later confirmed by Toutant[17].

It is thus still necessary to evaluate a child suffering from a moderate or severe head injury very carefully both clinically and with CT scan and to register all clinical data with clear definitions in order to improve the predictive value in giving prognostic statements in the acute phase after a head injury in children.

References

1. Berger S, Pitts NH, Lovely N, Edwards MSB, Bartkowski HM (1985) Outcome from severe head injury in children and adolescents. J Neurosurg 62: 194–199
2. Born JD, Albert A, Hans P, Bonnal J (1985) Relative Prognostic value of best motor response and brain stem reflexes in patients with severe head injury. Neurosurgery 16: 595–601
3. Bruce DA (1982) Special considerations of the pediatric age group. In: Cooper PR (ed) Head injury. Williams & Wilkins, Baltimore, pp 315–325
4. Choux M (1984) Head trauma in children. Lecture given at annual course, EANS, Edinburgh
5. Cooper PR (ed) (1982) Head injury. Williams & Wilkins, Baltimore
6. Dhellemmes P, Lejeune JP, Christiaens JL, Combelles G (1985) Traumatic extradural hematomas in infancy and childhood. J Neurosurg 62: 861–864
7. Espersen JO, Petersen OF (1982) Computerized tomography (CT) in patients with head injuries. Assessment of outcome based upon initial clinical findings and initial CT scans. Acta Neurochir (Wien) 65: 81–91

8. Gennarelli TA (1982) Cerebral concussion and diffuse brain injuries. In: Cooper PR (ed) Head injury. Williams & Wilkins, Baltimore, pp 83–97

9. Gjerris F (1976) Traumatic lesions of the visual pathways. In: Vinken PJ, Bruyn GW (eds) Handbook of clinical neurology, vol 24. North Holl Publ Comp, Amsterdam, pp 27–57

10. Gjerris F, Mellemgaard L (1969) Transitory cortical blindness in head injury. Acta Neurol Scand 45: 623–631

11. Humphreys RP, Jaimovich R, Hendrick EB, Hoffman HJ (1983) Severe head injuries in children. Concepts pediat Neurosurg, vol 4. Karger, Basel, pp 230–242

12. Jennett B, Teasdale G (1981) Management of head injuries. Davis FA, Philadelphia

13. Kølle-Jørgensen P (1971) Child accidents. A medico-social study of 4,820 accidents. Munksgaard, Copenhagen

14. Lindgren SO (1960) Acute severe head injuries. Acta Chir Scand [Suppl] 254: 5–49

15. Oddy M (1984) Head injury and social adjustment. In: Brooks N (ed) Closed head injury. Psychological, social, and family consequences. Oxford University Press, Oxford New York Toronto, pp 108–122

16. Snoek JW, Minderhoud JM, Wilmink JT (1984) Delayed deterioration following mild head injury in children. Brain 107: 15–36

17. Toutant SM, Klauber MR, Marshall LF, Toole BM, Bowers SA, Seelig JM, Varnell JB (1984) Absent or compressed basal cisterns on first CT scan: ominous predictors of outcome in severe head injury. J Neurosurg 61: 691–694

18. Zuccarello M, Facco E, Zampieri P, Zanardi L, Andrioli GC (1985) Severe head injury in children: early prognosis and outcome. Child's Nerv Syst 1: 158–162

Author's address: F. Gjerris, Department of Neurosurgery, Rigshospitalet, Copenhagen, Denmark.

Acta Neurochirurgica, Suppl. 36, 159 (1986)

Neurotraumatology

General Literature

Recent special symposias of interest for the medical profession:

Head and Neck Injury Criteria. A Consensus Workshop (Ommaya AK ed) Government Printing Office, Washington DC 20402. 1981.

The Biomechanics of Trauma (Nahum AM, Melvin J eds) Appleton-Century-Crofts, 1985.

Advances in Neurotraumatology (Villani R, Papo I, Giovanelli M, Gaini SM, Tomei G eds). Excerpta Medica, 1982.

Central Nervous System Trauma Status Report—1985 (Becker DP, Povlishock JT eds) NINCDS-NIH.

Transcranial Doppler Sonography

Edited by R. Aaslid

Contents: A. Eden: The Beginnings of Doppler. – P. Grolimund: Transmission of Ultrasound Through the Temporal Bone. – R. Aaslid: The Doppler Principle Applied to Measurement of Blood Flow Velocity in Cerebral Arteries. – R. Aaslid: Transcranial Doppler Examination Techniques. – R. Aaslid, K.-F. Lindegaard: Cerebral Hemodynamics. – K.-F. Lindegaard, R. Aaslid, H. Nornes: Cerebral Arteriovenous Malformations. – J. M. Gilsbach, A. Harders: Comparison of Intraoperative and Transcranial Doppler. – R. W. Seiler, R. Aaslid: Transcranial Doppler for Evaluation of Cerebral Vasospasm. – A. Harders: Monitoring Hemodynamic Changes Related to Vasospasm in the Circle of Willis After Aneurysm Surgery. – E. B. Ringelstein: Transcranial Doppler Monitoring. – T. Lundar: Transcranial Doppler in the Study of Cerebral Perfusion During Cardiopulmonary Bypass. – Subject Index.

From the Foreword by M. P. Spencer, M. D., Director of the Institute of Applied Physiology and Medicine, Seattle, Washington, U.S.A.: "Every few years a dissertation comes to the area of clinical application of medical technology which carries us forward as on a magic carpet into new regions of understanding and patient care. This book is such a magic carpet. It brings together, in a clear and incisive fashion, important hemodynamic principles with a simple non-invasive method of application to a part of the cerebral vasculature which has been relatively inaccessible. To the lucky and perceptive person who reads this book, a feeling of excitement and hope for progress is engendered. The diligent application of the potentials of transcranial Doppler ultrasound brings new power to our efforts in understanding the cerebral circulation and the causes, treatment and prevention of cerebrovascular disorders."

1986. 94 figures. XI, 177 pages.
Soft cover DM 68,–, öS 476,–.
ISBN 3-211-81935-5

Springer-Verlag Wien New York